A History of the Augustana Hospital
School of Nursing

# A HISTORY

## *of*

# THE AUGUSTANA HOSPITAL SCHOOL OF NURSING

## 1938–1987

With a Summary of A History of
The Augustana Hospital School of Nursing
1884–1938

*Compiled By*
JOYCE RABAUSCH HERTER '48, ETHEL JENSEN '47,
ESTHER FREDRICKSON LIND '47,
ELEANOR CARLSON SCHNIER '38, MARILYNN MOTZER STAMMICH '56
AND CLAUDIA LANGEBARTELS FRANZ '56

*Published by*
THE ALUMNAE ASSOCIATION

OF

THE AUGUSTANA HOSPITAL SCHOOL OF NURSING

1998

Publishers' Graphics L.L.C., Naperville, Illinois 60540
© 1998 by The Alumni Association of The Augustana Hospital School of Nursing
Book design by Patrick Falso
All Rights Reserved. Published 1998
Printed in the United States of America

01  00  99  98     5  4  3  2  1

ISBN 0-9665196-0-4

Parts of chapters 1, 2, and 3 of Part I and parts of Part III of the present work
appeared in *A History of The Augustana Hospital School of Nursing 1884–1938.* © 1939
by The Alumnae Association of The Augustana Hospital School of Nursing.

Library of Congress Catalog Card Number: 98-66180

*We dedicate this book*
*to all the graduates of*
*The Augustana Hospital School of Nursing*

# PREFACE

In 1938 a group of nine Augustana Alumnae published the book "A History of the Augustana Hospital School of Nursing" to preserve for the future the facts which were available regarding the origin of the Hospital in 1884, and the establishment and growth of the School of Nursing to that present time—1938.

Fifty years later, in 1988, a group of six Augustana Alumnae decided to write the second History Book. It has been a somewhat difficult task, but our desire was to leave something tangible in memory of the training we received. Our first meetings were held around the dining room table in the Lila Pickhardt Lounge. We sent out questionnaires and read through old minutes of Alumnae meetings, hundreds of issues of the "Augustana Nurse" and other publications the Hospital had put out through the years in preparation for writing the book.

Part one of our book was taken directly from the first history book with no editorial changes. The poetry section was taken mainly from year books and the first history book—in some cases we do not have the name of the author, but we are quite sure they were written by an alumnus.

Special thanks to the committee—Joyce Herter, Ethel Jensen, Esther Lind, Eleanor Schnier, Marilynn Stammich and Claudia Franz, for writing, compiling, editing, sequencing and selecting materials for the book.

We also want to thank Lois Kane for the many hours of typing and helpful suggestions.

Many thanks to Edna Thornblade '32 (who had helped with the first book) and Esther Nelson '28 who continued to keep notes on our history.

Our thanks to all others who contributed in any way to help in the writing of this book. If there are any omissions, it was not intentional.

# CONTENTS

# ILLUSTRATIONS

# PART I

A HISTORY OF THE AUGUSTANA HOSPITAL
SCHOOL OF NURSING 1884–1938

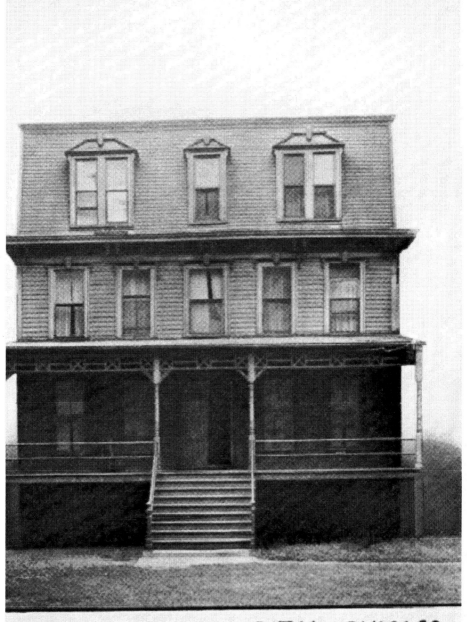

AUGUSTANA HOSPITAL, CHICAGO
ORIGINAL BUILDING, 1884

# CHAPTER I

## THE BEGINNING OF AUGUSTANA HOSPITAL

### AUGUSTANA

A-ngels of mercy who watch day and night;
U-niformed nurses in blue and in white.
G-irls ever cheerful, and ready to smile,
U-nselfish service, the kind that's worthwhile.
S-ympathy given to those in despair.
T-rusting, forgiving to those in their care.
A-lways wait patiently, ready to serve,
N-urses with sense and plenty of nerve.
A-ugustana Nurses, I bid you goodbye.
                                    —A FORMER PATIENT

THE DEACONESS INSTITUTION of the Swedish Evangelical
Lutheran Church was incorporated February 13, 1882, under the laws of the State of Illinois. The Charter states "that
the objects for which it is formed are as follows: the training
of well qualified nurses, the establishment and support of hospitals, the care of the aged, the education of the young, and
in general the exercise of mercy among the suffering—that said
corporation is not formed for pecuniary profit."

This was an extensive plan, but the immediate objective was
the establishment of a hospital which became known as the
Augustana Hospital. In 1924, the corporate name was legally
changed to Augustana Hospital. The name Augustana is taken
from the Augustana Synod, which is the branch of the Evangelical Lutheran Church in America which was established by
Swedish immigrants. However, "Augustana" was first applied

to the confession of the Evangelical princes of Germany laid before the Emperor, Charles V, at the Diet of Augsburg in 1530. "Confessio Augustana" means "The Great Confession." "Augustana" means great, august, imperial.

The Synod desired to erect the hospital in the Lake View district, and once wanted the site now occupied by the Columbus Memorial Hospital, but these deals did not materialize. Rev. Evald, Rev. Abrahamson and Rev. Ranseen drove with a horse and buggy looking for a suitable site. They found the one they wanted had been sold just thirty minutes before their arrival. In a disheartened mood, they drove back to the home of Rev. Erland Carlsson. There it was decided to rent his residence, a two-story frame building, facing Lincoln Avenue and adjoining a large vacant area on Cleveland Avenue.

This building was equipped to house fifteen patients. It was opened on May 28, 1884, with Dr. Truman Miller as Physician and Surgeon, Mrs. Hilda Carlson, wife of the Rev. A.B. Carlson, missionary to India, as matron, and Miss Lotta Frejd as her assistant. The first surgical patient was the wife of Rev. Vibelius. Dr. Miller performed the operation and Miss Marion Mitchell, an Illinois Training School nurse, came to assist him and remained to care for the patient. Miss Mitchell later became the wife of Dr. A.J. Ochsner.

Thirty-five patients were given care during the first year. Mrs. Carlson left after a short stay and Miss Lotta Frejd became the matron. In 1884, the building was badly damaged by fire; no one was injured, but the nurses lost all their belongings. The eighteen patients were carried by Miss Frejd and her assistants to a saloon across the street and later removed to the German Hospital, which is now Grant Hospital. Fire insurance covered the financial loss, and the hospital was soon rebuilt.

In February of 1885, the new three-story frame building was completed, having twenty six beds. On the first floor was a large reception room which also served as the operating room. When needed for that purpose, the rug was rolled up against the wall and an operating room table was improvised by putting some planks on the tables. The floor was cleansed with carbolic acid solution. Maternity cases were cared for in their own rooms, and once a case was given the necessary attention in the men's ward as no other space was available. The staff consisted of Dr. Truman Miller, Dr. John Chew, and Dr. Woodward, with Miss Lotta Frejd as matron. She and the cook each received three dollars a week and the two nurses each were paid two dollars a week.

Miss Frejd was a tall, strong woman, with unbounded energy. She had short hair, which was most unusual for that time, and this gave her an extremely masculine appearance. She did not always wear a uniform. Sometimes she wore black and sometimes a white shirtwaist with a black skirt. She had all the instincts of a pioneer woman. Her mind was very keen and she was quick to grasp a situation. When necessary she acted as cook, laundress, anesthetist, janitress, and carried patients up and down stairs. When help was scarce, she would arise at three o'clock in the morning, and have the hospital washing on the line by seven. In her spare time she made appeals to the churches and societies for aid. She carried a Bible with her and read the Scriptures to the patients. She did a great deal of work herself and expected her nurses to do likewise. She had very positive likes and dislikes and while she had many friends, she also had many enemies. Dr. A.J. Ochsner said that she was the first woman ever to give an anesthetic. He paid her the great compliment of saying that he would never forget what she had done for Augustana Hospital.

The Board of Directors was anxious to have the institution under deaconess supervision and control, and the nurses who came during that period were more of the deaconess type, deeply religious, self-sacrificing, satisfied with their lot, giving much and asking little.

The uniforms worn by the nurses were made of blue and white striped gingham, with a full gathered white apron. The nurses were supposed to work from 7:20 a.m. to 7:30 p.m., but they remained on duty until the work was completed, and were on call day and night if their services were needed. The patients had small hand bells with which to summon a nurse. A wash stand was placed in each room or ward; this contained a white basin and pitcher, soap dish, and some towels. Baths were given from heavy white crockery basins. No nurse was assigned to active night duty, as Miss Frejd said that the patients were supposed to sleep at night, but in the case of a very ill patient, the nurse slept in a rocking chair in the hall, ready to give any necessary attention, but she was required to be on duty, as usual, at 7:30 a.m.

Instruments for operations were boiled in a big kettle on the kitchen stove. Dressings and towels were sterilized in a small portable sterilizer. Heavy white crockery platters were sterilized and used as instrument trays. The nurses did all the dressings, removed packings, made their own iodoform and carbolated gauze, and sterilized catgut and horsehair. Carbolic acid and iodine came in crystal form, from which they made their solutions.

The hospital was becoming better known and the number of patients was gradually increasing.

In 1884 37 patients were treated
In 1885 97 patients were treated
In 1886 106 patients were treated
In 1887 103 patients were treated

In 1889 an attempt was made to start a few nursing classes. Mrs. Gilmore, who was in charge of Mrs. Porter's Children's Hospital, now Children's Memorial Hospital, came twice a week to give talks to Miss Frejd and the nurses, who numbered about three or four. These classes were soon discontinued, as nurses rarely had time to attend.

In 1890...the hospital had now reached the point where it must expand, having outgrown its present quarters. Dr. Ochsner's ability in diagnosis and surgery was making him well known in the city. The number of patients was constantly increasing and the staff wished better accommodations for them, and wanted modern operating room equipment.

The cornerstone of the new building [at the corner of Lincoln and Cleveland Avenues] was laid in September of 1892. It [the hospital] was to be 68 by 84 feet, of fireproof construction, six stories in height, with a capacity of 125 beds. Construction began at once and continued throughout the year. The south wing of Augustana Hospital was formally dedicated on September 17, 1893. The hospital was erected at a cost of $74,890.95.

The new building, for that period, seemed well equipped. The wards had white iron beds, with white bedside tables. The large wards had sixteen beds each, the smaller ones had two, three, or four beds. The private rooms were large, airy and comfortably furnished. Portable back rests were used. Crisp white sash curtains hung at the windows and the white iron screens had white muslin covers. Carts were used to carry patients to and from the operating room. The elevator was a real luxury. It was operated by Miss Frejd or the office girl, or the handyman. Walking to the sixth floor was not an uncommon occurrence. The diet kitchens were provided with gas stoves, new dishes and silver for the trays. The food was sent to the floors on a "dummy" elevator, which was pulled up and down by means of a rope.

The new hospital required an entire new set-up of rules and regulations. Considerable debate was conducted about its supervision. The Board of Directors was still desirous of adhering to the original plan of having it under Deaconess control, but the staff, headed by Dr. A.J.Ochsner, preferred a training school. Deaconesses were very difficult to procure, and the training school idea was proving very popular and desirable, so the Board of Directors decided in favor of a two year training course, with a graduate nurse in charge.

In 1880 there were fifteen schools of nursing in the United States, in 1890 there were thirty-five, and in 1900 there were

432.[1] Augustana Hospital, having begun its school in 1894, was included in the latter number.

The south wing consisted of six floors. The sixth floor was used for the operating room' kitchen, store rooms, children's ward, and rooms for student nurses. The fifth floor was at first unfurnished, but later was used for private room patients. Two rooms were given to the internes. Fourth floor had private rooms, all large and sunny, bathrooms, diet kitchen, clothes closets, and some semiprivate rooms. Third floor, which was reserved for women, had two large wards of sixteen beds each, two small wards, diet kitchen, bathrooms, and a large clothes closet. Second floor, arranged the same as third floor, was used for men. The first floor had a waiting room, business office, examining room, laboratory, a room for the matron, and the chapel. The latter also served as the office for the Superintendent of Nurses. The basement contained the boiler rooms, laundry, linen, sewing and ironing rooms, and drug room. As probationers began to enter they were housed on first floor. After fifth floor was furnished the internes were also given quarters on first floor.

During the first months in the new building Dr. A.J. Ochsner performed in a day four or five operations, three days a week. Miss Louise Bylander, who had spent some time in the frame building, became the first operating-room nurse. Dr. Ochsner personally taught her how to prepare for surgical operations, and planned the routine to be followed, which he had reduced to the simplest form. This simple routine is still followed as much as possible at the present writing [1938]. Dr. Ochsner also taught the nurses how to give the "Swedish Movements," a set of exercises for patients, and prepared a chart for their use, outlining the different steps to be taken. Miss Bylander had no assistant and used to arise at 4:00 or 4:30 a.m. to prepare the operating room. There was no limitation as to the length of time a student nurse spent in the operating room. If she did

---

1. American Journal of Nursing, November 1937.

good work the doctors were loath to dispense with her services. Miss Bylander, being a most capable and trustworthy nurse, served a whole year. She spent three years in the hospital [as a student], but received credit for only two years.

The skill of the Surgical and Medical Staff had placed the hospital on a high plane, and Dr. A.J. Ochsner's reputation spread so rapidly that the hospital soon had a marked increase in patronage. But the nursing staff had not increased in proportion, as nursing was not yet a popular or well-known profession for women.

Besides the surgical patients a great many typhoid patients were given care. During this time, Chicago water was considered very impure. Placards were posted everywhere warning people to boil their drinking water. At the hospital the water supply for drinking was carried over in open buckets from the artesian well at the brewery, then located where the new Augustana Hospital now stands [411 W. Dickens]. There was a water cooler in each kitchen, and one near the elevator. A common cup was used by all visitors. Nurses were forbidden to use the patients' glasses or cups, so they used a sugar bowl, labeled "Nurses," and all nurses drank from the same bowl. In Lincoln Park a tin cup for common use was chained to the drinking fountain.

The nurses wore the same style uniform of blue and white stripes that had been worn in the old building. They were made in the then prevailing style of leg o'mutton sleeves, long, tight basques, with a long, full skirt. The apron was gathered full and had a bib, but no shoulder straps; these were added in 1894. Miss Frejd introduced the little round organdy cap, made with rushing at the bottom, and a black velvet band tied into a little bow at the side. New caps had to be made every two weeks, as they were not washable.

The nurses slept on sixth floor, three in a room, and the night nurses slept in the same beds vacated by the day nurses. They were constantly being disturbed by noises from the kitchen, operating room, children's ward, and the ringing of the large school bell to announce dinner and supper. A maid stood on sixth floor, near the elevator, and rang the bell vigorously so that it could be heard on all the floors.

The nurses still went on duty at 7:30 a.m. and had a twelve hour day. However, they remained until their work was completed, which was often as late as 9 p.m. During the day one nurse was in charge of a large ward and a small ward. One bath a week was given to the ward patients, for which the nurse allowed herself fifteen minutes. Private room patients had two baths a week. One night nurse came on at 7:30 p.m. to care for the patients on all the floors. She ran up and down stairs all night, waiting on the patients. They had little tinkle bells with which to summon the nurse, and she often had great difficulty in locating a particular tinkle. She would run from floor to floor, from room to ward, trying to find out who was calling her. After a nurse had been on night duty a short while her legs became badly swollen from constantly running up and down the stairs. Inasmuch as the hospital had gas lights, the night nurses went about with candles.

The charts hung on the foot of the patients' beds in the wards, and were placed on the dressers in the private rooms and semiprivate rooms. The charting was very simple, consisting of temperature, pulse, respiration, daily evacuations, bedside notes, and a urinalysis sheet. An operating room sheet was added if the case was surgical.

The first year in the new building proved difficult in many ways. There was no one at the head with a hand firm enough to guide a rapidly growing institution. Miss Frejd did not approve of what she called "new fangled methods" and it was felt that an actual program to train and teach the nurses must be inaugurated. This required the services of a woman who had the necessary qualifications to organize and supervise.

In 1893, the year during which Augustana Hospital was opened, the Chicago World's Fair was held. This was also the year that the nurse executives of the hospitals throughout the country formed The Superintendents' Society, which was the beginning of the National League of Nursing Education. This organization made the first attempt to collect ideas on nursing and to use them for the benefit of all. Up to this time nurses and hospitals had been self-centered, working only for their own interests.

At this time the work was exceedingly heavy. Several probationers had entered during the year, so there were now about fifteen nurses. There was lack of cooperation; some bitter criticisms were directed at members of the personnel. The number of operations was steadily increasing. Nurses and help alike felt the strain of long hours, overwork, and lack of guidance.

Into this state of affairs, in the fall of 1894, one year after the opening of the new building, came Miss Lila Pickhardt, a recent graduate of the Illinois Training School. In the words of one of the nurses, she was "young, slender and pretty, with a twinkle in her eye."

Miss Pickhardt made an effort to organize the nurses' work. She changed the breakfast hour, the nurses having their breakfast before going on duty. More help was placed on the floors, releasing the nurses from much of the menial work. Previously a nurse would leave a pan full of dishes, wipe the soap suds off her hands, and go out to wait upon a doctor. Miss Pickhardt asked the doctors to give talks to the nurses on the surgical and medical care of patients. Dr. A.J.Ochsner, Dr. Oliver N.Huff, Dr. L.H.Prince, and Dr. Mellish gave these lectures in the evenings, but the nurses' hours were so long, and their duties so heavy, that it was difficult to plan time for them. The nurses took notes, and Miss Pickhardt gave them one examination. Some of the nurses still remember their poor grades.

Miss Pickhardt gave her personal supervision to a thorough cleaning of the whole hospital, going through the kitchen, store rooms, bathrooms, patients' rooms, and clothes closets. After a very hard winter's work, she felt that she was too tired physically. to continue, so she left in May of 1895, much against

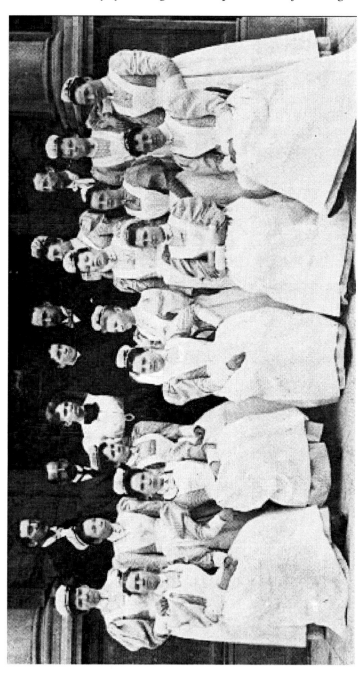

The Hospital Family 1895

the wishes of Dr. A.J. Ochsner and the nurses, who had learned to love and respect her.

Miss Frejd had gone for a visit to Sweden. Miss Christine Blomquist, who had been a nurse in the old building, and had entered as probationer in the new hospital, gave up her training to act as matron. She took complete charge until a new Superintendent of Nurses could be procured. Miss Blomquist was tall and dark and had a most pleasing manner. She wore a black uniform, with white collar and cuffs. She had charge of the housekeeping and linens, purchased supplies, planned menus, relieved the office girl, looked after the general care of the patients, and checked up on the nurses' work during the two months interval in which she was in charge. She was very efficient, quick and alert, with a keen sense of humor. The nurses, with whom she worked, were intensely loyal to her, thus there was splendid cooperation. Miss Blomquist remained as matron after the new Superintendent of Nurses, Miss Julia Andersen, arrived.

Miss Julia I. Andersen came to Augustana Hospital in July, 1895. She was a recent graduate from Illinois Training School, a school which has known the influence of such pioneer nursing leaders as Isabel Hampton, Isabel McIsaac, Lavinia Dock, and Edith Draper. Miss Andersen was a competent nurse, a remarkable teacher, and a splendid organizer. She was just and fair, but very stern and severe and simply would not tolerate poor work. She succeeded in making fine nurses of women who made up in zeal what they lacked in education. The first thing Miss Andersen did each morning was to make rounds to check on the night nurses' work, and she would appear at any time during the day to inspect the work of the day nurses. Before going off duty in the morning, the night nurses gave reports to her; these reports were given in the business office. They were given orally, and the nurses were expected to remember every detail of each patient's condition. In the evening Miss Andersen reported in the same manner to the night nurses before they returned on duty. She took a personal interest in the patients and knew each one by name.

A system of semi-military discipline was established, and the following rules and regulations for prospective probationers were formulated by Miss Andersen:

1.   The applicant must furnish a physicians certificate of sound health, a letter from her pastor, and the name of some reliable person for further reference.

2.   She must answer satisfactorily all questions in the application blank.

3.   She may leave the school at the end of the month of probation if she so desires.

4.   The applicant must pass, during her month of probation, an examination in English, reading, writing, and arithmetic; also, a satisfactory examination at the end of each year.

5.   Each nurse is entitled to two weeks' vacation each year. Further time lost by sickness or other accident must be made up at the end of the two-year service. The school diploma requires two full years of work and study.

6.   The nurse is to receive an allowance of eight dollars per month to pay for uniforms and books.

The form of the first application blank was:

1.   Name in full.
2.   Present address.
3.   Age ___ Height ___
4.   Have you any physical defects? If so, what are they?
5.   Have you always been well and strong?
6.   Are both parents living? If not, what was the cause of death?
7.   What is your present occupation?
8.   Can you read and write English? [At this time most of the student nurses came from Sweden.]
9.   To what church do you belong?
10.  Have you read, and do you clearly understand the Rules and Regulations?

Miss Andersen planned a course of lectures and class work. The following textbooks were obtained for the nurses: Kimber's Anatomy and Physiology, Dock's Materia Medica, and Hampton's Nursing Principles and Practice. The doctors gave lectures on Surgical and Medical Diseases, Obstetrics, Pediatrics, Physiology, and Materia Medica; and Miss Andersen gave lectures in Practical Nursing. A dietitian came twice a week to give lectures on dietetics and to teach cooking. The classes in dietetics were conducted in one of the diet kitchens during the afternoon hours, and the other lectures and classes were given in the chapel, two or three times a week, at 7:30 in the evening.

Several probationers entered during the first year. The senior class now numbered eight nurses. Miss Andersen endeavored to establish regular hours on duty, but nurses still worked long, hard hours. A night nurse was assigned to each floor. A maid was employed for each diet kitchen. The nurses swept the ward floors with a common broom, and once a week the maid scrubbed them on her hands and knees.

It was planned to have a senior nurse in charge of each floor. Her duties consisted of putting up and passing medicines, giving out linens and supplies, doing all the special orders, and supervising the younger nurses' work. The older nurses taught the younger ones, and therefore the training of the latter depended much on the quality of the work done by the older nurses.

In the spring of 1896 the first class of nurses graduated. They had entered under Miss Frejd, had eight months with Miss Pickhardt, and one year's training under Miss Andersen.

The graduation exercises took place in the chapel, and Miss Andersen presented each nurse with a bouquet of roses. Refreshments consisting of coffee, cake and ice-cream were served to all present. The nurses wore their old striped uniforms, but they had new aprons and new caps. They rushed off duty for just a few minutes to brush up a bit before going into the chapel for the exercises.

A committee composed of some board members and nurses had designed the school pin, which in shape resembles that of the Illinois Training School, and has as its seal, "The Good Samaritan." The idea was adopted from the name of the little church paper which had been edited to interest the public in hospital affairs. The nurses each paid $7.50 for their pins.

Although the nurses put in long, hard hours, they also had many good times. Miss Andersen wanted them to have parties and helped to plan them. At one time they gave a taffy pull in the chapel, and once a mock wedding. At another time they played "Blind Man's Buff." To these parties nurses, internes, and the whole household, were invited. Dr. and Mrs. A.J.Ochsner were kind and sympathetic to these early nurses, and often gave them parties at their home. During the first years, while the school was small, an undertaker sometimes took them for a sleigh ride, later to stop at a restaurant for sandwiches and coffee. Christmas was always a merry time. The old customs established by Miss Frejd were carried out.

In 1897, ten nurses graduated, with exercises in a church. Two nurses of this class, Alice Holmberg and Hedwig Wahlberg, became missionaries. A registry for the graduate nurses doing private duty now appeared in the hospital office. Private duty nurses received $15.00 per week, but when on duty at the hospital they were required to pay $5.00 a week for their board. Telephones were not common in those days. The doctor would call the hospital, and a messenger would notify the nurses who lived in the neighborhood. The nurses decided among themselves which one was to go. Nurses often drove ten miles or more out to a farm home. For such trips, Dr. A.J. Ochsner advised them to put newspapers over their chests and backs, inside their coats, to keep out the cold. Besides caring for the patient, they had to help with the cooking and general housework, especially if the mother was the patient. Nurses slept on the floor, on stiff leather couches, or on a trunk and chair placed together. Then, by contrast, in a wealthy home, they had a luxurious room next to the patient's, and were treated as guests.

In May of 1897, at Dr. A.J. Ochsner's suggestion, the first apartment for Augustana graduate nurses was established; it was located on Garfield Avenue, near the hospital and near Dr. Ochsner's office. This home was made possible through the generosity of Miss Louise Bylander, who was willing to advance the necessary money for the first month's rent, and for furniture, linen, and bedding. All the members of the class of 1896, and two of the class of 1897, shared the apartment. Also at Dr. Ochsner's suggestion, a telephone was installed almost immediately after the apartment was organized. This was the first home to be established by private duty nurses in Chicago, and was the origin of the idea that nurses establish themselves in groups for the sake of convenience, economy and sociability. Miss Bylander maintained such a home for a period of forty years, in various locations near the hospital.

The Spanish-American War occured in 1898. Although the war was short, lasting only three months, the mortality was great; the camps were filled with soldiers ill with malaria and typhoid fever. Miss Josephine Oberg, 1896, was the only Augustana nurse who enlisted for service in the Spanish-American War. She reported for duty at John Blair Gibbs Hospital, Camp Hamilton, Lexington, Kentucky. Later she served at the Military Hospital, District of Matanzas, Cuba. She cared for soldiers who had contracted typhoid fever. The salary paid to such "contract" nurses was $30.00 a month.

Bed linens were changed only about once a week [at Augustana Hospital]. Beds were brushed out every day with a whisk broom to free them from crumbs. When a nurse went into the ward to care for her patients, she did not enter with an armful of clean linen, but with a whisk broom in one hand and a bottle of alcohol in the other. The patients' backs were rubbed if they did not get a bath.

Cathartics were used very freely. The "Augustana Cocktail" was the most famous. This consisted of castor oil served in beer foam; cups were used for the cocktail so the patients could not see the oil. On Sunday afternoons, one nurse spent several hours making and giving these "cocktails" to patients preparatory to operations the next morning. The head nurse was always on duty on Sunday afternoon to admit the new patients.

For the past two years the nursing staff had been slowly but steadily increasing. The graduates, called in on special cases, helped to lighten the load on general duty, so that more individual care could be given the patients. More interest in nursing as a profession was seen by the increasing number of applicants. More time was being given to class work, but during these early years a nurse's work was always hard and her hours very long.

Nurses always wore their white cuffs to chapel, in the dining room, to classes, when serving trays, when taking temperatures, and when going to the office. When not worn they were tucked inside the bib, ready for use at any moment. Nurses always put on clean aprons to meals, but never were they to appear on the street wearing either their aprons or their caps. This rule was strictly enforced. The nurse who took temperatures always wore her cuffs; she was not supposed to answer bells, and, of course, there was not time, for she had to take the temperatures of all the patients on the entire floor. Mischievous patients enjoyed asking her to do little things for them, knowing beforehand that she would have to refuse. The hours off duty from one to three were very desirable, because a nurse could have a nap and come back, don her cuffs and take temperatures with a calm, aloof air, ignoring the bells. A nurse who insisted upon wearing her cuffs all the time was looked upon by her co-workers as affected and possibly a little lazy. Nevertheless, while they preferred to see a nurse with rolled up sleeves, ready for any action, they secretly longed for a task at which they could wear cuffs.

On Sunday mornings, nurses appeared on the floors in clean dresses, aprons and cuffs—they fairly rattled as they walked. Nurses were allowed one uniform, four aprons and one set of underwear a week in the laundry. They were required to launder their own hose and cuffs. Handkerchiefs were sent at their own risk.

A night nurse was on duty from 7:30 p.m. until 7:30 a.m. The first thing she did after coming on duty was to read the orders, then put on a kettle of milk to heat while she took the eight o'clock temperatures. All the patients were served a cup of hot milk or cocoa at bed-time. After a month of night duty, the nurse was supposed to have a day for recreation, but was frequently called to return for day duty at noon.

There was only one telephone in the building located in the main office on first floor. The night nurse on second floor was obliged to run down to answer the telephone, and to admit night patients, and to unlock the door for doctors if they came in late. Most nurses at that time had their first experience with a telephone after they entered the hospital, because telephones were not in evidence in private homes. Telegrams were rarely received. When they did come they were opened with fear and trembling, as they were usually messengers of sad news.

Night nurses relieved each other for midnight lunch and for four o'clock coffee. They had special dishes and silver which were kept in a cupboard in the diet kitchen on sixth floor. Night duty was often exciting. There was no night supervisor. The senior nurse took the responsibility; the younger ones went to her for aid.

In 1898, twelve nurses were graduated. In this class was Miss Anna Heistad, who had become one of the most prominent graduates of our school, due to her untiring work at Marcy Center, a Jewish settlement house in Chicago.

In 1899, ten nurses were graduated, of whom one, Miss Andrea Hanson, became a foreign missionary. The graduates, upon their return from the graduating exercises at church, were entertained with a little party given on the veranda of the Nurses' Home. Place cards were used for the new graduates, and on each was written some humorous incident of their training days. These cards were read aloud to the enjoyment of all.

The applicants for nurses' training during these formative years of the hospital were required to be recommended by their pastors, and to be at least twenty-one years of age. It was considered that a woman under this age was not capable of accepting the responsibility of nursing.

In July of 1899, Miss Julia I. Andersen resigned her position as Superintendent of Nurses to become the wife of Dr. Edward H. Ochsner.

After the resignation of Miss Julia Andersen, Miss Pickhardt was again asked to become the head of the training school. As she was unable to leave her position at the City and County Hospital, St. Paul, Minnesota, until a later date, Miss Barbara Jensen, a graduate of the Illinois Training School, became Acting Superintendent of Nurses for a period of seven months. Miss Jensen had served in one of the camps during the Spanish-American War.

In July 1899, Mrs. Tillie Rydell, a graduate of the class of 1897, succeeded Miss Blomquist as matron. She was especially interested in obstetrics, and made arrangements for the graduate nurses to take a post-graduate course at the Chicago Lying-In Hospital which was then located on South Ashland Avenue. The course was not compulsory.

In 1900 when Miss Pickhardt returned, the school had graduated thirty-three students.

The nursing service at this time consisted of the Superintendent of Nurses, two surgical nurses, one septic dressing room nurse, one night nurse on each floor, a senior day nurse in charge of each floor, and others who gave bedside care. The latter nurses were each responsible for sixteen to twenty patients.

Very little attention was given to a sick nurse, unless she was ill enough to enter the hospital. Nurses were afraid to report illnesses, often coming on duty when they were physically unable to do so, greatly fearing that they would be sent home if unable to work.

One nurse on each floor was assigned to take the eight o'clock temperatures. Generally temperatures were taken only once a day, at 3:00 p.m. Nurses furnished their own thermometers, carrying them in little cases. A nurse usually owned two. When she borrowed another from a co-worker she could take temperatures more readily. Bichloride of mercury and alcohol were used as disinfectants.

Each nurse served breakfast to her own patients. After breakfast, the beds and bedside tables were put in order for the awaited rounds of the doctors. This group consisted of Dr. A.J.Ochsner, Dr. Edward Ochsner, the internes, and Miss Pickhardt who carried a little notebook in which she wrote the doctor's orders and later copied in the order book at the nurses' desk in the diet kitchen. Rounds were always dignified and rather solemn affairs upon which the nurses looked with awe and respect.

Dinner was served at noon, and supper at 5:00 p.m. The old dinner bell was still rung to announce the serving of meals. Hours off duty were from one to three or three to five, with a half day a week and another on Sunday. Miss Pickhardt appeared on the floors just before noon to announce half days and hours off duty. A nurse could never make any definite plans. Miss Pickhardt used to say, "No appointments, no disappointments."

Miss Pickhardt wished the "specials" who were on twenty-four hour duty to wear a blue striped gingham night wrapper, buttoned up to the neck. They were also to wear hose, sleep behind a screen, and practice the utmost decorum.

In 1900, ten nurses graduated and in 1901, twelve nurses were graduated. The classes of 1900 and 1901 called a meeting of the graduate nurses in the chapel, with Miss Pickhardt presiding. Only a few nurses were present, but they decided to unite for mutual benefit, pay an initiation fee of one dollar and dues of one dollar a year; they formally adopted a resolution to begin their Alumnae Association.

The need of a permanent surgical nurse was being manifested. Miss Jennie Gummeson, who had spent twelve months of her training in the operating room, was chosen by Dr. A.J.Ochsner and Dr. Edward Ochsner to become the head surgical nurse. She had one assistant. They worked from twelve to sixteen hours daily and were subject to call day or night in case of emergencies. Miss Gummeson's salary for the first years was twenty-five dollars a month, but later this was increased to forty dollars. The doctors were constantly commending her for excellent work.

The operating room was old-fashioned and inconvenient; instruments were sterilized in a small enamel fish boiler on a gas plate. Visiting doctors stood on wooden benches to witness the operations. There were about a dozen of these benches, which the nurses had to scrub at the close of an operating day. The linens, surgical pads, and bandages were sterilized in a somewhat primitive contrivance about forty inches square. Later on, a copper autoclave was installed which was a vast improvement, but a big task for the nurses to keep bright and shiny. Up to this time, gloves had not been worn at Augustana. But one day as Miss Gummeson was cutting bandages, she cut one of her fingers quite badly. Dr. A.J.Ochsner told her to put on rubber gloves and go right on working. This incident introduced the use of rubber gloves at Augustana Hospital. Dressings were washed and resterilized for drainage cases; large gauze bandages were washed and rerolled.[2]

In 1901, the style of uniform was changed from the tight fitting basque to the shirtwaist type with the leg o'mutton sleeve. The nurses carried their watches in little pockets on the waists; the watches were attached to a black silk cord worn around the neck.

Some of the leaders of nursing began to urge a State Association for Nurses. A meeting of the graduate nurses was planned, but having no list of hospitals or training schools to whom notices could be mailed, letters were written to postmasters containing an announcement and return postage. The letters were all written in longhand. This was the first attempt to obtain a formal list of hospitals in the State. The postmasters were asked to mail the letters to hospitals in their towns. These notices reached forty-one training schools in Chicago, sixteen

---

2. The information regarding the operating work of this period was contributed by Jennie Gummeson Lundquist.

hospitals in other cities, and three nurse registries. This led to many discussions among the various groups of graduate nurses. About one hundred nurses came from fourteen schools in the city to meet and consider the proposal. The organization to be planned was to be called The Graduate Nurses' Association of the State of Illinois. Its main object was to bring about State registration of nurses. It was incorporated on August 22, 1901. The first regular meeting was held in September 1901, when the draft of the bill that was to be sent to Congress was discussed.[3]

Miss Johanna Nelson of the class of 1901, was chosen by the Board of Directors and the Staff to become Miss Pickhardt's assistant, and to take her place while she had a much needed vacation. In January 1902, Miss Nelson came to the hospital to relieve Miss Pickhardt, who went to her home in Milwaukee for a needed rest as her health had not been good for some time. She came down once a week to give class work to the Seniors and Juniors and also to complete the program for the graduation of the class of 1902.

In May 1902, sixteen nurses were graduated. This was the first class honored with a banquet by the Alumnae. It was given at the Stratford Hotel, on the corner of Jackson and Michigan Boulevards where the Straus Building now [1938] stands.

On May 17, 1902, a notice was sent out recommending that applicants for membership in the State Association of Graduate Nurses should be graduates of a general hospital of fifty beds giving two years of hospital training with systematic classes in instruction.

It was urged that a state inspection of schools be made, and that there be an examining board made up of nurses to determine who was eligible. A fee of ten dollars was to be asked of the nurse who was applying for the State Board Examination.

---

3. Information was obtained from The History of the Illinois State Nurses' Association, Chap. 1, pp. 2-3-4.

Any nurse who had been practicing for five years before the law went into effect could be accepted for registration without examination provided the application was made within six months of the passing of the bill.[4]

In October 1902, Miss Pickhardt had a very serious illness. Miss Emelia Dahlgren, a senior nurse, was assigned to take Miss Pickhardt's place during her illness and absence from duty.

The "Augustana Nurse" was originated in January 1903, by members of the class of 1901. At the time of the organization of the Alumnae Association, Miss Jennie Gummeson from the class of 1900 had suggested such a publication. Miss Hilda Hedin was editor-in-chief, and Miss Mary Youngren, assistant editor.

Miss Hedin was very near-sighted, so sat patiently with her eyes close to her work, writing these first copies of The "Augustana Nurse" in a beautiful old-fashioned script. A copy was written in longhand for each alumnae member.

In 1903, Miss Hattie Nelson served as the first Night Supervisor, at the urgent request of Dr. A.J.Ochsner and Dr. Edward Ochsner who felt there must be more supervision during the night; this became a permanent position. At first, nurses who were making up time lost by illness or other causes held this position, but were paid no salary.

The nurses were still working hard to ensure the passage of the bill called, "An Act to Regulate the Practice of Professional Nursing in the State of Illinois." If it should be passed it was planned to hold examinations twice a year to determine the fitness of the applicant to practice professional nursing.

The subjects in which the applicants were to be examined were materia medics, physiology, anatomy, chemistry, obstetrics, urinalysis, children's diseases, hygiene and sanitation, dietetics, and practical nursing. The applicant must be of good

---

4. Information obtained from The History of the Illinois State Nurses' Association, Chap. 1, pp. 6-7-10.

moral character, twenty-one years of age, and a graduate of a two-year training school in a general hospital approved by the board.

After passing her State Board Examinations and paying a fee of ten dollars, she would receive a license to practice professional nursing, and would be known as a registered nurse.

The bill finally passed the assembly on April 22, 1903, and was sent to Governor Yates for his approval, but he considered it unconstitutional and vetoed it.[5] The nurses, while they were disappointed, did not lose courage, but began at once to plan for success at the next session of Congress.

In June 1903, Miss Johanna Nelson returned from Columbia University. Miss Pickhardt was given a leave of absence and left at once for Europe. She wished a long rest from the strain of so much responsibility. Miss Nelson brought to the hospital many new ideas on nursing. She personally taught the nurses how to bathe a baby, holding it in her lap, which was the approved method of that time. She gave the nurses demonstrations in the giving of hypodermics and various treatments. These demonstrations were given individually, and not in groups. She also introduced the method of making cotton pledgets and putting them in mason jars to be sterilized. Prior to this, the nurse tore off small bits from the roll of absorbent cotton as they were needed. Miss Nelson gave more personal supervision to the nurses' work in the wards.

The nurses' lectures for 1903, were as follows:

Dr. Edward Ochsner, Surgery, Gynecology and Bacteriology
Dr. C.O. Young, Medicine and Dietetics
Dr. C.E. Blomgren, Materia Medica
Dr. Josephine Jackson, Pediatrics, Medical and Surgical Emergencies
Dr. Emma Hackett, Obstetrics
Dr. Oscar Dodd, Eye and Ear

---

5. Information obtained from The History of the Illinois State Nurses' Association, Chap. 1, pp. 8-9-10-14.

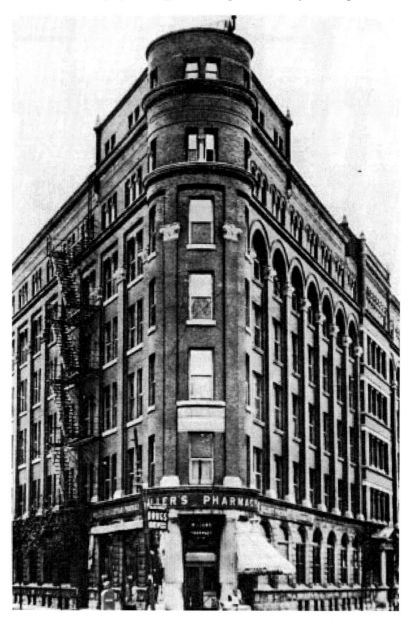

Augustana Hospital 1904–1937 at the corners of Lincoln,
Garfield (Dickens), and Cleveland Avenues,
which later became the President Hotel

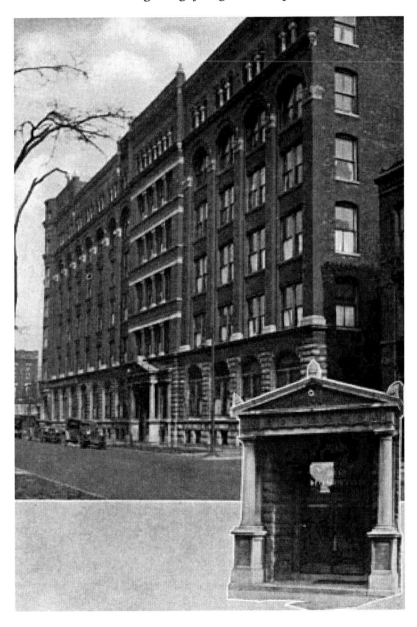

The former Augustana Hospital 1904–1937
looking south on Cleveland Avenue toward Lincoln Avenue

Dr. G.W. Green, Urinalysis
Dr. N.M. Percy, Hygiene and Nervous Diseases
Dr. T.R. Spears, Physiology and Anatomy

The class to be admitted in 1904, was to be the first three-year class. A month of probation was to be given, during which time the nurse was on duty full time after the first two or three days.

Miss Nelson planned to admit the nurses in a class instead of one by one, as had formerly been done. Two classes were to be admitted; one in the spring, and the larger class in the fall. This was a great step forward in the nurses' education, as all received the same class work from the beginning.

Miss Nelson also introduced the probationers' uniform, which consisted of a plain blue chambray dress, white collar and white apron. This was a big improvement on the variety of gingham dresses worn by former probationers. This uniform was in mode until the fall of 1929.

There were only a few obstetrical cases in the hospital, so Dr. Hackett often took nurses with her to a nearby Maternity Hospital. Miss Pickhardt tried to have a nurse see one case while in training.

The nurses in Children's Ward never had any hours off duty, as the work was usually very heavy. The night nurse in Children's Ward cooked the midnight lunch. She was also required to polish the operating room needles, a very unpopular task.

The new addition [to the hospital], costing $117,000.00, was ready for occupancy in December of 1904, with a bed capacity of 225. The Board of Directors allowed $5,000.00 for new furnishings. The building was fireproof, the partitions were either hollow tile or solid brick walls. The different floors were separated by hollow tile, supported by steel beams. There were fire escapes on the south and north sides, accessible from all the floors.

The first floor contained the administration rooms, library, waiting room, consultation rooms, chapel, laboratory, locker rooms, room for matron, and quarters for internes.

The second, third, fourth, and fifth stories comprised four large wards, twenty-four smaller wards, three children's wards, and thirty-five private rooms, twenty of which had private baths. On the sixth floor were three modern operating rooms, three dressing rooms, two anesthetizing rooms, and two sterilizing rooms. Here the floors were of flake mosaic laid on hollow tile. There were two recovery rooms, the maternity ward, one nursery, one confinement room, general kitchen, diet kitchen and general dining rooms.

The basement contained boiler, engine and dynamo rooms, steam laundry, ironing rooms, linen rooms, sewing room, drug room, and general store rooms.

On each floor was a large diet kitchen, general bathrooms, store rooms and linen rooms. There were two elevators, one for passengers and one for general service.

All sick rooms were equipped with signals of colored electric lights to be operated with a push-button by the patient. This simultaneously lighted an electric lamp over the door of the patient's room and one in the diet kitchen, in which the nurses' desk was located. The old bells were no longer in use, much to the joy of the nurses. The hospital operated its own electric light plant. Distilled water was used for drinking purposes and in the operating rooms.

Miss Tillie Rydell resigned to be married; her place was taken by Miss Minnie Peterson, who served for one year as matron.

With the beginning of the three-year course the work was divided into the Probation Period of one month, the Junior, Intermediate, and Senior Years. The classes were formed during the spring and summer months, and many applicants had to be refused admittance because the waiting list was so large. The course of study was graded: the first six months demonstrations were given, also lessons in cooking, bedside care of ward patients, both male and female, including one term of night duty; later came the care of private ward patients, children, post-operative patients, operating room service, special diet kitchen service, and obstetrical service. Classes were held daily; doctors lectured three times weekly.

The corps of lecturers were as follows:

Dr. C.R. Blomgren, Materia Medica
Dr. R.W. Holmes, Obstetrics
Dr. E.H. Ochsner, Surgery
Dr. E.O. Benson, Pediatrics
Dr. Anders Frick, Medicine and Dietetics
Dr. M. Wahlstron, Parliamentary Law and Psychology
Dr. J.L. Yates, Bacteriology
Dr. F.M. Horstman, Elementary Materia Medica
Dr. N.M. Percy, Hygiene
Dr. C. Ranseen, Bacteriology
Dr. H.W.Abelmann, Urinalysis

Miss Johanna Nelson conducted the class work and carried on her duties as Superintendent of Nurses, with the assistance of a graduate night supervisor and a graduate surgical supervisor, until the fall of 1904, when Miss Pickhardt returned after her leave of absence. There were seventy nurses in training at this time.

The schedule of classes was rearranged to give the student nurses a definite number of hours in each subject. Miss Nelson taught the probationers and gave them demonstrations, and Miss Pickhardt taught practical nursing and ethics. The doctors gave lectures on which the nurses took notes to be handed to Miss Pickhardt for correction.

The class schedule was as follows:
Probationers
    20 Classes:
        Nursing Ethics 10 hours
        Nursing Clinics 10 hours
Junior year
    20 Lectures:
        Bacteriology 10 hours
        Hygiene 4 hours
        Urinalysis 6 hours

48 Classes:
   Cooking classes
   2 divisions—24 in each division
52 Recitations:
   Elementary Anatomy and Physiology
   Use and care of sick room appliances
   How to observe, report and record bedside symptoms
   Baths, emenata, douches, catheterizations, gastric
   lavage, couterirritants, charting, administration of medicines
   Preparations of patients for operations and aftercare
   Special nursing
Intermediate Year
  32 Lectures:
    Bacteriology 7 hours
    Elementary Materia Medica 8 hours
    Medical Diseases 10 hours
    Dietetics 10 hours
    Hygiene 4 hours
  38 Recitations:
    Anatomy and Physiology continued
    Nursing of fever patients and general diseases
Senior Year
  55 Lectures:
    Advanced Materia Medics 4 hours
    Obstetrics 11 hours
    Eye and Ear 3 hours
    Surgery 6 hours
    Pediatrics 8 hours
    Dietetics 10 hours
    Parliamentary Law 5 hours
    Psychology 8 hours
  36 Recitations:
    Obstetrical Nursing 10 hours
    Pediatrics 10 hours
    Care of nervous and insane 8 hours
    Private Nursing 4 hours
    Training School Administration 4 hours

The nurses' records were kept in a large ledger, one page being devoted to the record of each nurse. This contained the name of nurse, address, relative, church affiliation, by whom recommended, a record of class work, attendance, grades, doctors' lectures, and usually a remark, such as "noisy," "forgetful," "heedless," "careless," "good," "excellent," which described the nurse.

There was a new central diet kitchen where nurses prepared the general diets for the private patients, and any special diets ordered by the doctors; there was also a central supply room where the nurses prepared the surgical supplies as they were ordered, and put them up in properly labeled packages ready for sterilization.

In 1905, Miss Charlotte Johnson became matron. The diet kitchens were then placed under her supervision.

In 1905, the Illinois State Association of Graduate Nurses became a member of the Nurses' Associated Alumnae of the United States. The "Nurses' Bill" was introduced to the Senate in February, 1905, and was passed on March 23, but was later vetoed by Governor Deneen, who felt that it was unfair to many nurses. The third "Bill" was drafted, trying to overcome all objections to the other two "Bills." On May 2, 1905, Governor Deneen signed the "Nurses' Bill," and State Registration became a law.[6]

In 1905, seventeen nurses were graduated: they were the first Augustana nurses to wear white at their graduating exercises.

In this year the first non-Scandinavian student was admitted to the training school. Miss Frances Heinrich had been especially recommended by Dr. A.J.Ochsner because of her ability to speak German. Her admission marked the beginning of admitting others who were not Scandinavian or not Lutheran.

The general health of the nurses was given more attention. A nurse was allowed two days off duty after being on night duty, and was also given relief when on a difficult special case. She was encouraged to report any illness at once to Miss Pickhardt.

In 1906, sixteen nurses were graduated. The need for taking the course at the Chicago Lying-In Hospital was not deemed

---

6. Information obtained from the History of the Illinois State Nurses' Association, p. 34.

necessary at this time because a splendid course was being given at Augustana Hospital under the capable supervision of Dr. Rudolph Holmes, who was Chief of Obstetrics.

The hours on duty [in the operating room] were from seven to seven, with two or three hours off during the day and a half day during the week and on Sunday.

The nurses prepared all their own suture material. The clinics were large and well attended by visiting surgeons from various states and Europe. Miss Munson [O.R.Supervisor] visited hospitals in Chicago and eastern cities, finding out many things that improved her technique. Classes were held with each group in preparing and scrubbing for operations.

In those years, no student was permitted to actually scrub for any operation. All laparotomy pads were counted seven times before the surgeon received them, and three times after coming from the abdomen.

At one time the surgical nurses gave a demonstration for the Illinois Training School for Nurses showing the method that Augustana Hospital used in making and counting laparotomy pads. There were two operating rooms and three dressing rooms.[7]

In 1906, Miss Pickhardt, for the first time, sent a monthly report of the training school to the Board of Directors. She stated that the nurses were to be given a month in the laboratory, and that lectures on the Eye and Ear were to be added to the class schedule.

The nurses were rapidly outgrowing their quarters. The other side of the building at 344 Garfield Avenue was rented in order to obtain more rooms. Life in the Nurses' Home was happy. Nurses often cooked coffee over a gas jet, a one burner affair. They took turns holding the coffee pot, as they had to stand on a chair in order to reach the gas jet. One night Miss Pickhardt caught them toasting marshmallows over a one-ring gas

---

7. Taken from 8 letter written by Mrs. Beda Munson Lundgren, January 18,1938.

stove. Ten or twelve nurses were sitting on the floor, and Miss Pickhardt stood in the doorway watching them without saying a word; suddenly someone looked up, saw her, and gave a gasp of astonishment.

In 1908, Miss Pickhardt gave a report that 120 lectures had been given, 222 recitations, besides the cooking classes. The senior nurses wrote formal papers which showed study and preparation, and gave gratifying results. This year Miss Johanna Nelson left to be married. Miss Anna M. Jorgenson of the class of 1907 took a post-graduate course at the Cook County Hospital and later returned to become Miss Pickhardt's assistant.

# CHAPTER II

## THE TWENTY-FIFTH ANNIVERSARY
## AND BEYOND

O N MAY 28, 1909, Augustana Hospital completed the first twenty-five years of its existence. A marked progress had been made in every department. A far step had been taken from the boarding house type, such as was found in the old frame building, to the institution of 1909 where modern business methods had been adopted. The progress was due to the efficient work of Dr. A.J.Ochsner, Dr. Edward Ochsner, and the other eminent physicians and surgeons connected with the hospital, as well as the corps of well trained nurses.

In 1909, the three months' probationary period was introduced. After the first week the probationers were on full duty. Demonstrations were given by Miss Jorgensen in the class room; all practical work was demonstrated before the probationers appeared on the wards. The records of the nurses were kept in a large ledger. The general requirements for entrance were: twenty-one years of age or over, a common school education, and a high school education was preferable.

The qualifications of the applicants for admittance were determined by Dr. Wahlstrom and Miss Pickhardt. The school now consisted of seventy-two nurses. A two weeks' vacation was given during the first and third years, and three weeks during the second year. In her annual report, Miss Pickhardt stated that 252 inquiries had been received regarding the training school. Twenty-seven inquiries were made regarding nurses for hospital positions.

On May 1, 1910, the nurses moved from the white brick building at 344 Garfield [Dickens] Avenue to a four-story apartment building across the street at 351 Garfield [Dickens] Avenue. One apartment on first floor was set aside for the home use of the students. There the parties, teas, musicals, and bazaars were held. There was no elevator service, and no telephone service until 1916, when one telephone was-installed on first floor. Already the nurses were planning and dreaming of the new Nurses' Home which had been promised to them. That year twelve nurses were graduated.

Miss Pickhardt resigned to go to California for a long needed rest, and Miss Anna M. Jorgensen became her successor. Her assistants were Elizabeth Proctor, 1909, and Mayme A. Gunderson, 1909.

In that year the nurses' records were changed from the big ledgers to a card system containing full data about the nurses, their attendance, record of work, rotation of service, number of classes and lectures, and grades on all subjects. These cards were filed in alphabetical order in a cabinet provided for that purpose.

Augustana Hospital became eligible in 1910, for State Registration in New York. Miss Pickhardt had made plans for this before she left, for she wished to make available further training and education to the Augustana Hospital nurses. This was a marked step forward for the training school.

Admittance to the Training School now required one year of high school or its equivalent.

Lecturers and instructors for 1910, were as follows:

Dr. E.H.Ochsner, Surgery
Dr. Anders Frick, Internal Medicine
Dr. R.W.Holmes, Obstetrics
Dr. E.O.Benson, Pediatrics
Dr. A.T.Lundgren, Gynecology and Eye and Ear

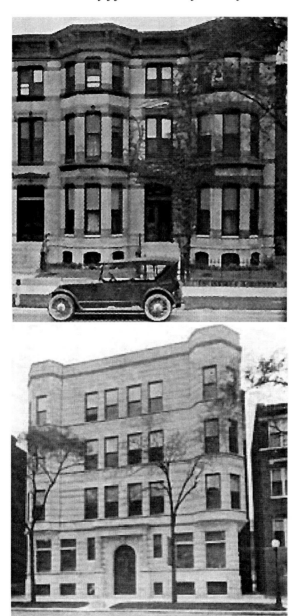

Nurses' Apartments at 344 Garfield Avenue and
351 Garfield Avenue, Circa 1912

Dr. Geo.W.Post, Jr., Venereal Diseases and Moral Prophylaxis and Materia Medica

Dr. G.H.Wynecoop, Dietetics

Dr. Emil Ochsner, Bacteriology

Dr. Lister Treholske, Hygiene

Dr. A.F.Grove, Urinalysis

Dr. M.Wahlstrom, Psychology and Parliamentary Law

Dr. Caroline Hedger and Social Hygiene Committee, Moral Prophylaxis

Miss Anna Jorgensen, R.N., Nursing Ethics, Care of Children and Practical Nursing

Miss Olga Hultman, Massage

Miss Laura T. Osman, Physical Chemistry and Diet Cooking

Miss Beda Munson, R.N., Surgical Demonstrations

Miss Elizabeth Proctor, R.N., Physiology and Anatomy

Miss Mayme Gunderson, R.N., Materia Medica and Practical Nursing

During the winter of 1911, Miss Proctor, due to ill health, resigned as Miss Jorgensen's assistant. Miss Mary E. Nelson, 1911, while not yet finished with her course of training, was asked to fill the vacancy.

That fall Miss Gunderson resigned as assistant to Miss Jorgensen. The vacancy was filled by Miss Margaret Saenger, 1910.

During this year [1911] the following types of cases were treated:

    1,836  surgical
      461  medical
       83  nervous and mental
      374  obstetrical
       46  eye and ear
      119  nose and throat
      383  pediatric

In 1911–1912, the hospital comprised the following departments:

General Surgery
Ophthalmology and Otology
Rhinology and Laryngology
Dermatology
Pathology
Dentistry
Internal Medicine
Neurology

Obstetrics
Gynecology
Pediatrics

In 1912, the name of the "Superintendents' Society" which had been formed in 1893, became changed to "The National League of Nursing Education." The membership was small but steadily increasing, and growing in influence. The dues were one dollar a year. The change in name indicated what it hoped to accomplish. A few of the officers of the old Superintendents' Society were women who had left their mark in the nursing worlds, such as Linda Richards, Lavinia Dock, Isabel McIsaac, M. Adelaide Nutting, Helena McMillan, Isabel Hampton Robb and Mary Wheeler. All of these helped to lay the foundation on which our present practice is built.[8]

This year thirty-three nurses graduated-the largest class to date. An extra apartment at 545 Garfield [Dickens] Avenue was rented for the student nurses. A new Nurses' Home was badly needed and the idea was being seriously discussed.

In the fall of 1912, the districts of Illinois had become organized and Chicago became part of the First District. A mass meeting attended by 300 nurses was held at the Palmer House.

In order to take the State Board Examination, the applicant must be a graduate of a school having a three-year course, and she must be twenty years of age. The Nurses' Practice Act of 1913, provided for an inspector of training schools, a standard curriculum and a penalty for not recording the Certificates of Registration.[9]

In 1913, Augustana Hospital became one of the six Chicago Hospitals to require four years high school of its applicants. The other hospitals were Mercy, Presbyterian, St. Luke's, Wesley, and Evanston. The State required that the applicant must have one year of high school. Augustana Hospital for a number of years did not adhere closely to this requirement.

---

8. Trained Nurse—Hospital Review, June 1928, p. 687.
9. History of the Illinois State Nurses' Association, p. 43.

The total number of graduates from the school since 1896, was 296. Dr. Wahlstrom in his yearly report stated that the income from student special nursing was $12,218.00 for one year. The cost to patients for a student nurse in training was three dollars a day for twenty-four hour duty, with three hours off during the day. The graduate nurses were receiving $30.00 a week, and the patient paid one dollar a day for her board.

It had been the custom of each hospital to manage the employment of its own nurses, and calls were received through the various nurses' apartments. A movement was now begun to establish a Central Registry for Nurses, so it was planned to have a combination Club and Registry. An old apartment at 10 East Huron Street was the first home of the Central Registry. Miss Lucy Last, later Mrs. Van Frank, was its first registrar. Soon the old building was found to be inadequate and the Registry was moved to 1910 Calumet Avenue, the beautiful old Caton residence. [10]

A list of required reading was given to the nurses in training by Miss Jorgensen:

The American Journal of Nursing
Tooley's Biography of Florence Nightingale
Dock & Nutting's History of Nursing
Hampton Robb's Nursing Ethics
Selected Articles from Medical and Nursing Journals and Books

General admission required good health and physique, good moral character, age not less than twenty-one and not more than thirty-five, love and aptitude for the work; two years of high school or its equivalent. Preference was given to women of broader education.

Theoretical instruction closed with the month of May. During the summer months only the practical work and demon-

---

10. Information regarding the Central Registry for Nurses was taken from History of Illinois state Nurses' Association, 1901–1935, pp. 94–95.

strations were carried on. The theoretical instruction was again resumed with the regular classes in September.

Miss Emma J.Ochsner, a sister of Dr. A.J.Ochsner and Dr. Edward Ochsner, gave instructions in the giving of drop ether. The student nurses gave drop ether in the operating room under the supervision of an interne. Miss Ochsner was the first lay person to be appointed to a government position as anesthetist. After leaving Augustana Hospital in 1914, she worked for two years in the Philippines.

In 1914, Miss Mary Nelson resigned as assistant to Miss Jorgensen. Miss Ella Linder, 1911, was Miss Nelson's successor.

Woman's suffrage was coming to the front. Six Augustana nurses marched in the big suffrage parade June 7, 1916.

Miss Ella Linder resigned her position as assistant to Miss Jorgensen, and Mrs. Julia Flikke, who had just recently returned from Columbia University, succeeded her. Miss Jorgensen also resigned and Miss Esther T. Jackson of the class of 1904, was chosen to be her successor.

In spite of the rumblings of war and the unsettled condition of our country, the training of the pupil nurses and the hospital routine had to be continued.

Two classes entered every year, one in the spring and one in the fall. The first three months were devoted to the probationary courses of instruction. During this period the beginner was assigned to the men's and women's wards of the hospital. After the fourth month she acted as assistant to an older student on night floor duty, and gradually was advanced to more responsible duties such as private ward patients, children, post operative patients, diet kitchen, supply room, laboratory, operating room and obstetrical service.

The practical work of each year was accomplished by courses of lectures and demonstrations. The course of instruction conformed with the rules and regulations of hospital service, and the requirements of the Illinois State Board of Registered Nurses.

CURRICULUM OF STUDIES AND LECTURES
PROBATIONARY COURSE 1917–1918

Nursing Clinics ............................................................................ 50 hours
Nursing Ethics ............................................................................ 15 hours
Observation of Symptoms ............................................................ 4 hours

The Probation Period of three months covered fifty practical demonstrations about such conditions that might arise with and around a patient. These demonstrations were made to the whole group in the class room.

JUNIOR YEAR - RECITATIONS

Chemistry ................................................................................... 12 hours
Bacteriology ............................................................................... 14 hours
Hygiene ...................................................................................... 12 hours
Urinalysis ..................................................................................... 6 hours
Elementary Materia Medica ......................................................... 14 hours
Anatomy and Physiology ............................................................. 30 hours
Practice of Nursing ..................................................................... 16 hours

INTERMEDIATE YEAR - LECTURES

Therapeutics and Internal Medicine ............................................. 10 hours
Emergencies and First Aid ........................................................... 10 hours
Roentgen Treatment .................................................................... 12 hours
Surgical Technique ....................................................................... 4 hours
Pediatrics .................................................................................... 4 hours
Administration of Anesthetic (Ether and Chloroform) .................... 3 hours

INTERMEDIATE YEAR - RECITATIONS

Principles and Practice of Nursing ............................................... 18 hours
Advanced Materia Medica ........................................................... 25 hours
Nursing Ethics ............................................................................. 6 hours
Chemistry
Analysis of Food
Diet Cooking ...............................................................................36 hours
Dietetics

SENIOR YEAR - LECTURES

Obstetrics .................................................................................... 11 hours
Gynecology ................................................................................... 6 hours

Diseases of Eye, Ear, Nose and Throat ......................................... 6 hours
Surgery ...................................................................................... 10 hours
Psychology ................................................................................ 6 hours
Parliamentary Law ..................................................................... 6 hours
Medical Jurisprudence ............................................................... 5 hours
Social Service
State Registration ⎫ ............................................................... 6 hours
Nurse Associations ⎭
Tuberculosis .............................................................................. 3 hours
Venereal Diseases and Moral Prophylaxis ................................... 2 hours

### SENIOR YEAR - RECITATIONS

Obstetrics................................................................................. 20 hours
Care and Feeding of Children ..................................................... 4 hours
Surgical Demonstrations ............................................................. 6 hours
Nursing Ethics and Private Duty ................................................. 3 hours
Hospital and Training School Administration .............................. 4 hours

### LECTURERS AND SUBJECTS 1917–1918

Dr. N.M.Percy ............................ Surgery
Dr. Anders Frick ......................... Therapeutics and Internal Medicine
Dr. Rudolph W. Holmes ............. Obstetrics
Dr. E.O.Benson .......................... Pediatrics
Dr. E.A.Gray .............................. Tuberculosis
Dr. A.T.Lundgren ....................... Gynecology and Eye, Ear, Nose and Throat
Dr. E.H.Ochsner ⎫ ............... Diseases of the Nervous system
Dr. Edward Foley ⎭
Dr. Y. Joransen ⎫ ................... Materia Medica
Dr. G.B.Parker ⎭
Dr. G.B.Parker ........................... Urinalysis and Laboratory Work
Dr. Y. Joransen ........................... Chemistry
Dr. Lipkoe ................................. Anaesthesia
Mr. G.B.Anderson ...................... Medical Jurisprudence
Dr. M. Wahlstrom ...................... Psychology, Parliamentary Law, Analysis of
                                                          our Government

Lectures were usually given in the evening, after the nurses were off duty. One of the graduate nurses always attended the lectures. A formal paper on an assigned subject was written by each senior and was read and discussed in class. Chapel services were conducted every morning by Dr. Wahlstrom, or in his absence by Miss Jackson or Miss Saenger.

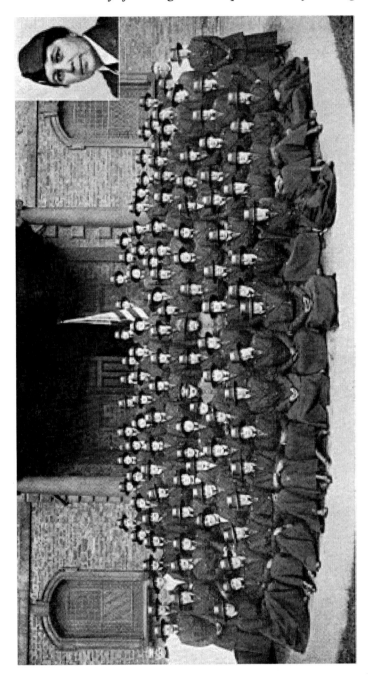

Nurses of Army Base Hospital Unit No. 11 World War I
Inset: Major Julia O. Flikke

The probationers wore plain blue gingham dresses and full gathered aprons and white Peter Pan collars. After probation the nurses wore blue and white striped uniforms with the skirts four inches from the floor, and high Bishop collars buttoned in the back. Black shoes and black cotton hose were worn. The aprons had full gathered skirts and large bibs with shoulder straps. The students had three hours off daily besides two half-days a week. Two late leaves were given each month. They received an allowance of four dollars per month the first year, six dollars the second year, and eight dollars the third year. Applicants were required to be nineteen years of age at the time of entrance. By special arrangement between Miss Jackson and Miss Mary Wheeler, Superintendent of Nurses of the Illinois Training School, a number of the senior students (class of 1918) were sent to the Cook County Hospital for a month of affiliation in obstetrical training. Not only did these nurses gain knowledge and experience insofar as this particular field was concerned, but the association in a hospital of a different type with patients of a different status was invaluable.

On April 6, 1917, the United States declared war on Germany. Signs appeared in the Nurses' Magazine—"Wanted, Nurses for the U.S. Army," "Your Country Needs You." Dr. A.J.Ochsner began to organize Unit No. 11, Mrs. Julia Flikke, 1915, was appointed chief nurse and the enrolling of Augustana nurses began in earnest. Mrs. Flikke published the following notice in the "Augustana Nurse" of May, 1917:

If our fathers, brothers, and others dear to us are called to fight for our country, should we nurses not be happy and thankful that our training has been preparing us also to render some service to our country in its hour of need? How better could we serve than by serving in battle? All women who love our country should be stirred with a desire to do some active relief work at this time; nurses should feel it not only a duty but also a privilege to serve in the Military Hospitals. Let it never be said that Augustana Nurses were slow to respond to the call—"Enroll today in Base Hospital No. 11."

Miss Jackson, Superintendent of Nurses, had suggested to

Dr. Wahlstrom and to the Board of Directors that the training school pin should be given to each nurse at graduation. Prior to this time each nurse had purchased her own. When the twenty-six nurses graduated that spring, for the first time the presentation of the pin was made part of the graduation program. Miss Jackson presented the pins. The wearing of the beautiful school emblem now took on a new meaning which linked the graduate in closer bonds with the hospital, its official staff, and Alumnae.

In the meantime nurses were being urged to <u>enroll</u>, EN-ROLL, <u>ENROLL</u>. The student nurses presented a beautiful new flag for the Nurses' Home. At this time Dr. A.J.Ochsner and Dr. Nelson M. Percy were each given the rank of Major in the U.S. Army. Miss Mabelle Sundblad, 1913, chief surgical nurse, and Miss Margaret Saenger, 1910, assistant to Miss Jackson, were given leave of absence to join Unit 11.

In May 1918, the graduating exercises for a class of twenty-seven nurses took place at Ebenezer Church. The Alumnae banquet was held at the Parkway Hotel and was attended by eighty nurses. The Alumnae Association presented to the Nurses' Home a Service Flag representing the fifty-one graduates in service. The doctors of Unit 11 were in camp at Des Moines, and all but six nurses of the Unit were in cantonments [a group of more or less temporary structures for housing troops].

In the summer of 1918, practically one-half of all the registered nurses of Illinois were in military service. Nurses were leaving for service [to live] in cantonments and later overseas. In their absence came the epidemic of influenza, creating a demand for skilled nursing. During the epidemic all available nursing was pressed into service. Unused buildings were turned into temporary hospitals, and persons who had not been afflicted volunteered to assist caring for the sick and dying.

In the hospital, at one time about forty student nurses were ill. As the "flu" cases increased, extra night nurses were placed on each floor. The students were supposed to have three hours off at night, but at times they worked the whole night through from 7 p.m. to 7 a.m. The term of night duty was for four weeks. The night nurses took turns cooking supper for the entire force. Some were very good cooks, others very poor. When the poor ones were discovered, they were not again asked to prepare the food. It was most difficult to find the time to prepare the meals.

There was no night operator at the switchboard; the night supervisor and the second floor nurses had to contend with that additional work. Some nights, just answering phone calls took up all one nurse's time.

The last two weeks of October revealed the greatest shortage of assistance due to much illness among doctors and nurses. Never in the history of Augustana Hospital had there been so many critically ill patients at one time. Class work for nurses came to almost a standstill during these trying times. War and influenza took up most of everyone's time and thought. Miss Jackson said that the more sick nurses there were, the harder everyone else worked. They were all thankful they remained well and were able to give assistance. All surgical work in the hospital, except emergency cases, was temporarily postponed. The order of the Health Department restricting visitors nearly caused a riot one evening when an unusually large number of visitors demanded to see their sick friends or members of their families. Two officers were stationed at the door, and after explaining the situation, succeeded in restoring order and calming the excited crowd.

In the meantime, interesting letters were received from those who were overseas. Those at home were conserving flour, sugar and butter. Prices were high and steadily soaring higher. Graduate nurses were given $6.00 a day. Skilled and unskilled labor received big wages. Women were taking the places left vacant by the men. Then came the great day of November 11, 1918, when the Armistice was signed and peace again reigned over the earth.

On July 26, 1919, Miss Pickhardt, accompanied by Miss Hildur Blomstrand, 1898, returned from California to Augustana Hospital for her last stay. She was very weak and suffered intensely. Although the best medical care was given her, it was of no avail. Two student senior nurses were selected to serve as her special nurses, and many times she expressed her appreciation for the splendid care given her. After her condition improved somewhat she was able to see her old friends for short visits. She was deeply interested in the hospital, its nurses, and the plans for the new building. At times there were hopes for Miss Pickhardt's recovery, but she passed away suddenly on August 26, 1919. It has been aptly said, "Death loves a shining mark." Miss Pickhardt possessed wonderful executive ability, great devotion to her friends and to her work, and had a self-sacrificing spirit. She was a power wherever she appeared. The good report that our training school and nurses have enjoyed can be traced to her efficient supervision.

During Miss Pickhardt's last illness, Miss Jackson enjoyed many little talks with her regarding the training school. One of the main questions at issue was to secure permission from the Board of Directors to employ an instructor. Many of the hospitals were now employing one or more full-time instructors. Miss Pickhardt spoke to Dr. A.J.Ochsner, and secured his approval and that of Dr. Wahlstrom. It was finally decided to have a full-time instructor of nurses. The need of more graduate supervision for the floors was also discussed.

On October 1, 1919, Miss Lillian Olsen, 1915, was appointed instructor, remaining in that capacity for two years, conducting classes during the school year from September to June. Miss Olsen relieved in the office of the Superintendent of Nurses during the summer vacations. Miss Jackson taught all classes in ethics; Miss Saenger, anatomy; and Miss Tweeton, advanced practical nursing. The instructor taught preliminary subjects in practical nursing and materia medica to probationers; to the older students she taught hygiene, care and feeding of children, obstetrics, materia medica and history of nursing. Because of the World War and influenza epidemic of 1918, class work had practically ceased. This necessitated double work for instructors and students for the following year. Miss Olsen, after giving the probationers demonstrations, also did the follow-up work on the floors.

Miss Jackson obtained graduate head nurses for second and third floors, and one to serve between fourth and fifth floors. Prior to this, senior nurses had acted as head nurses.

During this time for one year, the Public Health Nurses' Association of Chicago started a course for the training of Public Health Nurses. This was given to a group of selected students for a period of six weeks. The students lived at the South Side Nurses' Club, had their theoretical work there, and during the days accompanied some Public Health Nurse on her rounds. Several senior Augustana nurses were chosen and were much pleased with the arrangement, but the Public Health Nurses' Association found it too expensive to continue.

At Augustana Hospital the main problem was to obtain room for patients. Scores of patients were turned away every month. For many years the hospital had been filled to capacity. Single rooms were made into two and three-bed wards, and even the corridors were used for patients. The great need for a larger hospital and a new home for nurses was apparent to everyone. The Board of Directors was making plans for a greater Augustana Hospital.

Miss Esther Jackson was the first Superintendent of Nurses to use the Florence Nightingale Pledge at the graduating exercises:

I solemnly pledge myself before God and in the presence of this assembly to pass my life in purity and to practice my profession faithfully. I will abstain from whatever is deleterious and mischievous, and will not take or knowingly administer any harmful drug. I will do all in my power to maintain and elevate the standard of my profession, and will hold in confidence all personal matters committed to my keeping, and all family affairs coming to my knowledge in the practice of my calling. With loyalty will I endeavor to aid the physician in his work and devote myself to the welfare of those committed to my care.

In January 1920, an additional nurses' home was opened on

Cleveland Avenue where Miss Lillian Olsen and fifteen students lived until the new home was completed.

During the school year of 1920–1921, all class work was taken over by the instructor, with the exception of ethics, which Miss Jackson continued to teach, and dietetics, which was taught by Miss Williams. Classes were reorganized so that all subjects could be completed during the first two years of training, leaving the third year for lectures, and for a review of all nursing subjects in preparation for State Board examinations. At this time, each class was divided into two sections so that at no time was an entire class away from its duties in the hospital. The instructor chaperoned all lectures conducted by the doctors, consequently her duties began at eight in the morning and were not completed until nine at night. Lectures were conducted by doctors on the staff of the hospital, internes, and Dr. Wahlstrom.

In 1920, forty-five students were graduated, the largest class so far to graduate from Augustana Hospital. The Alumnae banquet was a most enjoyable affair, especially with so many happy, hopeful, new faces.

The Central Registry for Nurses had been rapidly growing; the need of a central location was felt, so the Registry was moved to the fifteenth floor of the Lake View Building at 116 South Michigan Avenue. The Residence Club at 2710 Prairie Avenue never did become a financial success. Mrs. Lucy Van Frank still continued as Registrar. All Augustana graduates were now receiving their calls through the Registry. The fee was ten dollars a year, and nurses were receiving six dollars per day for twenty-hour duty.

On January 7, 1920, the Augustana Alumnae Association decided to raise a Lila Pickhardt Memorial Fund, the money to be used in furnishing a recreation room in the new Nurses' Home whenever that dream would become a reality. Miss Esther B. Olson wrote letters to all the Alumnae members to remind them of Miss Pickhardt's outstanding qualities, and to urge them to help furnish a recreation room as a memorial to Miss Pickhardt.

The present Nurses' Homes were very crowded, so a new flat for eleven nurses was rented at 2056 Lincoln Avenue. All the flats had many inconveniences. Cots and beds were placed everywhere, old pantries served as closets, and kitchen sinks as washstands. Sometimes there was hot water and sometimes there was none.

The flats were all badly in need of repairs; but all these hardships were cheerfully borne for the building plans were being freely discussed, and the "Great Day" was coming when a modern Nurses' Home would be erected; therefore, a general spirit of cooperation existed. Dr. Wahlstrom announced that the financial campaign was on in earnest, and that the fund had reached the $163,000.00 mark.

Dr. A.J.Ochsner wished to have student special nurses for his surgical patients. In order to distinguish them from the other nurses, they wore dark gray uniforms with white collars and cuffs. They had four hours off duty every afternoon and extra days after coming off a case. These nurses enjoyed the distinction of being called Dr. Ochsner's gray nurses. The hospital received four dollars a day for the services of senior nurses, and three dollars a day for intermediate nurses. This money was placed in a fund reserved for the Nurses' Home. At this time, the Illinois State Board passed rules discouraging student specials, or at least limiting the practice to the senior year, and then to be only for a month.

There was some talk about the feasibility of spreading vacations over a period of twelve months, but the nurses protested against such a ruling.

Miss Charlotte Johnson resigned to be married, and Miss Vina Allen, 1906, took her place for a short time until Miss Emma Carlsted, 1916, became matron. Miss Margaret Saenger and Miss Marie K. Peterson continued as assistants to the superintendent of nurses.

The World War had deferred the erection of the new hospital, but the delay gave the Board of Directors time to study and perfect the plans. The old buildings had been removed from the proposed hospital site, and everything was in readiness for a modern hospital and training school for nurses.

It was planned to erect a building with a frontage on Garfield [Dickens] Avenue of 379 feet, with two seven-story pavilions extending to the south, and to have a sun porch on each floor on the south end.

The financial campaign of 1920 netted the sum of $116,894.04. This money was used to pay for the new hospital site and to apply on the cost of building the Nurses' Home. The Alumnae Association pledged $3,410.00, and individual classes pledged $3,525.00 towards the furnishings of the home.

[In 1921] two students at a time were being given a month of service in the laboratory to obtain instruction from the interne then on duty. It was found that he was usually too busy to devote much time to them, so they received very little instruction and very little supervision. Miss Jackson wished the school to be progressive, and urged the employing of a full time technician. In the summer, Miss Marie Fredrickson, 1903, accepted the position of laboratory technician. Dr. Gaillardo, a former interne, came to take charge of surgical specimens, pathological sections, Wassermans, cultures, etc. Previous to this time the pathological work had been in charge of Dr. John Nazum.[11] Two or three student nurses came in for half-day periods to help with blood counts, urinalyses, and examination of sputum for tubercle bacilli and of feces for blood. No maid was assigned to the laboratory; the nurses were obliged to keep the room presentable, as well as to wash specimen bottles and glass slides, to label and file all tissue slides, and to pass report sheets to the different floors.

Miss Jackson now made a change in the style of collar, apron,

---

11. From a letter written by Marie Fredrickson, 1903.

and cap. The nurses had always worn high collars. During the warm weather these collars wilted, and besides, on off duty hours when low necked dresses were worn, there was always visible a discolored neck. On very hot days the nurses were allowed to wear large handkerchiefs worn kerchief style. The full, gathered aprons were changed to gored aprons and separate bibs; these could be laundered more easily and were also more practical in other ways.

Miss Jackson and Miss Saenger found it more and more difficult to teach the student nurses to make the organdy caps. Everyone liked the old caps because they were pretty, dainty and distinctive, but many of the young nurses did not know how to sew. The graduates were also asking for a change; many outside of Chicago found it difficult to obtain the organdy and rushing. A cap was desired that could be laundered and could be packed flat in a suitcase. Samples were brought to the Alumnae meeting, and the style designed by Matilda Anderson, 1915, was accepted and has been in use ever since [to 1987].

In 1921, twenty-one nurses were graduated. This was the first class to wear the new caps and the low collars on their uniforms. The skirts had been four inches from the floor, but whereas dresses were being worn extremely short, the nurses were permitted to wear uniforms seven inches from the floor. This class was also permitted to wear white Oxfords. The student nurses could wear black Oxfords during the summer, but wore high black shoes in the colder weather. During the winter months it was necessary to arise earlier to allow time for lacing or buttoning high shoes. Graduate nurses wore high, white shoes.

The Annual Alumnae Banquet which was held at the Parkway Hotel on May 6, was one of the most enjoyable in the history of the training school. Covers were laid for 125; this included the honor guests, the class of 1921, and the class of 1896, which was celebrating its twenty-fifth anniversary. Of the eight members of the latter class, five attended: Miss Louise

Bylander, Mrs. Hilda Hedin Rydell, Mrs. Josephine Oberg Lofgren, Mrs. Ingeborg Johnson Fowler and Miss Louise Wensjo. Mrs. Edward Ochsner, their former superintendent of nurses was also an honor guest. The menu cards were tied with the Augustana colors of blue and gold.

The committee on arrangements, Miss Ida Burkhalter, chairman, with the chef of the Parkway Hotel, planned the farewell to the old cap. A round form of ice cream was covered with a perfect replica of the organdy cap made of spun sugar, complete even to the black velvet ribbon and ruching. When it was time for dessert, the lights were turned low and the waiters lined up at one end of the room, each holding a tray on which was a fancy cap. Lights were directed on the caps and Miss Esther Holmgren, 1919, recited the poem composed by Mabell Holm, 1918:

PASSING OF THE CAP

> Here's to the cap we know so well.
> The memories it brings, no words can tell,
> Memories of days we shall never forget,
> Recollections so tender, no thoughts of regret.
> This cap is our emblem, it stands for one thing,
> To humanity's suffering, relief I will bring.
> Though we bury our treasure, our memory still clings,
> Fond memories, fond longings, our yearning hearts swell.
> Staunch, faithful friend, We must bid you farewell.

It was a most effective and touching scene, and a very pretty sight. The ribbons were removed, the caps were cut and each nurse served a portion; the ice cream was also sliced and served, and—the old organdy cap was a memory. [12]

The erection of the Nurses' Home was now in progress. The building was to have seven stories and a basement, and to house 240 nurses. The construction was to be concrete, reinforced

---

12. Story of 1921 banquet from letters written by Miss Ida Burkhalter and Miss Mabell Holm.

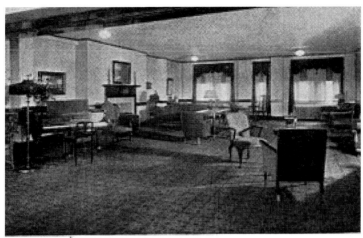

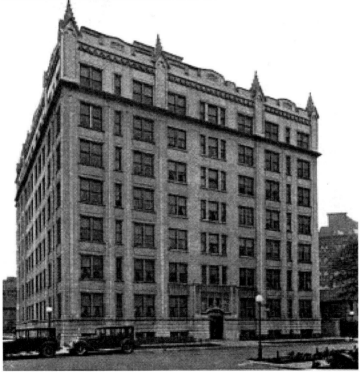

Lila Pickhardt Memorial Room
Nurses' Home erected 1922

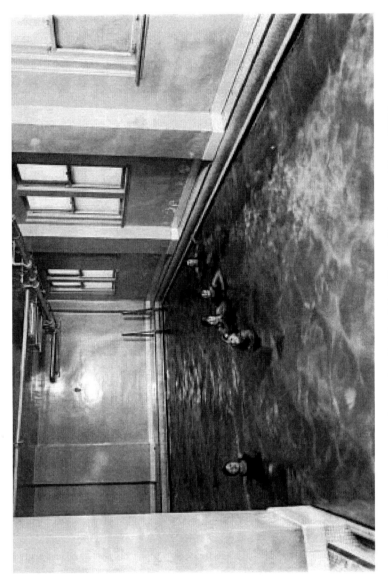

Basement Swimming Pool of the Nurses' Residence Circa, 1922

steel, faced with cut stone, light brick and terra cotta, all fire-proof; each floor to have a south veranda with connecting iron stairways. The estimated cost of the building, without the furnishings, was $325,000.00. A large assembly or living room 27 by 53 feet, with a sun parlor and an adjoining kitchen, were on the first floor; also the office, small reception rooms, the class rooms, library, reading rooms and suites for the Superintendent of Nurses, and for the Directress of the Home. A large recreation room, 27 by 53 feet, with an adjoining kitchen, and a swimming pool, were in the basement. The open space in the rear which was enclosed with a brick wall was to have a sunken garden.

The Alumnae Association decided to give a Bazaar to aid the Lila Pickhardt Memorial Fund. There were $1,685.00 in the fund, but that was not sufficient to furnish a room 27 by 53 feet. The mother of Miss Sara Liljegren, 1914, offered to weave rag rugs if supplied with sewn rags. At the November meeting, the Alumnae members brought scissors, needles and thread. Old striped uniforms and white aprons were torn into strips and many balls of carpet rags were made. A prize was given to the one who sewed the largest ball. The bazaar was most carefully planned. Every Alumnae member was asked to contribute, and to attend if possible. Each class was represented by a chairman who contacted each of her classmates, and the proceeds from the gifts of the individual classes were accounted for and credited. Mrs. Helen Yoerg Thulin was chairman of the bazaar, which was held on December 2 and 3; it was a splendid success and netted $3,600.00. The nurses felt repaid for their faithful hard work.

This spring [1922] Miss Esther Jackson resigned her position as Superintendent of Nurses to resume her old position at the Iowa Lutheran Hospital in Des Moines, Iowa. She was succeeded by Miss Ida Ehman, 1915. Miss Marie K. Peterson remained as Miss Ehman's assistant. Miss Margaret Saenger was appointed Directress of the Nurses' Residence.

Students had been receiving an allowance of four, six and eight dollars a month. The seniors were given an increase of two dollars a month at this time.

September 15, 1922, was the last night spent in the old Nurses' Homes. Nurses in the various flats celebrated with the wildest parties they could plan. No one interfered, so they did just as they pleased; they had been told that the new home was to be more quiet and reserved. When the next day dawned, trunks, boxes and bags were packed. Everyone was in readiness for moving. Each nurse carried her own belongings over to a room all newly furnished with two cots, dresser, library table and two chairs. The senior nurses had the preference of rooms. Mrs. A.J.Ochsner had much to do with the planning of the furnishings of the home. She especially asked for comfortable beds with good mattresses.

Then came a great change into the life of the Home. Lunching in the rooms was prohibited. Any four girls who occupied the same suite of rooms could have a good time, but they had to dress and go down to the kitchen if they wanted a lunch. The kitchen next to the recreation room in the basement was completely equipped and was for the use of student nurses; the one adjoining the living room on first floor was for the use of the supervisors. Through an arrangement with the hospital authorities the Alumnae Association received permission to use the living room for its monthly meetings. All classes were held in the class room. Everyone was permitted the use of the swimming pool, gymnasium and living room. The doors were locked at ten o'clock, and late leaves were strictly enforced. A student was fined twenty-five cents if the shades of her room were not drawn after dark.

Until the erection of the new hospital, the two upper floors of the new home were reserved for the exclusive use of Dr. A.J.Ochsner's surgical patients, thus relieving the crowded condition of the hospital, and making a combined hospital capacity of 260 beds. The patients' department in the Nurses' Residence, which became known as "The Extension," was kept entirely separate from the nurses' quarters.

On sixth floor, all rooms were used as two-bed rooms with the exception of the corner room, 612, which was a private room with bath. There were thirty-seven beds on sixth floor. Room 618, which later became the general bathroom for the nurses, was the main kitchen where all the food for the patients was prepared by the cook. Room 620 was the diet kitchen, a very small room, but it contained the gas stove, sink, ice box, ice chest for chipped ice, medicine cupboard, water cooler and tray rack. On seventh floor there were fourteen private rooms and five two-bed rooms. Room 720 was the diet kitchen. A bungalow-like addition above the seventh floor served as the operating room. Special duty was entirely supplied by the student nurses who wore gray uniforms.

The swimming pool was now ready for use; graduates were invited to come and bring their swimming suits and towels. After one of the nurses had been pulled out of the pool by her hair, it was decided best to receive some instructions on "How to Swim." Miss Hartwick of the University of Chicago came to teach a class of twenty students and twelve graduates. After fifteen lessons they secured a letter "A" on their bathing suits, provided they had accomplished the following:

Perfect stroke, length of tank
Treading water
Back stroke
Side stroke
Australian crawl
Floating
Bobbing
Kick-off

Students were taking calisthenics twice a week under the direction of Miss Neeb of the Chicago Normal School of Physical Education.

It had become increasingly difficult for the nurses to find time to prepare the midnight meal. Through the suggestion of Miss Carlsted, Dr. Wahlstrom engaged a night cook. This new change was a great boon to the nurses, who now had properly prepared meals served at the right time; likewise, dishwashing was eliminated.

In September, Miss Carlsted resigned as matron to become instructor of nurses at the Swedish Hospital in Minneapolis. Miss Nettle Hoff, 1912, succeeded her.

At this time [1923] there was installed on each floor a chart room with a gray desk. Charts were now removed from the beds. All the nurses wanted to chart at once, and how exciting it was. Also a new system was introduced in checking up and keeping an accurate account of narcotics.

Twelve-hour duty for graduate [private duty] nurses was being discussed; opinions varied greatly. These were some of the arguments:

> A tired nurse is a dangerous nurse.
> A twenty-four-hour nurse is simply an endurance test.
> Two nurses make two personalities for the patient to contend with.
> Patients cannot afford two nurses.
> Most older nurses have been alone on a case, except when patient was very ill.
> A good nurse should not care to share the care of her patient.

The matter was tabled for the time being.

The graduating class of 1925 was making plans for the first Annual. In discussions about the name of their Annual, they decided that one of the most interesting books they had read was the "Hour Book" which showed their hours off duty, so it was decided to call the new Annual the "Hour Book." To make it more possessive, it was named the "Our Book." The year book of 1925 concerned members of the entire student body, contained numerous pictures, and inspirational articles which tended to foster class spirit and school loyalty.

In 1924, the bobbed hair craze reached Augustana Hospital. This was the so-called "Flapper Age" when everywhere women, young and old, appeared with bobbed hair; but all training schools looked upon it with marked disapproval. Some nurses were bold enough to have their hair bobbed, but came on duty with "buns" or "rolls" pinned on. Some hospitals refused to employ graduates who had short hair. This craze caused the superintendents a great deal of grief; in some places whole classes were reprimanded and special meetings of the Boards of Directors were called. Training schools had extra sessions with their training school committees, but nevertheless bobbed heads continued to increase. The hospital boards declared it lowered a woman's dignity, that it was unprofessional, and that loose hair would get into the food. Newspapers and magazines wrote editorials and articles about this most vexing problem.

On September 25, 1924, Miss Ehman organized the Jenny Lind Chorus and placed it under the leadership of Mr. Paul Hultman, of the Bush Conservatory of Music. The class that entered that fall was the largest class ever to enter the school, and was the first complete class to be all high school graduates. Miss Ehman discovered that many of these students could sing and her suggestion of a chorus met with enthusiasm. She felt that it would be both an educational and recreational activity and hoped it would become a permanent part of the school. To foster interest, Mr. Hultman brought artists from various studios to give short concerts.

In January 1925, the Jenny Lind Chorus gave its first public concert. It was given at the Irving Park Lutheran Church, and proved to be a great success. In February they gave another concert at the Ebenezer Church; in March at the Saron Lutheran Church; and in April, at the Trinity Lutheran Church.

On December 5, the Senior Bazaar, given to raise money for the first "Our Book," netted $500.00.

The Seniors experienced a new privilege, one late leave a week. They pledged themselves not to overstep their good luck.

The following rules applied to the Nurses' Home:

Outer door locked at 10 p.m. on week days and at 10:30 p.m. on Sundays.
Late leave key once a week after the preliminary period.
Each nurse responsible for her own room.

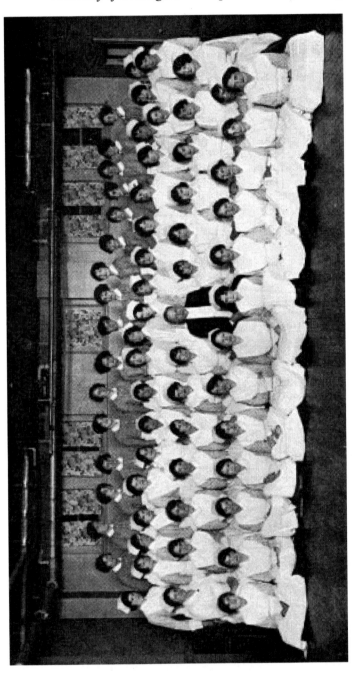

Jenny Lind Chorus 1925

Preliminary period four months, included in the three-year term.

Nurses on duty fifty-six hours a week, from 7 a.m. to 7 p.m., with three hours off; three days off for rest and recreation after being on a term of one month of night duty.

Four weeks vacation allowed each nurse each year.

The large class of students who entered in October, 1924, received their caps at a special ceremony on February 6, 1925. This was the first class to have the four months preliminary period and the first nurses to receive their caps at a special ceremony.

Miss Helen Olson wrote the following regarding the Nurses' uniform:

As all of you know, this is the first time we have made an occasion of the wearing of the cap and uniform. All graduates will tell you that the first day they appeared in caps and stripes was much more thrilling than any subsequent day in their nursing career, superseding even the day of graduation.

We must first remember that we are to be uniform in our uniforms and are also to take pride in our appearance as nurses. So look to your caps—the fold should be three inches wide; wear it uniformly. See that your sleeve bands have buttons, keep uniforms mended. If your apron bands are too wide, sit down and sew in a tuck. Wear bone collar buttons in the aprons. Do not wear fancy, clocked, or chiffon hose; use plain black Oxfords with rubber heels.

Twenty-eight nurses graduated on April 30 [1925], with exercises at the Trinity Lutheran Church. The Hospital reception was held April 28 in the beautiful Lila Pickhardt Memorial Room. The Alumnae dinner was given at the Belden Hotel. The honor guests were the class of 1925 and the class of 1900 which was represented by Katherine Knudson and Mrs. Hilma Johnson Anderson of Albert City, Iowa. One hundred forty nurses were present.

The first edition of the "Our Book" was presented at the Alumnae Banquet. It was a splendid effort and showed true pioneer spirit. The class of 1925 dedicated the first "Our Book" to Dr. A.J.Ochsner, "...whose influence and direction have been largely responsible for the development of a greater Augustana and for its present rank among Schools for Nurses,..." Dr.

Ochsner was much pleased when a copy was presented to him. In Memoriam they honored Dr. Wahlstrom "...whose paternal guidance and love for twenty years has upheld Augustana in its brightest light, the memory of whom still lingers with us as an idea, a follower of the best morals and standards."

Miss Marie K. Peterson, 1920, assistant to Miss Ehman, resigned her position to be married. Miss Agnes Bergh, 1916, became her successor.

On May 12, 1925, the Jenny Lind Chorus presented a musical program in commemoration of Florence Nightingale; this program was broadcast from Station WEBH at the Edgewater Beach Hotel. The following day the newspapers reviewed the broadcast as follows: "The Jenny Lind Chorus, consisting of seventy nurses from the Augustana Hospital, appeared on Station WEBH last evening. The selections were delightful, and the smooth blending of their voices carried with it something of the ethereal." Congratulations poured in from our Alumnae members, doctors, and former internes, from all over the country, much to the delight of Miss Ehman and the nurses. Miss Ehman stated, "The Chorus has cultural value for it develops the nurses' appreciation of good music, encourages the musically talented and stimulates group spirit. They take pride in singing."

The corner stone for the new hospital was laid on June 21, 1925, on a Sunday afternoon at three o'clock. In the corner stone were placed many papers and pamphlets, and among these was a copy of the 1925 "Our Book."

On Saturday, July 26, 1925, Dr. A.J.Ochsner passed away. He had served from 1888.

The Board of Directors in their Resolution said:

THEREFORE, BE IT RESOLVED:

That we express in unstinted words our appreciation of the brilliant services of Dr. Ochsner during all the years he was connected with the hospital, from 1888 to 1891 as Assistant Chief of Staff, and since 1891, for a period of 34 years, as the Chief of Staff.

The completion of the Augustana Nurses' Residence marked the beginning of new recreational activities among the student nurses. The library became the center of educational recreation. The Augustana Alumnae Association provided periodicals of general interest as well as professional literature. Class parties and informal gatherings had also gained in popularity since the nurses had suitable social rooms. Holidays, such as Christmas, St. Valentine's Day, St. Patrick's Day and Halloween were celebrated with appropriate parties. Each New Year's Day there was a large reception, and open house was held on Hospital Day. There were the usual class banquets at graduation time; these were managed by the students themselves. Weekly sandwich sales were often the source of revenue for financing such parties. A group of nurses made sandwiches and sold them to the nurses in the home, going through the corridors between the hours of eight and ten in the evening.

The craze for bobbed hair was continuing, and superintendents of nurses were undecided whether or not to permit it. One night Miss Helena McMillan, Superintendent of Nurses of the Presbyterian Hospital, Chicago, and also President of the League of Nursing Education, addressed a meeting and said she felt it wrong to make any further protest; she urged all training schools to permit the bobbing of hair. At Augustana Hospital, after nurses were permitted to appear with bobbed hair, they were required to wear nets. The skirts at this time were growing shorter and shorter, and at the urgent plea of the nurses, uniform skirts were shortened to fourteen inches from the floor. A few nurses came on duty with skirts to their knees. The short skirt fad caused upheavals in many training schools.

Miss Ehman had at one time visited Peter Bent Brigham Hospital, Boston, and had become interested in its method of having a senior nurse assist with practical demonstrations and then do follow up work on the floors. She decided to put this method into effect at Augustana; it proved to be most successful. It was a splendid experience for the seniors, and most helpful to the young students. Miss Ehman was much pleased with the result.

In February 1926, the probationers, who were now being called "Preliminary Students," were given their caps at a special service held in the chapel. The service was conducted by Rev. Nelson and consisted of a hymn sung by all the students, a prayer, a Scripture reading, and a special welcome to the new nurses who were, for the first time, wearing their striped uniforms. The capping ceremony was conducted by Miss Gaulke and was most impressive. Each junior student received the emblem of responsibility, the Augustana cap, from a senior or intermediate student who recited a quotation as she pinned the cap in place, and then extended congratulations. Thereupon the new juniors recited the Florence Nightingale Pledge.

In this year, the old card system used in keeping the nurses' records, was discontinued and new, modern records were begun with files and cabinets; each nurse's record was then complete in her separate envelope. Student nurses were no longer put on special duty; graduate nurses were called for all special cases. There were 158 nurses in training at this time. The nurses received six dollars a month the first year, eight dollars a month the second year and ten dollars a month the third year. The preliminary students wore plain blue gingham uniforms with white collars and cuffs and aprons without bibs. All uniforms were made with long sleeves, skirts fourteen inches from the floor. Black Oxfords with black cotton hose were still being worn.

On April 1, Miss Amelia Loerhke, '11, became the first paid anesthetist at Augustana Hospital. Dr. Ben Morgan had been coming in occasionally for many years to give gas anaesthesia.

Registration with New York State had been discontinued, and Miss Ehman had been striving for three years to have it restored. Miss Bailey, one of the Regents of the New York State Board made a general inspection. She devoted a whole day to the inspection of both the old hospital and the Extension, and interviewed the nurses of the school. In order to be reinstated, it became necessary to have four months' affiliation with Children's Memorial Hospital, and four months' work at the Chicago Lying-in Hospital. The affiliation with the Children's Memorial Hospital began on the first of May. This necessitated a change in the teaching schedule, as most of the class work had to be completed during the first two years, reserving the last year for special subjects and affiliation.

On May 12, another great sorrow came to the Augustana Hospital Training School; Miss Mabelle T. Sundblad, who had been the surgical nurse for thirteen years, passed away after an illness of a few hours. She was a member of the class of 1913, and shortly after her graduation accepted the position of surgical supervisor in our hospital. She was a most able and competent surgical nurse, and taught many of her students to become efficient surgical nurses. Visiting surgeons often watched Miss Sundblad as she waited upon Dr. Ochsner, and marveled at the ease she displayed, and at her cool, calm, collected manner in conducting a long schedule of operations. It was most difficult to find someone to replace her, but Miss Trine Schmidt, '20, with the cooperation of the other assistants carried on until the vacancy was filled.

Sixteen months after construction began on the new hospital, it was ready for occupancy. The dedication service was held on June 24, 1926, in the presence of His Royal Highness, Crown Prince Gustav Adolph of Sweden, the Crown Princess Louise, and many thousands of spectators. A platform had been erected for the occasion along Garfield [Dickens] Avenue in front of the hospital.

The Crown Prince spoke in both Swedish and English, paying a special tribute to Dr. Albert J. Ochsner.

In June 1926, the Alumnae Association decided to furnish a room in the new hospital at a cost of $300.00. This room was to be called "The Alumnae Room." Twelve hour duty for graduates was instituted at Augustana Hospital at this time. It was a welcome relief not to have cots standing about in the patients' rooms, and nurses going through the corridors dressed in kimonos. Also, it enabled the nurses to obtain proper rest. At first the patients protested somewhat, but soon became accustomed to the change. They could have either a day nurse or a night nurse or both. Six dollars a day was charged for twelve hour duty at the hospital plus $1.50 a day for the nurse's board; seven dollars was charged for twenty-four hour duty in the homes. Only graduate nurses were employed as "specials." Lockers for private duty nurses were placed on each floor; the nurse to obtain a key from the Superintendent of Nurses' office when first assigned to a case. All calls were arranged through the Central Registry; each nurse paid a yearly fee of $15.00 to the registry.

To Miss Ehman, who had had the task of opening the new Nurses' Residence, came also the task of moving into the new Hospital. As the building was nearing completion, the nurses became anxious to move. All the equipment was on hand; the nurses assigned to make up the beds were thrilled to be using all new supplies. They went happily from room to room, from floor to floor, until all was in readiness. Every chair, table and dresser was put in place, curtains hung, and rugs were laid. The bedside tables were equipped with everything needed for the patients' bedside care.

Only the patients from the Extension were transferred to the new hospital or East Building as it came to be called; the old hospital now became officially known as the West Building. The plan was to have medical and obstetrical patients at the West Building, and all surgical patients at the East Building. The combined capacity of the East and West Buildings, not including bassinets, was 450 beds. The first five floors of the new building were used first, and by the end of a year, all seven floors were in operation. The upper floors of the Nurses' Residence were now used as a part of the nurses' quarters, so the "Extension" became a thing of the past.

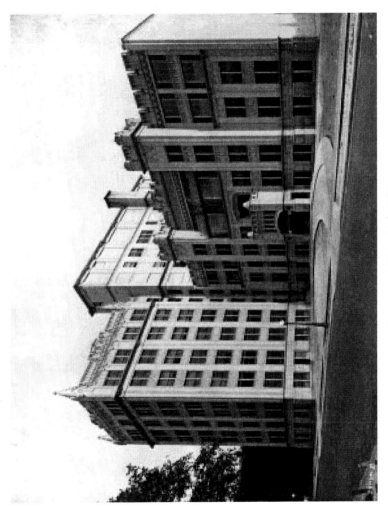

Augustana Hospital 1926

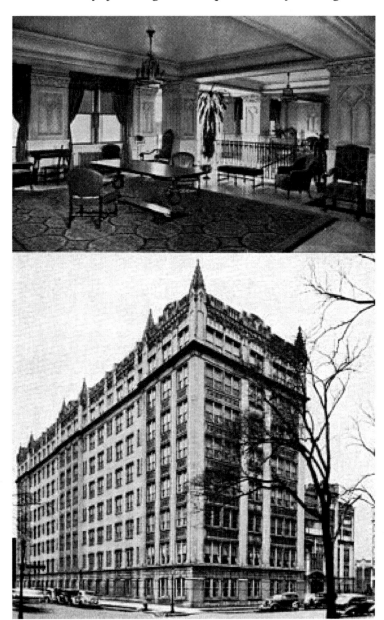

Hospital Lobby
Augustana Hospital 1926

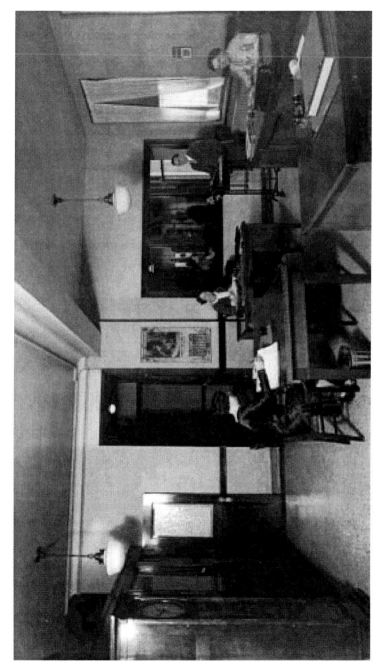

Business and Administration Office at Augustana Hospital

The X-ray department was under the direction of Dr. David S. Beilin. Miss J. Annyce Hummel, '18, served as technician. Two courses in the principles and practice of X-ray technique were offered to registered nurses—a three months' and six months' course. A tuition fee was charged for the three months' course, but the six months' course was given free because the nurse was required to assist the technician with the work. The hospital also offered a four months' course in anaesthesia under the direction of Miss Amelia H. Loehrke. The student received both practical and theoretical work in the various types of an-aesthesia, namely, ether, chloroform, nitrous oxide and ethylene. Only two students were taken at one time; a fee of $100.00 was charged for the course.

This autumn [1926] the preliminary students entered in two divisions, a group of fifty came September 1, another group of twenty-five on September 30. This was the largest preliminary class thus far to have entered the training school.

Miss Margaret Saenger organized the Big Sister's Movement. The purpose of this was to provide a friend for the new student nurse. The name of each prospective student was given to an older student who wrote to her "little sister" and gave her all the information she could concerning the hospital, the home and the various activities. When the new student arrived she found her big sister ready to help with the problems that arise during the first few months of training. The Big Sister organization was a great help to the younger nurses; it was an example of the friendly spirit that prevailed among the nurses of the Augustana Hospital Training School.

In December of 1926, a laboratory was equipped on the eighth floor of the Nurses' Resident in the room previously used as an operating room during the days of the Extension. This laboratory was to be used in teaching chemistry and bacteriology to the student nurses. Provision was made for twenty-four students as a laboratory group, each nurse having individual equipment. It was here that Dr. Rudolph Kremer devoted one or more hours weekly in lecturing to the students. He was a splendid teacher. After this time no students have received training at the clinical laboratory in the hospital.[13]

In the fall of 1926, remodeling was done to make a modern obstetrical department in the West Building. Rooms 402 to 408, and 502 to 508 were made into nurseries. The remainder of fourth and fifth floors was used for the obstetrical patients. On sixth floor the main operating room was kept intact for gynecological surgery. The operating room near the passenger elevator, formerly number three dressing room, was fitted for a main operating room to be used for any other patients. The remaining space in the old surgical department and the delivery rooms was remodeled for birth rooms and labor rooms. Dr. F.H.Falls, who had succeeded Dr. Rudolph Holmes as chief of the obstetrical department, used this department for all of his gynecological surgery. The obstetrical personnel had charge of this surgery as well as the post-operative care of the patients. The surgical personnel from the East Building had charge of any other surgery, but there were only a few cases each month.

The chapel now was used for a demonstration room and devotional services were conducted each morning in the nurses' dining room. All of the laundry work from both hospitals continued to be done in the old laundry at the West Building. Trucks were hired to transport the large baskets of linens.

In January 1927, began the task of making a complete survey of nursing in the United States. A grading committee had been composed of a group of nurses, representing the various organizations; of doctors, representing the medical organizations; a lay woman, representing the public; and educators for giving technical advice on educational problems. The committee had taken its function to be the ways and means for insuring an ample supply of nursing service of whatever type and quality was needed for adequate care of the patient, at a price

---

13. Miss Marie Fredrickson, '03, laboratory technician.

within his reach. The heads of this committee were Dr. William Darrack and Dr. May Ayers Burgess of New York City. [14]

In March 1927, Miss Agnes Bergh, following a serious illness, resigned as Assistant Superintendent of Nurses. Her successor was Thyra Larson, '20.

At this time a steel display frame for the pictures of our graduation classes was procured for the Nurses' Residence. It was hoped it would prove to be interesting to the nurses of the future as well as to those of the present. Miss Annabel Alberts, '27, gave much of her time to do the lettering on the pictures as they were mounted.

On Saturday, May 7, the Alumnae Banquet was given at the Drake Hotel; 170 nurses attended. The graduating class and the class of 1902 were guests of honor. Two members of the latter class were present—Mrs. Rosala Freeman Lewis, St. Cloud, Minnesota and Mrs. Rebecca Johnson-Mellin, Marquette, Michigan. The following toast was given to the class of 1927 by Miss Helen Olson, '16:

> It is my pleasure to convey to you the sincere good wishes of all of those who have gone before you, extending back thirty-two years. This body of women, The Augustana Alumnae, have a peculiar interest in you-their youngest arrival, their latest child. Everyone of them has trod the same road as you, had the same long weary hours and footsore bodies along with the joy and satisfaction of work well done and difficulties overcome; the same dogged tenacity to their goal. Now to you, the child of our Alumnae, I am going to read a little children's verse written by A.A. Milne. Someone said of this poet that he wrote children's verses for grown-ups to read. It is called "The End."
>
> > When I was one
> > I had just begun.
> > When I was two
> > I was nearly new.
> > When I was three
> > I was hardly me.
> > When I was four
> > I was not much more

---

14. Committee of the Grading of Nursing schools, Nursing Schools Today and Tomorrow, pp. 15–16.

When I was five
I was just alive.
But now I am six
I'm clever as clever,
So I think I'll be six
For ever and ever.

You smile at this as I did the first time, but, as is usual with the most simple things, it has a much deeper meaning. How many of you are going to be six now "for ever and ever?" How many, now that you are graduated, are going to call this "the end" and be content to stay as you are now? After the novelty of being a graduate wears off, are you going to remain as you are now "for ever and ever?"

If I were your fairy godmother and now, on the evening of your birth, could give to you the gift which would be most prized and useful to you in your life, the gift I would choose for each one of you, I am afraid you would think rather queer. It has no definite name, just as it cannot be definitely explained—for I would give you the double gifts of the inward vision and inward dissatisfaction. I do not want you to be dissatisfied with externals and other people and always rumbling and complaining. But I said an inner dissatisfaction; sit down and with this inner vision examine yourself and say to yourself a year from now, "Am I still six, or have I grown in the past year?" And I hope that you will find in yourself a dissatisfaction which will spur you on for your second mile, to not be content with whatever education or training you have, but to seek more to keep abreast of the times and not be six when other people are twelve; to attempt to improve yourself in whatever manner needs improvement, and we all need it. And as time passes on we will meet again some day, with you as our honored twenty-five year class. May your accomplishments be great and your inner dissatisfaction be somewhat satisfied, and each of you be a true. "Lady of the Lamp" in that you tended faithfully the inner light which God places in the souls of every one of us to lead us onto higher things.

At the end of May, Miss Ida Ehman resigned her position as Superintendent of Nurses. Before Miss Ehman left she had arranged for four months' affiliation in obstetrical training at the Chicago Lying-In Hospital; this went to effect June 1, 1927.

August 1, 1927, Miss Mabel E. Haggman, a graduate of the General Hospital, Kansas City, Missouri, came to Augustana as the new Superintendent of Nurses. For the previous ten years Miss Haggman had been the Superintendent of Nurses at Grace Hospital, Detroit, Michigan and Hurley Hospital, Flint, Michigan. Miss Helen Olson, instructor, and Miss Thyra Larson, had carried the responsibilities of the Training School office during the summer months. Miss Larson remained as Miss Haggman's assistant.

On September 1, 1927, twenty-six students enrolled; a second group of twenty-six entered on October 1, and a third group entered on October 31; making a class of about seventy-five. This class, upon entrance, was asked to make a deposit of $25.00 to pay for books. A students' service room was equipped adjoining the small parlor at the Nurses' Residence. This was fitted with an electric plate and dishes so that the nurses might prepare a light lunch for their friends if they so desired.

On November 15, a Central Service Room in conjunction with the old supply room was opened with Miss Vera Sifford, '22, in charge. The personnel consisted of four nursing students and two maids. With the exception of Dr. Edward Ochsner's and Dr. Lundgren's patients, who continued to have their dressings done by the operating room personnel, all other dressings were now being done on the floors by the Service Room personnel. Dressing carts had replaced the market baskets for dressings when the East Building was opened. The Service Room maintained tray service: hypodermoclyses, infusions, intravenous injections, etc. Inhalators and all rubber goods were dispensed from this department. During the first year of its existence, 15,323 dressings were done. The Service Room was kept open from 6:30 a.m. to 11:00 p.m., after which the night supervisory cared for any service needed. All surgical supplies with the exception of sponges used in surgery were made in the supply room.

In July, 1928, Dr. Burgess, the director of the Committee on the Grading of Nursing Schools, published a complete report in a book entitled "Nurses, Patients, and Pocket Books." The findings of the Grading Committee would seem to lead to four suggestions:

1. Reduce and improve the supply. Raise entrance requirements high enough so that only properly qualified women will be admitted to the profession.
2. Replace students with graduates. Put the majority of hospital bedside nursing in the hands of graduate nurses.

3. Assist hospitals in securing funds for the employment of graduate nurses.
4. Get the public support for nursing education. Place schools of nursing under the direction of nurse educators instead of hospital administrators; awaken the public to the fact that if society wants good nursing it must pay the cost of educating nurses. Nursing education is a public and not a private responsibility.

The Committee on the Grading of Nursing Schools was a cooperative National organization officially sponsored by the American Medical Association, the American College of Surgeons, the American Hospital Association, the National League of Nursing Education, the National Organization for Public Health Nursing and the American Public Health Association. The Chairman of the committee was William Darrach, M.D., dean of the College of Physicians and Surgeons, Columbia University; the twenty-one members consisted of nurses, physicians, hospital and public health administrators, educators, and laymen of national prominence.

In 1928, there were two thousand members in the National League of Nursing Education. This body may now be said to control the nursing standards of the country. Since it is composed of representative and influential women, their opinions must be accepted as the best thought of the time.[15]

Twenty-three preliminary students were admitted on September 5. The following day the Big Sisters entertained them with a picnic in Lincoln Park. On October 5, twenty-two students were admitted, and on November 1, twenty-five were admitted. A $35.00 deposit was required from all students this year.

In the fall of 1928, the Thalian Drama Club was organized "to help bring joy, happiness and a little playful fun to those who may have forgotten how to play." This was an honor society, whose order consisted of elective members of a certain scholastic standing. If their grades became lower than eighty-three, members could be carried only for one year. All new candidates were chosen by club members. The object of the club

---

15. Trained Nurse & Hospital Review, June 1928, p.687.

was to arouse and maintain a real, intrinsic interest in dramatic art, and at the same time provide the necessary facilities for developing individual talents. In carrying out these objects they gave several one-act plays for the students and faculty. They endeavored to give one big play a year. Under the efficient leadership of Miss Saenger and the direction of Miss Current, a dramatic teacher, the work became gratifyingly interesting and progressive. There were twenty charter members: Hortense Fortney, '30, was President. The membership was limited to twenty-five nurses who had been approved by Miss Haggman. Dues were fifteen cents a month. The first play, "Gift," was given at Christmas time at the Trinity parish house. The second play, "Pin Money," was given at the Club rooms of the Daughters and Sons of Sweden.

The nurses at the Residence were enjoying a fine Zenith radio. Staff doctors and friends of the nurses and the hospital made this radio possible. Mrs. A.J.Ochsner, who was always interested in the progress of the hospital and school, sent many books for the school library. Often she sent the nurses tickets for the Symphony Orchestra and other splendid concerts. Many friends helped to give the students a happy Christmas. Dr. Henry Kleinpel never failed to give them ten dollars for their Christmas party. Dr. Frick also remembered them by sending candy. Early on Christmas morning the Chorus sang Christmas carols at both the East and the West Building.

The Alumnae Association requested the members to submit words and music for an original school song; three prizes were to be given for the best songs; ten, five and three dollars, respectively. This was later changed to a grand prize of $25.00. The Association also passed a resolution that married nurses were to be carried on a separate registry, and that they were to be called only after the supply of single nurses was exhausted; also, that they were expected to take night duty as well as day duty. A Private Duty Section of the Alumnae Association was started; monthly meetings were held in the Sun Room on the eighth floor of the East Building.

The preliminary students who entered in September, 1929, were the first to wear green uniforms made on straight lines, with cuffs three inches wide on long sleeves and a white Buster Brown collar. A white "butcher" style apron and black Oxfords worn with black hose completed the uniform.

Miss Thyra Larson resigned her position as Assistant Superintendent of Nurses to become the wife of Mr. Eric Lindstrand. She had been a faithful, competent nurse, and a loyal Alumnae worker. She helped to inaugurate the Scholarship Fund, which is the outstanding contribution of the student body. Miss Larson was succeeded by Miss Amy Chamberlain, '12.

In November, 1929, a great many influenza cases were admitted and quarantined on second and third floors of the West Building, where Mrs. Nora Smith, '26, was the supervisor. This epidemic, while not of the virulent type of the war period, was very severe, and as graduate nurses were unable to fill all the demands, the student nurses carried a heavy burden; they worked long hours, but were rewarded by the fact that most of the patients recovered.

Affiliation with Cook County Hospital for obstetrics began on April 1, 1929, and continued to December 1, 1929. The affiliation with the Chicago Lying-In Hospital terminated March 1930. By that time the Augustana obstetrical department had grown to such an extent that students were receiving the required amount of obstetrical training in our own school.

Nursing in the sky became another field of activity for graduate nurses. In the early spring of 1930, the Boeing Air Transport, Incorporated, were inaugurating their big twenty-eight passenger tri-motored bi-planes on regular passenger service. It was decided to have a crew of three: a pilot, a co-pilot and a steward. Miss Ellen Church, a graduate of a Minneapolis hospital, persuaded the officials that the position as steward could be adequately filled by nurses. Doubtful that women could fill the bill, they granted her a year's probation; Miss Church was immediately dispatched to Chicago to find the nurses. Among these pioneers was Miss Alva Johnson, '28. There were several requirements of which the important ones were: to be a registered nurse of good standing, to weigh less than 118 pounds; to be less than five feet and five inches tall; and be between twenty-one and twenty-six years of age.

The nurse's uniform was a forest green serge tailored suit with a double-breasted, brass-buttoned coat and plain skirt with a side kick-pleat. The blouse, a gray cotton broadcloth, was worn with a plain green tie. Black Oxfords completed the uniform. On the lapel was fastened a pin spelling out Boeing, with wings projecting from the sides of the "B" to form the shape of an aeroplane. In addition to the uniform the nurse had a skirt-length green cape lined with French gray flannel and a green beret. In the winter, a leather sport coat with removable flannel lining was added to the uniform.

The duties aboard the plane were variable for the sky nurse. They were most dependent upon her aptitude to meet each situation as it arose. She sold tickets and collected tickets; kept the cabin record; checked the cleanliness of the ship; made passengers comfortable with pillows and blankets; served light lunches; provided magazines, chewing gum, maps and cards. In short, she endeavored to make each passenger's trip so interesting and pleasurable that he would want to continue air traveling in the future.

Actual nursing was truly negligible, but an occasional case of air sickness required treatment and there were infrequent times when nursing was essential. A sensible, dependable and level headed person was required. The work was interesting and very enjoyable.

Alva Johnson, '28, was the first Augustana graduate to be a sky nurse. After a year in the air service, she met with instantaneous death in an automobile accident. Martha Dalin, '30, replaced her. Three months later Hilda Zwicky, '30, joined the sky nursing force and in the late fall of '31, Genevieve Zwicky, '29, also joined. Later, the Augustana nurses became well represented on the various air lines. However, none have served long in this branch of service due to activities of Dan Cupid. Marriage automatically cancelled the services of air nurses. [16]

The depression was beginning to be felt. It affected the nursing profession from the first, because people could not afford to pay for special nurses. Daily someone would find himself without work; factories were closing one by one; the newspapers were full of comments regarding unemployment; everything became shrouded with uncertainty, and confusion reigned in everyone's mind. All were hoping and struggling for security. The calls for graduate nurses became less and less, and frankly, nurses were becoming disturbed over the situation.

In June 1931, the remaining patients at the West Building— medical and chronic—were moved to the East Building. Later, several graduate nurses occupied the rooms on the fourth floor of the West Building; they shared kitchen privileges and found it a most convenient and economical way to live. A few of the hospital employees lived on the first floor. The laundry was still in use at the West Building.

In September 1931, a new class of students entered our school; the entrance fee was increased to $45.00.

In October a Young Woman's Christian Association was organized within the student nurses' group. This provided a source of new recreation, new thought and fellowship for all those taking advantage of membership. The nucleus of the organization was the executive committee which was composed of six students who met with representatives and secretaries of the Chicago Metropolitan Y.W.C.A. student department. A membership drive was launched, officers and a cabinet were chosen, and the organization was under way before a month had passed. Much was accomplished the first year. A constitution was drawn up and accepted at the National Y.W.C.A. Convention in the spring of 1932. Activities included social events, and hours of quiet inspiration, and worship. In this way

---

16. Information given by Martha Dalin Heath, '30.

the members were striving toward rounding out their lives as students and living the student purpose as follows:

> We united in the desire to realize a full and creative life through a growing knowledge of God.
> We determine to have a part in making this life possible for all people.
> In this task we seek to understand Jesus and to follow Him.

The membership of the Augustana Y.W.C.A., since its advent, has represented about seventy-five percent of the student body. Girls have worked and planned together without class distinction; hence, this brings about a friendly acquaintanceship and cooperation between the students. Especially those whose homes and friends were not in the city have learned to know students from other schools through interscholastic events, and thereby enriched their own lives as students.[17]

At this time [1932] the depression was keenly felt by everyone. People could not afford to become sick, or think of having special nurses, thus making the oversupply of nurses appalling. The average daily assignment of nurses from the Central Registry was only thirty. During the first quarter of 1932, there was an average of seven days' work a month for each nurse. The public did not have proper medical attention, people waited until an acute emergency arose before they called a physician. Our nurses took turns in being called for gratis nursing, and no patient in the hospital lacked the necessary nursing care.

The private duty nurses seemed most reluctant to ask for or to accept financial aid during those depressing times. Very few requests were received through the individual nursing organizations. Many of the nurses forfeited their high standards of working and living; they accepted what was offered in the way of work, and at whatever price was offered; some of the nurses

---

17. Information of Y.W.C.A. activities contributed by Mary Falk, '32.

cared for sick in their own home towns, accepting whatever the patient could pay, and were happy just to be occupied. Chronic patients were cared for on a salary basis, thereby giving the nurse a home. Most of the nurses moved into smaller quarters; in fact, into crowded quarters. Many returned to small towns and lived with their families while waiting for a call. The registry cooperated with these nurses who lived in Wisconsin, Michigan, Illinois, Indiana, or Iowa, by sending notification of their approaching turn. When they came in for a call they could get rooms at the Nurses' Residence for a minimum price. At this time there was usually a wait of five or six weeks for a call, and sometimes even three months. Each nurse, however, was entitled to four days' work before she lost her place on the registry. The rates at this time were five dollars for eight-hour duty, six dollars for ten-hour duty, and seven dollars for twelve-hour duty. Several of our nurses accepted positions for general duty in various hospitals; they were then assured of room and board. Others were on call for general duty to help out at busy intervals in the hospitals. Fewer students were accepted in the nursing schools, thereby creating a demand for this type of service. Few nurses remained idle between cases; many of them studied domestic arts, some attended free sewing and knitting classes; many went to night school to study English, history and the languages; they made use of the free golf links, tennis courts and swimming facilities; two of our nurses made dolls that sold for fifty cents apiece; two others made candy; still another knitted caps to match the popular knitted suits. The nurses helped each other whenever possible, especially in cases of illness and in sharing apartments. Nurses doing institutional work, public health, etc., had several cuts in salary, and vacations were forfeited. Many institutions had to dismiss some of their staff to reduce expenses.

During the depression the hospital, by reason of the great drop in business, found it necessary to close one semi-private and one private room floor for long periods of time. This was due to the fact that with the great amount of unemployment and great losses taken by individuals in all walks of life, they could not patronize private hospitals. This was true not only of Augustana Hospital, but of all other hospitals in the city, as well as those in all parts of the country. Of course those institutions which were fortunate enough to have large endowments and other forms of unearned income were able to take care of a large number of free patients. But their private accommodations were not patronized nearly so much as they were previous to the depression.

Graduate nurses were receiving four dollars a day for eight-hour duty, five dollars for ten-hour duty and six dollars for twelve-hour duty. The registry fee was ten dollars a year.

On March 18, 1933, during morning devotionals in the hospital chapel, twelve preliminary students were accepted as regular students in the School of Nursing. Miss Haggman gave an inspirational message to the group, after which she placed the school cap upon each student's head. Six senior nurses who were to act as advisors and "big sisters" to the new members stood with the class during the service. The new students repeated the following pledge:

In becoming an accepted nurse at the Augustana Hospital School of Nursing I promise that I will always appear on duty in complete uniform as now; that I will wear my uniform for duty only; that I will be obedient to the rules of the School; that I will take an intelligent interest in all of its activities; that I will give my loyal support while in training and after my graduation to any policy that may be deemed for its best good, and realizing that all graduates should become registered nurses, I will take the registration examination at such a time and place as shall be determined; that I will at my earliest opportunity become a member of the Alumnae Association, and that I will upon all occasions and by every means at my command, and especially by my own personal conduct as student and a graduate, endeavor to raise the nursing standards in the professional world.

Due to the opening of the Century of Progress at the end of May, graduation festivities were delayed to allow visitors attending graduation the opportunity of also visiting the Fair. The

exercises took place at Trinity Parish House on May 31. On
June 3 the annual banquet was given at the Edgewater Beach
Hotel in honor of the thirty graduates. Six nurses of the class
of 1908 were also guests. The sum of $107.10 was given by the
class to the Hospital Fund instead of to the Scholarship Fund.
Miss Bertha Klauser was given the Alumnae Scholarship for that
year. Miss Josephine Anderson was awarded a scholarship from
the First District.

Miss Margaret Saenger won the prize in the song contest for
the following song:

### HAIL TO THEE!
### Tune: Blessed Assurance

Hail Alma Mater We sing to thee-
Praises to thee thy daughters do sing;
Thine are the laurels, thine is the crown;
On waves of song our voices ring.

Chorus:
Hail! Alma Mater, we honor thee,
We raise on high the blue and the gold.
Old Augustana, we promise thee,
Until we die our hearts you hold.

Teacher and mother, dearest and best,
In thy kind arms, we shelter knew;
With thy wisdom thou didst endow
And thou has kept us loyal and true.

And all thy children every year
Come home like pilgrims to honor thy shrine,
Catching the spark which in thee glows,
Thy faithful service to all mankind.

A motion was passed that after the Alumnae Fund allotted
for that purpose had been exhausted, and until some of the
loans were repaid, any nurses applying for relief should be referred to the First District. Miss Haggman provided needy

nurses with work whenever possible. Conditions in the nursing field were not showing much improvement.

Thirty young candidates entered September 6, 1933. The classes which had been admitted previous to September were given a monthly allowance which continued throughout their entire course. After this date the monthly allowance was discontinued.

On Easter morning [1934], the Augustana student nurses participated in the Easter Sunrise Service held on the Century of Progress grounds. It was estimated that about 80,000 people were in attendance.

At this time there were only fifty-eight nurses in training, which was the smallest number in many years. About twenty-five graduates were being employed as general staff nurses. The graduating class of 1934 numbered twenty-nine. Graduation exercises were held on May 31 at Ebenezer Church. Home-coming Day was June 2, with luncheon at noon and Open House in the afternoon. In the evening the Alumnae Banquet was given at the Oriental Room of the Knickerbocker Hotel. The graduating class and the class of 1909 were honor guests. Miss Viola Hawkinson, president of the graduating class, presented the Alumnae Association with a check for $121.69 for the Scholarship Fund. The Alumnae scholarship this year was awarded to Miss Vera Leaf, '24. Miss Bertha Klauser, '33, was awarded a scholarship from the First District.

At this time the Illinois Emergency Relief Commission offered to place nurses under the Civil Works Project, and several Augustana nurses took advantage of the offer. The visitors to the Century of Progress were helping somewhat to restore prosperity in Chicago and by the late fall of 1934 a noticeable improvement was seen in the nursing profession. The West Building was being used as a Tourist Home under the supervision of the Hospital Board. Rooms were rented for 75c, $1.00 and $1.50 a day.

Forty new students entered the school of Nursing in September, the preliminary period at this time was six months. The first six weeks were spent in the classroom; after this time they began to wear their uniforms and to do floor duty for a few hours a day, the time on duty being gradually increased. Besides class work, these new students, conforming to previous custom, also received instruction in swimming and gymnastics. This was the first class to wear the preliminary uniform of stripes having short sleeves with three-inch detachable white cuffs, and white Buster Brown collars. They also wore the white butcher style aprons, and after receiving caps at the end of six months they were given the gored aprons with shoulder strap bibs. Black Oxfords and black hose were worn until their graduation, after which they wore white Oxfords and white hose, even though still in training.

# CHAPTER III

## THE FIFTIETH ANNIVERSARY AND BEYOND

On October 31, 1934, the hospital held its golden anniversary services at the Central Lutheran Church, corner of Sedgwick and Hobbie Streets. The program was opened with an organ prelude by Mr. Harry T. Carlson, followed by a scripture reading and prayer by the Rev. J. Helmer Olson. Addresses were given by the Rev. Gottfred Nelson and the Rev. Peter Peterson. The Augustana Nurses' Chorus sang several selections. It was stated that: since the first patient was admitted, May 28, 1884, over 140,000 patients had received care; approximately 2,000,000 days of hospital service had been provided; 1,015 nurses had graduated; the hospital had accommodations for 350 patients.

A class of fifty preliminary students entered the School of Nursing on September 4, 1935. Two of the new students were daughters of Augustana Hospital graduates: Alice McDaniel, daughter of Ellen Carlson McDaniel, '99, and June Porlier, daughter of Jeanette Warner Porlier, '12. The entrance fee was increased to $75.00 this year.

The Annual Convention of the Illinois State Nurses' Association was held at Danville, Illinois, on October 25, 26 and 27. At the regular banquet the American Journal of Nursing celebrated its thirty-fifth birthday. One of the original subscribers, Miss Josephine Oberg, '96, now Mrs. Lofgren, was present.

Miss Minnie Carlson of Rockford, Illinois, where the eight-hour day for private duty nurses had met with great success, stated that: the eight-hour day is being freely discussed for private duty nurses; the eight-hour day schedule only, is endorsed by the American Nurses' Association; every group must work out its own problems in its own community; better working conditions for the nurses must be for the patient's good; the arguments for long hours are based on habit, not on reason; instead of charging more pay, such a nurse should charge less, for her services are worth less; and a sleeping nurse has no place in a sick room.

It was a great surprise to the entire Nursing School when Miss Saenger announced that she intended leaving Augustana. She left to make her home with a sister at Janesville, Wisconsin. Miss Saenger "grew up" with the Nurses' Residence. Her duties were manifold; she performed them all cheerfully. When she left, the best wishes of all the nurses followed her. Miss Clara Belle Anderson, '31, took over the duties of the Residence until a permanent director could be obtained.

In 1936 the Registry dues were $14.00 a year, with a $2.00 discount if paid on or before date due. Graduate private duty nurses received $5.00 for eight-hour duty, $6.00 for ten-hour duty, and $7.00 for twelve-hour duty. The Alumnae dues were $8.00 for active members and $4.00 for associate members, payable in January.

At the October [1936] meeting of the Alumnae Association, reports of the Biennial Convention at Los Angeles, California, June 21-26, were given by Clara Oberg, Ruth Williamson, and Ida Burkhalter; these members shared the responsibility of a delegate to represent the Alumnae Association.

Some of the ideas presented and discussed at The League of Nursing Education section were:

Students entering schools of nursing should have two years or more of college work. This will bring to nursing more mature women, with greater breadth of culture and a more adequate fund of general knowledge.

Most of the advances in medical science have been made since the time of Florence Nightingale, and what was adequate training at that time no longer meets the demands placed upon nurses. The course of study for schools of nursing is being revised to meet the exacting requirements of the community and to keep abreast of medical practices. These changes are not revolutionary. The committee wishes to include only those changes which can be made by the good schools, within a reasonable length of time, and to set up the best standards for schools that want to do a good job.

Nursing is becoming more highly specialized and techniques are more involved. If nursing be considered a profession, preparations must be on a par with other professions. If not, we assume that nurses are mentally incapable of mastering subjects expected of other professional groups.

The prime objective of all changes in the course of study, and in the organization of schools of nursing should be to improve training in bedside nursing, and to train nurses to meet the health needs of the community.

When a hospital sets itself up as a school of nursing, it must organize itself accordingly, and keep in mind that the main purpose of a school of nursing is the education of a nurse. The reason for lack of progress in many schools is that they have been established primarily for the nursing service they could render the hospital, and the proper training of students has been a minor concern. The number of students should be determined by the educational facilities of the hospital, rather than by the number of patients. The supervisors have the most important role in teaching nursing procedures because they come in contact with the students more than any other member of the faculty. Only through adequate training and supervision of its nurses can the hospital hope to render the best type of nursing care to its patients.

To provide students with opportunities for the amount of experience they need in the various departments of the hospital, at the time it will do them the most good, the hospital should have a staff of general duty nurses. It should be made clear that the general duty nurse is not inferior to the head nurse or supervisor. Hers is the greater opportunity for service in bedside nursing, which requires all the qualifications of any branch of nursing. It is not to be wondered that there is such a rapid turnover in general duty nurse staffs throughout the country. As a general rule such positions do not pay a living wage, involve undesirable hours, too many patients to care for, many duties which should rightfully be assigned to maids, and the necessity of living in an institution. Good general duty nurses might be retained longer by paying higher salaries, providing opportunities for new experiences, by assigning no more patients than can be given good nursing care, and relieving nurses of maids' duties.

The motive force behind all these efforts in nursing education, Miss Effie Taylor expressed most effectively: "We want a place for our selves in the educational program of the country—not for ourselves, but so that we might better serve others. We want to keep in mind that bedside nursing is our objective!"

On February 24, 1937, the West Building was sold to a Chicago Syndicate which planned to remodel it into a hotel. When this transaction became known, many experienced sadness in losing this last tangible evidence of the happy memories of the old hospital. The nurses who had been living there found other quarters, inasmuch as the building was to be vacated by April 1, with the exception of the laundry which was to be used until the hospital could make other arrangements. The pre-natal clinic, which had remained in the West Building, was transferred to four rooms at the north end of the second floor in the patients' pavilion of the East Building.

In March 1937, ground was broken at the rear of the main building for a new laundry. Besides the laundry, the new building has a two-story wing; the lower floor is used for a linen room, and the upper floor is used as a demonstration room for the School of Nursing and has its own entrance and stairway.

In March, Mrs. Nettie Hoff Johnson resigned her position as Matron of the hospital and left for her new home at Bridgman, Michigan. She was succeeded by Miss Blanche Lauger, '22.

Vera Leaf, M.D., started her interneship at Augustana Hospital on July 1, 1937. She had graduated from the Augustana School of Nursing in 1924, and since that time had studied at the Lewis Institute, Chicago, Augustana College, Sioux Falls, South Dakota, and Rush Medical College, Chicago. She was the first Augustana nurse to earn a medical degree.

On July 1, 1937, the eight hour day for private duty nurses went into effect at our hospital. Hours of service were 7:00 a.m.3:00 p.m.; 3:00 p.m.-11:00 p.m.; 11:00 p.m.-7:00 a.m. It was found that the eight hour day had increased the demand for private duty nurses. The nurse soon learned that she was more alert and rested when she began her day, and felt better equipped mentally and physically to meet the requirements of the sick room. This arrangement also allowed her more time to read, to study, and to keep abreast of the times.

The nurses of today cannot comprehend the old days of private duty, with the long hours, mental strain, hard physical work, little rest, sleeping on cots or on floors or with the patient. Oftentimes, the patient required the full twenty-four

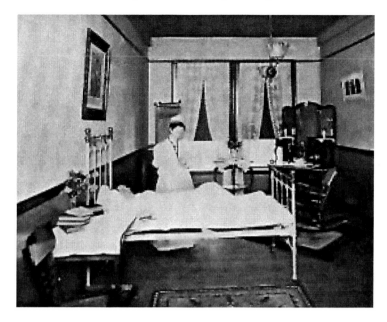

Private Room, Circa 1897

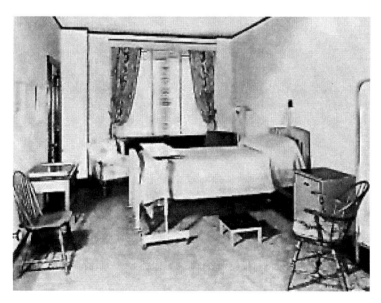

Private Room, Circa 1937

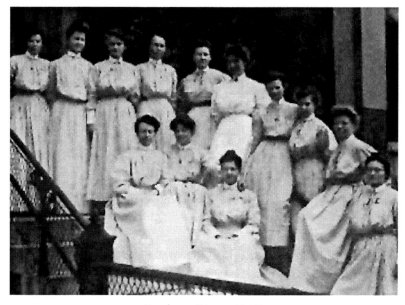

Student Group 1907

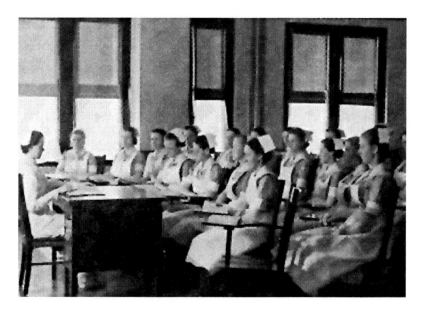

Student Group 1937

hours of the nurse's time, and the whole family depended upon the nurse for their meals. After a nurse came off a case, she did nothing but sleep, so as to be ready for the next hard case. In spite of all its hardships, many liked bedside nursing. Some of our Augustana nurses have done only private duty because they preferred it to any other branch of nursing.

On July 23 [1937], Charles A. Swanson, engineer of the West Building for thirty-four years, served his last day on duty. He was retiring from active service in which he had been a faithful and devoted worker, giving his best to the hospital he loved to serve. After he had drawn the shades of the West Building and with tears in his eyes handed the keys to Mr. Erickson, the old hospital was no more. This fine old building in which medical and surgical history had been made, was left to stand as merely a vacant building. Another change came when Garfield Avenue was changed to Dickens Avenue. The older nurses were proud to say that their hospital was located on the presidential corner, at Garfield, Lincoln and Cleveland Avenues.

When the East Building was opened in 1926, about 300 operations were performed a month. The work gradually increased until in 1929 the peak was reached; the monthly average was 505 operations. Then there was a gradual decline until in 1933, when the monthly average was 305. Again there was a climb and the average for 1937 was 376 per month. About fifty percent of the surgical work consisted of major operations. The foregoing figures did not include the "street cases" of which there had been an average of fifty a month. The surgical department did the sterilizing for the entire hospital. Most of this was done at night.

At this writing (May 1938), Martha A. Rohrbeck, '15, is the Surgical Supervisor; she has three graduate assistants. There are four anesthetists, Amelia Loehrke, '12, is in charge. With the exception of night duty, all students receive the same training during their three months' service. Only one out of four is given night duty—these nurses must prove themselves especially adapted for that service. Before receiving surgical training the students are given ten on-hour lectures and demonstrations in surgical technique, and further demonstrations in conjunction with their practical work in the surgical department. Students "scrub up" with a graduate nurse, until they feel confident they can manage by themselves. Each nurse "scrubs" for thirty or more major operations. After a year of general work in surgery many of the general duty nurses have had the opportunity to obtain good surgical positions.

Amy B. Chamberlain, '12, is Assistant Superintendent of Nurses. Ruth Williamson, '31, until her resignation in March, 1938, was the Educational Director; Josephine Anderson, '32, and Mary Elizabeth Falk, '32, are her assistants. Agnes Carlson is Director of the Nurses' Residence.

The School of Nursing Committee is composed of:

Dr. Rudolph Oden, Chairman

Rev. C. A. Lindvall

Dr. Anders Frick

Mr. E. I. Erickson, Superintendent of the Hospital

Miss Mabel E. Haggman, Superintendent of Nurses

The entrance requirements to the School of Nursing are: high school education including one year in Chemistry; good health; good character; 18-1/2 years of age. If the application is favorable, the candidate is sent a blank which she completes and sends to the Department of Registration and Education at Springfield, Illinois. This entitles her to a Qualifying Certificate which is necessary for entrance to all accredited schools of nursing in Illinois. Augustana requires an entrance fee of $100.00 to cover the cost of text books, breakage fee, and physical education. Students are given a careful physical examination upon entering, then again at the end of the Preliminary Period, and annually thereafter. A four weeks' vacation is given each student annually.

The Preliminary Period is six months. Two months of intensive class work is given before any student goes on duty. During the three year period, classes are held during the day, with one hour allowed off duty for each hour of class work over one hour. There are three "in nights" a week during the preliminary period. This means that the students must be in at eight o'clock. One late leave is given every two weeks. After the completion of the preliminary period, there are no "in nights" and one late leave is given every week. A "late leave" means that the students may stay out until twelve o'clock. The front door is locked at 10 p.m.

The preliminary students' uniforms now worn were inaugurated in 1937. They are made of the same stripe material as the school uniform, and have short sleeves. Instead of the Buster Brown collar, a narrow band of the stripe is worn, fastened in front with a small brooch. The preliminary apron is the regulation gored apron, worn with a small bib which is fastened in place with buttons. When a student is accepted as a regular student, she received a cap and wears the regulation school uniform.

Religious services are held every morning before breakfast in the Recreation Room of the Nurses' Residence, conducted by Rev. Julius Lincoln, successor to Rev. Alfred Nelson. During the school year courses in Bible Study are available to the students, and they also have the opportunity of joining the Y.W.C.A. group, the chorus, or any other extra-curricular activities of the school.

Each student works eight hours a day. Relief service, 3:00 to 11:00 p.m., is given at intervals for a period of four weeks; and night duty, 11:00 p.m. to 7:00 a.m., is also given at intervals for a period of four weeks. Day nurses work from 7:00 a.m. to 3:00 p.m.

During the second and third years the student continues her work in the diet kitchen, service room, surgery, obstetrics, medical and surgical services, with graduate supervision in all departments. A four months' affiliation in Pediatric Nursing is given in the senior year at the Children's Memorial Hospital, three blocks distant.

Courses of lectures and demonstrations accompany the practical work of each year. A case study is completed every six weeks. Written examinations are given at the completion of each lecture course, and at intervals during a recitation course. The passing grade is 75.

Summary for the Graduation Class of 1938 [follows in Table 3.1.]

The service in the dietetic department is six weeks. This course covers a study of foods, including classification, source and function; also caloric values, and balanced diets. Practice is given in the preparation of foods, care of utensils and necessary equipment. Miss Aile Beckman is in charge of the dietetic department.

The School of Nursing has a most interesting library, to which new books are added at regular intervals. At present there are about seven hundred copies of reference books including the Encyclopedia Britannica. There are five hundred books in the fiction department; forty-three books on history and government: also books on religion, psychology and ethics. The library is always a very popular department with the students.

The housekeeping of the hospital is under the able direction of Miss Blanche Lauger, '22, who has complete charge of the personnel, including all those employed in the kitchen, laundry, linen room, diet kitchen, floors, lounges, and dining rooms. Miss Lauger also plans the regular menus and purchases all food supplies.

[The 1884–1938 history closes with these words.]

The days and months and years have passed along, and to the older nurses it is a pleasure to hand the torch over to the younger nurses who will in turn hand it over to those who are yet to enter our School of Nursing.

May the fine standards established in the early days of our school and so faithfully carried on through the years, ever be maintained.

Table 3.1
Class Work

| | Recitation Hours | Lecture Hours | Demonstrations and Practice Hours |
|---|---|---|---|
| Preliminary Course | | | |
| Anatomy | 90 | 10 | |
| Chemistry | 15 | 30 | |
| Bacteriology | 15 | 30 | |
| Drugs and Solutions | 15 | 15 | |
| Ethics | 15 | | |
| Hygiene | 27 | | |
| Sanitation | 12 | 16 | |
| History of Nursing | 24 | | |
| Nursing Arts | 70 | 60 | |
| Freshman Course | | | |
| Materia Medica | 45 | | |
| Psychology | 30 | | |
| Case Study | 10 | | |
| Advanced Nursing | 30 | | 20 |
| Nutrition | 15 | | 30 |
| Massage | | | 16 |
| Junior Year | | | |
| Medical Diseases | 10 | 26 | |
| Surgical Diseases | 10 | 16 | |
| Dietotherapy | 15 | | |
| Communicable Diseases | 15 | | |
| Obstetrics | 22 | 14 | |
| Surgical Technic | 10 | | |
| Gynecology | 6 | 10 | |
| Emergencies | | 15 | |
| Eye, Ear, Nose, and Throat | | 6 | |
| Dermatology | | 4 | |
| Psychiatry | | 20 | |
| Senior Year | | | |
| Modern Social Conditions | | 24 | |
| Professional Problems | | 8 | |

# PART II

A HISTORY OF THE AUGUSTANA HOSPITAL
SCHOOL OF NURSING 1938–1987

*The year is now 1993 and we again have picked up the pen to finish the History of the Augustana Hospital School of Nursing. The School of Nursing graduated its 91st class, the last class on July 11, 1987, and then closed the school. Augustana Hospital was taken over by Lutheran General Foundation on December 31, 1987, and closed Augustana on December 8, 1989. At this writing, our beloved Augustana Hospital and Nurses' Residence is being demolished. To help keep the memory alive, we will continue the history, for from its beginning, Augustana nurses have distinguished themselves the world over.*

# CHAPTER I

## THE END OF THE THIRTIES

Nurses training at Augustana was more than just classes and clinical work. We learned to live together in the Nurses' Residence, look out for each other and developed a great deal of camaraderie.

In September of 1938, forty-five students entered training and they were immediately introduced to the "Big Sister" program which was one way that they were helped with problems or questions. Many friendships developed that would last a lifetime.

Some fun activities that were available were swimming in the pool located in the basement of the Nurses' Residence and playing tennis in the courts that were behind the Nurses' Residence.

One of the extracurricular activities was the Jenny Lind Chorus which was organized in 1924 by Miss Ida Ehman '15. Our first director was Mr. Paul Hultman who directed the Chorus until 1929 and Dr. Harry T. Carlson directed it from 1929 to 1965. Performances were given at National Nurses' Conventions before audiences of 10,000, the Sunday Evening Club, World Flower and Garden Show, radio, church and hospital functions. Money collected was used by the hospital to buy new equipment or used to benefit the Free Bed Fund.

The Alumnae Association continued to be active. Regular meetings were held in the Lila Pickhardt Lounge of the Nurses' Residence at 8:00 p.m. on the first Wednesday of each month excepting July and August. Programs or lectures, refreshments and a social hour followed the business meeting. A monthly newsletter was published and sent to each member. At the September meeting the History Committee presented the newly bound volume of the first issue of the "Augustana Nurse" which was recorded by hand. The first president of the Alumnae Association, begun in 1901, was Anna Johnson Helt, class of 1896.

The annual Alumnae Christmas party was held on December 7th with 156 present. Following the business meeting, the program portion was introduced by the reading of the "Saviour's Birth" by Miss Haggman. Members of the student nurses' Thalian Drama Club presented a one act play, "The Last Christmas," after which a candlelight service of carols was rendered by the Preliminary students. A delicious buffet lunch was served in the lounge by members of the Refreshment Committee. The collection for sick nurses amounted to $74.00.

A Hess Incubator was purchased by the Alumnae and installed in the Hospital Nursery at a cost of $361.00. The present cost of an incubator (1993) is approximately $3,000.00.

A very enjoyable evening was spent in the Nurses' Home, December 22, when the nursing staff and the 1938 graduates entertained Dr. Vera Leaf, '24, at an informal party. She was the first Augustana nurse to become an M.D. It was a surprise to Dr. Leaf, who had been invited in for the evening with the intern staff to sing Christmas carols. During an intermission, she was presented with a monetary gift from the nurses. This was but a token of the love and esteem they all had for Dr. Leaf and they wished for her happiness and success as she went on to assume the duties of practicing her profession at her office at 2051 Sedgewick Street.

The students were very busy working on the Mardi Gras which the Juniors were sponsoring on February 17th. There were to be sideshows, prizes, games, eats, orchestra and raffles.

In February, Miss Bertha Klauser '33, accepted the position to act as the Alumnae Association representative to the Central Council of Nursing Education. Also in February, on the recommendation of the Board of Directors, it was decided to establish the Educational Scholarship Committee. The work of this committee was to outline the general plan for the functioning of the Scholarship Fund begun in 1928, and to present these plans to the Board of Directors.

A letter was read from the First District at the March Alumnae meeting, stating that $125.00 scholarships were available in three nursing groups, (1) Institutional, (2) Public Health, and (3) Private Duty. Many of our nurses attended the Fourth Annual Institute sponsored by the Private Duty Section of the First District which was held on March 30 and 31, 1939. The sessions were divided among Illinois Research and Educational Hospitals, the Cook County School of Nursing and Presbyterian Hospital. Just as in the past, the program was arranged to meet the needs of all nurses and all nurses were invited. There was a conducted tour through the Orthopedic Building of the Illinois Research Hospital, where the most up-to-date equipment was demonstrated. Dr. Henry B. Thomas, well-known orthopedic surgeon, spoke on the development of orthopedic surgery. Dr. Howard Haggard, professor of Applied Physiology at Yale University and author of "Devils, Drugs and Doctors," was also a speaker.

In April, 1939, Mrs. Nancy Ekstrom Amour, '04, of Stockholm wrote that she won second prize in a radio contest for writing a play on the life of Florence Nightingale; it was one of 100 manuscripts submitted. It was decided to use her play as a text book in the public schools.

The following was taken from Edith Belden's '41, article in the "Nurse," regarding the capping ceremony in April:

"Friends and relatives of the pre-clinical students of the Class of 1941 gathered in the Recreation Room of the Nurses' Home at 8:00 p.m. The Preliminary students escorted by their 'Big Sisters' entered singing 'Rejoice, Ye Pure In Heart' and took their places at the front of the room. Addresses by Miss Haggman and Dr. Julius Lincoln and two solos by Miss Viola Lofquist ['40], emphasized the solemnity of the occasion and made it an unforgettable one. After the capping,

Miss Wickman [Mildred '38], again played the hymn 'Rejoice, Ye Pure In Heart' and the students left the room, their heads held high with their newly acquired crowns."

April was a very busy month for the students. The Senior Minstrel Show was held Thursday, April 20th, the Supervising Staff of the Hospital entertained the Seniors on Monday evening, April 24th at an informal party, and the Junior Class again carried out the traditional entertainment of giving a dinner to the Senior Class on Wednesday evening, April 26th, at the Swedish Club.

Baccalaureate Service was held at the Saron Church, Shakespeare Avenue and Richmond Street, at 11:00 a.m., Sunday, April 30th. Dr. Carl Christenson, pastor of the church, conducted this service. The Graduating Exercises were held at the Ebenezer Church, Paulina Street and Foster Avenue, at 8:00 p.m. on Tuesday evening, May 2nd. This was followed with the Reception in the Nurses' Residence for the families and friends of the Graduating Class.

Saturday, May 6th, was Alumnae Association Day. The Hospital cordially invited all out-of-town guests to come early enough to have luncheon at 12 noon with the Hospital staff. This was always a very happy occasion. The Luncheon was followed with the usual Afternoon Alumnae Tea in the Nurses' Residence, to which all graduates of the School were invited and urged to bring their children as well. These children were cared for in the Recreation Room of the Nurses' Residence by student nurses so that the mothers had ample opportunity to visit. The climax of these activities was reached with the Annual Dinner, which was at the LaSalle Hotel, at LaSalle and West Madison Streets. Tickets were $1.75. The Senior Class and the Class of 1914 were guests of the Alumnae Association.

At long last in May of '39, the publishing of the History Book was a reality and it was a beautifully illustrated book. The Association voted to have 1,000 copies printed and the contract was let to the Robert O. Law Company. The price of the book was set for $2.50 a copy. It was to be off the presses in October. Every issue of the "Augustana Nurse" advertised the book and Alumnae members were encouraged to buy it. This article appeared in the May, 1939 issue.

- FLASH -

History of the Augustana Hospital School of Nursing by Miss Amy Schjolberg. 246 pages, 40 illustrations. Price $2.50.—We do expect our History to go off the press in October. May we ask that you send in your subscription and advance payment by postal or express money orders to the History Committee, Augustana Alumnae Association, 427 Dickens Ave., Chicago. Make the money orders payable to Genevieve Peterson, Treasurer.

Please contact Augustana graduates who are non-members of our Alumnae in cities where you live. We do know that every graduate will want this fascinating book which will be a lasting heritage to the Hospital and School we love.

Of the many nurses who distinguished themselves in many fields, this is an article about one of them. The following article was taken from an April edition of the "Evening American" (a former Chicago daily newspaper):

'ANGEL' OF WEST SIDE
CLOSING 40 YEARS OF WORK AS NURSE

"The Red-Headed Angel of the West Side" was what they used to call Anna Heistad in her early days as visiting nurse in the ghetto section of Chicago.

On Sunday, April 16, she completed 40 years of social service. Of this time she has been for 20 years, superintendent of Marcy Center, a settlement of the Woman's Home Missionary Society at 1539 South Springfield Avenue. Though today her hair is silver-white and her head holds reminiscences of hundreds she has comforted, the 'Red-Headed Angel' has no wish to linger over bygone days.

"What's the use in reviewing the past when there's so much to be done right now?" she asks, showing a courteous annoyance that fuss should be made over her anniversary.

40 Refugees Enrolled

She referred specifically to the plight of Jewish refugees, 40 of whom recently enrolled for Americanization classes at the Center. Marcy, one of 106 settlements of the Methodist Episcopal Church, is perhaps the largest Christian charitable institution in the world situated in a Jewish community.

Miss Heistad was born 70 years ago in Kraga, Norway, and came to Chicago at the age of 3 years. Nursing was her one desire, and by 1901 she was named a director of the Illinois Association of Graduate Nurses. (Augustana graduate 1898.)

As she showed a visitor about the Center, opening doors to neat workshops, kindergartens and social halls, she walked with Viking erectness. She gave her ideas on social work — 'a well-rounded program at once educational, recreational and medical.'

Some years before the present Marcy Center was built in 1930 (the first was at Maxwell Street and Newberry Avenue), Miss Heistad had passed a particularly harassing day. All day long the broken-hearted, the consumptive, the deserted had trailed into her office. She felt weary in spirit.

### Gets Satisfying Poem

A knock at the door, and three ragged little girls, entering with a 'please, Ma'am,' handed her a poem called 'Recompense.' A neighborhood school teacher had composed it in tribute to her, and she forgot her fatigue. She calls it one of her most satisfying experiences.

But sentimentalism is not one of Miss Heistad's marked qualities. Her practical nature urges the young people who flock to the Center to 'fight for a higher education.'

'There's nothing extraordinary in my life,' she says. 'Just steady work. I've had a good time and a wonderful response both from Jews and Gentiles.'

### RECOMPENSE

I daily toil down in the dirt and grime
Amid the busy city's rush and roar,
Great iron masters bellow past my door;
Not far away are haunts of lust and crime,
Yet, I pass a rare enchanted time.
Here little children take me by the hand,
'Tis mine to lead them to the promised land.
And thus I know my task to be sublime.
The water-lily grows from mud and slime,
The sturdy oak springs from the blackest soil,
The muddy earth yields luscious fruit for food.
I ask but this, that out of dirt and grime,
Some little human plant may by my toil,
Spring up in beauty, strength, and all things good.

—EMMA M. HOERR

(Printed in a little pamphlet called "Recompense" by Lillian B. Lavin. Written as a tribute to Miss Anna Heistad.)

In December, 1942, Anna passed away. Following is the eulogy written by Katherine Knutson 1900:

"Our dearly beloved friend and Augustana Alumnae, Miss Anna Heistad has bid her last farewell. It was my privilege to meet and to know her before she entered the nursing profession. Her nobility of soul and appreciation of values as well as her deeply spiritual nature made a lasting impression. The nursing profession provided a marvelous channel for growth and we who knew Miss Heistad were privileged to see this spiritual development in her activities. As a nurse, Miss Heistad served in many capacities. She did bedside nursing; served as Superintendent of Nurses at St. Mary's Hospital; served as a visiting nurse when the VNA of Chicago numbered only 12 nurses; and her long and faithful service at 'Marcy Center' where she was greatly appreciated and from whence she departed December 26, 1942, for her final resting place. Long will we cherish her memory."

Many events stayed in the minds of our nurses. Edna Thornblade, '32, shared her happy memories of May Day 1939.

### MAY DAY—A SCHOOL EVENT

R-i-n-g-g-g-g-
A slow awakening and finally a realization that the alarm clock was again making itself heard. A glance in its direction—what—5 o'clock. Oh yes—May Day Breakfast at the lake. Ah me!

I laid back on my pillow and tried to plan a way I might tell everybody I was absent because I had turned off the alarm in my sleep.

But no—I didn't want to miss this traditional event. Raising on my elbows and looking out my window due East the first accents of dawn were to be seen, and the lake, what a beautiful sight it was. With a rush I was out of bed and dressed.

Shall we ever forget that glorious walk to the lake in the calm freshness of early morn? An uninhabited world it seemed with only the stir and twitter of waking birds and the whir of mallards and sea gulls flying overhead. Good fortune was ours, the sun had not yet arisen when we mounted the rocks along the lake shore. We sat as sentinels, awaiting—. Yes, it was beautiful and breathtaking, a great glorious red sun, illuminating the lake like gold and awakening us to the reward of an early rising.

The cool breeze and tang of the water made us soon conscious of our physical well being. The serving of breakfast proved quite a task but we were generously fed and how good it tasted.

Time—we couldn't stay it tho' we would. Soon we were on duty, but with a new zest and a feeling of satisfaction despite our early awakening.

Another notable event was graduation on May 12, of the Class of '39, when Dr. Nadeau gave the following very inspiring message.

The sort of influence each class and each student has in forming the tone of the school depends upon how fully ethical principles are accepted and used as the basis of conduct, or to what extent they are ignored.

From widely separated communities all over the United States and in nearly every country of the world, groups of young women of many nationalities, creeds and colors, having similar interests and animated by a like purpose, have entered and are entering schools of nursing. Because the schools are not for the purpose of general education but are maintained with a definite and comparatively simple end in view toward which all the teaching is directed, rapid changes are necessarily wrought in the habits and the thoughts of the pupil who follow the course. Conscientious and exacting care of the body is inculcated; worthy ambitions and inspiring ideals are fostered.

The money-making possibilities of nursing have been much advertised and a profession cannot fail to suffer when this happens. We have heard much more of this since the economic depression. The question of earning a living confronts an increasing number of girls and, having chosen nursing from among other gainful occupations, or having been thrust into it with no choice at all, one is expected to give unselfishly of her best efforts and to consecrate herself to her work as did the saints of old. On her side, she has a right to expect that a work which demands hard bodily labor, mental exertion of a high order, the possession of a pleasing personality, and good character, should be well paid. She should be able to live decently, and to make provisions for the proverbial rainy day. She should be able, without anxiety about money, to devote a reasonable amount of time to further study, rest, recreation and travel. However, she is headed straight for serious trouble if the money to be earned is her chief consideration. For our comfort, we should remember that some of the world's best work is prompted by the necessity of earning more money. It is good work, because, forgetting the economic compulsion, the doer throws her heart and soul into it.

It is unfortunate and harmful that nurses are so often called "Angels of Mercy," instead of honest, painstaking workers. A class of beautifully uniformed young women, giving earnest attention to the orator on commencement night affords a thrill which may and does tempt one to extravagant speech. Instead you should be told that you are fortunate in ranking among the workers of the world and that there could be no better rank. Your work is much needed and it should be work worth the payment asked for and received. That is the first essential in any work. The man who puts the best of himself into whatever he does is serving mankind just as truly as is the nurse, and he too is making the world a better place in which to live, whether he be occupied in sweeping a street, or ruling a state. After all, the reason why you chose nursing is not important in comparison with the sincerity with which it is followed and the thoroughness and effort which go into all its details.

The moral and intellectual tone of the school whose diploma she hopes to earn, whose teaching will probably change the trend of all her thoughts and influence the conduct of her future life, and by those whose reputation and standing in the community she will always be judged, cannot fail to be of surpassing importance to the graduate nurse. This is true in marked degree when the pupil is enrolled in a technical school whose object is to prepare its pupil for a special and rather limited field of work, a field in which character, scholarship, behavior, a disciplined mind, and a trained body with skillful hands, all have important parts. The tone of a school is acquired from its teachers and students, past and present. It is a composite photograph of the intellectual traits and the dominating characteristics of all the members of the miniature world which comprises an organization such as the Augustana Hospital.

In May, Agnes Carlson '24, who had served as Matron of the Nurses' Home for some time, resigned her position and assumed the responsibility of supervising the first floor of the Hospital. Margaret Saenger '10, who had been living in Janesville, Wisconsin for the last three years, returned to be the Matron of Nurses' Residence.

Margaret Saenger, Martha Rohrbeck '15, and Amy Chamberlain '12, were guests of Miss Anna Naegel, the starring actress in "Nurse Edith Cavell." Miss Naegel had expressed the wish to meet with twelve World War I nurses on her arrival in Chicago. Mrs. Ada Crocker, Chairman of the Chicago Red Cross Nursing Committee arranged the gathering which included luncheon in Miss Naegel's apartment at the Blackstone Hotel. The afternoon was spent in reminiscing over the experiences the nurses had had during the first world war and the visitors were shown a collection of pictures and correspondence from the Cavell family. Shortly after this meeting, Miss Naegel left for her home country, England, where she felt she could serve her people in their hour of apprehension for there were rumors of war.

In September, a wedding of interest to the hospital family took place at the Irving Park Lutheran Church when Ellen Graf, '31, became the bride of Fred Hartman on September 9. It was interesting because Mrs. Hartman's mother was Jennie Nilsson Graf, '06, and she had three aunts, all Augustana graduates, namely, Anna Nilsson, '18, Julia Nilsson Baggeson, '19 and Martha Nilsson Ruzek, '27. Dr. John Graf, father of the bride was a former Augustana intern.

Miss Marguerite McNall assumed the duties of Educational Director of the School of Nursing. Miss McNall was a graduate of the Mercy Hospital of San Diego, California and of the

University of Chicago. Besides teaching Anatomy, Physiology and Chemistry, she was a talented woman who taught ballet to some of the students, held exercise classes and assisted in swimming class. She was the press advisor for the student newspaper, "The Augustinian," published every 3 weeks by the students, begun in September, 1941. She also achieved recognition in the art world after leaving Augustana, marrying and moving to New York.

With the entrance of the September class of '39, Mantoux testing and chest X-ray became part of the admission physical of student nurses. Social events at the School included weekly teas at the Residence arranged by Margaret Saenger whereby the students were privileged to be hostesses to other students and staff members. The chorus organized for the year and rehearsals were every Monday evening. Their first engagement was for Reformation Day, October 29 at Concordia Lutheran Church. The Senior Class play cast was chosen and rehearsals started. The play was presented December 8.

A Lutheran Student Association was organized in the School, with Edna Thornblade, '32, as their advisor. Every Thursday evening they met for devotions with the students in charge. The plan originated with interested people in our school and of Lutheran Deaconess Hospital. It later became a National Organization. The aims of the Lutheran Nurses Guild were as follows:

1. To encourage daily devotions as well as private and group study of the Bible.
2. To foster a conscious Christian attitude in facing personal and professional problems.
3. To emphasize and to arrange for services of worship and the celebration of Holy Communion.

Friday evening, October 6th, the Association entertained the Nurses Guild of Chicago. Supper was served to 125 guests followed by a program.

Indirect lighting was installed in the classroom, offices and study rooms before the School season opened. The students and personnel found a real joy in this intervention.

In October of 1939, a typhoid epidemic broke out at the State Hospital for the Insane (known as Dunning, now called Reed Mental Health Center for the Mentally Ill and Developmentally Disabled) and several of our nurses were called to assist at the hospital.

The Illinois State Nurses' Association and the Illinois State League of Nursing Education held their 38th Annual Convention at the Pere Marquette Hotel in Peoria, October 19–21, inclusive.

The following report on the Convention was written by Edna Thornblade and printed in the November, 1939 "Augustana Nurse."

One guest speaker was Miss Virginia Dunbar, Washington, D.C., assistant director of Red Cross Nursing Service. She stated that the action of the Red Cross is determined by need and not by America's conduct with respect to the war. She said that there were 41,000 nurses in the U.S. on the reserve list of the Red Cross, 2,139 of them reside in Illinois. She explained that a commission of three Red Cross executives, headed by Ernest Swift, vice chairman in charge of foreign relations, was in Europe studying conditions, investigating needs and preparing to make recommendations regarding the future policy of the Red Cross. War clouds were gathering over Europe and already Great Britain, France, Germany and Poland had appealed for help for her needy. People were becoming alarmed and one of the great problems of the big countries in Europe was the refugee situation. American citizens abroad were returning fearful of a war in Europe. One serious problem arose in the flight of 100,000 refugees to Rumania, Latvia and Lithuania. Funds were not given, though asked for, but supplies and equipment were sent to these countries. Continuing with an account of Red Cross activities brought about by the war, Miss Dunbar said every ship that docked at New York from Europe was met by nurses rendering assistance to returning travelers who were in poor health. In closing, she stated, "We are not interested in the causes of war, but we are interested in helping suffering caused by marching armies."

Dr. Lena Madesin Phillips, president of the International Federation of Business and Professional Women was another speaker. Dynamic and forceful, she gave us a challenge which we shall not soon forget. She said, "To you who have done so much good for the world, I ask an additional demand—that you help America know that it must fight subversive 'isms', or it may be your duty to close the eyes of the dead on the field of battle." She warned that we in America must make democracy so perfect that there will be no room for subversive doctrines, and asked the nurses to rededicate their lives to a living patriotism and not one which is evidenced by only the conventional flag salutes and cheering at the mention of Americanism. Real patriotism goes deeper than that. "We sit placidly by," she said, "as if our nation was in no danger. This idea we must purge from our minds, for we are not isolationists, and foreign 'isms' will attempt to undermine true Americanism." Declaring that the women of America have a great duty to perform during this crisis, Dr. Phillips urged the nurses to study current events and to distinguish between facts and malicious propaganda. "Analyze the things you hear carefully and then back your convictions firmly. Don't base your conclusions on false promises." Dr. Phillips related an interesting incident of a visit to Europe a few years ago. She had an audience with Premier Mussolini in which she asked him if he could give her any promising message to take back to the peace-loving women of America. The dictator answered her, "There can be no peace without justice."

The second day was a program of round tables and luncheons of the different sections. In order to be brief, I will summarize the pertinent thoughts gleaned from them:

### The Illinois League of Nursing Education:

All nursing education should be done with the firm conviction that all nurses must be prepared for community service.

Health nursing is just as essential and fundamental as sick nursing. The prevention of disease at least is as important a function of the nurse as the comfort, care and cure of the disease. These functions cannot be separated.

The community has a right to expect that nurses have some conception of what it means to maintain community health. Therefore, the community has a duty to the student nurse—that of informing her of problems to be faced and methods to be used in solving them.

### Private Duty Section:

Dr. A. A. Hayden of Chicago, an advocate of the 8-hour day for nurses, stated that they should have a diversified living program of cultural attainment and recreation so that they would better take care of the responsibilities of their position. He urged a more widespread usage of the 8-hour day, in order to reduce unemployment among nurses, especially in the large cities.

Miss Lenore Tobins in her annual report also stressed the great need of the 8-hour day in order that nurses might maintain good health for themselves. Especially did she feel it was necessary for the older nurses who had reached the peak of their usefulness through much experience. She felt that long and difficult hours would prove their premature retirement.

[The October Nurse carried a request to the private duty nurses to adhere to the new 8-hour rule of duty. It states: We have noted a few cases where nurses are not adhering to the rule of working the regular 8-hour shifts: 7 to 3, 3 to 11 and 11 to 7. This does not seem such a big offense at the time but it does cause hard feelings among other nurses and it really is breaking a rule.]

The Public Health Nursing Section:

Dr. Louis Sauer of Evanston, Illinois in speaking on "Whooping Cough Prevention," attacked the present method of quarantine which does not confine the child until he has fully contracted the disease. The disease is most communicable about a week before the child develops the serious cough. "No one will go around the child when he has the cough, but where was the child the week before?" Dr. Sauer proved through statistics that whooping cough was more fatal to children under two years of age than diphtheria, scarlet fever and measles, combined. He outlined the progress which has been made by the medical profession in combating this disease through the development of vaccine. In records which he has compiled since the double strength vaccine was introduced in March, 1938, he showed that there had been no failures out of the 571 children inoculated.

Some of the year end activities included "Nora Nobody," the three act comedy which was presented by the Senior Class, December 8, and was well attended. The proceeds were given to the Student Scholarship Fund.

An orchestra was organized in the School and its members consisted of students talented in music. Mrs. Elizabeth Fisher, formerly instructor of cello at the University of Nebraska, coached the orchestra. They played at various School activities and surprised the Alumnae Association by playing music during the dinner hour at its annual Christmas party.

The Y.W.C.A. of the Metropolitan Area held their annual tea at the Nurses' Residence in November, with a fine attendance. They also planned a "Scavenger Party" for Wednesday, December 13.

Miss Margaret Saenger again planned a gay Christmas Season at the Residence. Wednesday, December 20, prior to the departure of many of the students to their homes, the Lutheran Students Association gave a program. There was "The Hanging of the Greens" (in other words, everyone assisted with the decorating of the Residence). A tea followed and there was the usual tour to the various rooms to view the many Christmas trees. A Lut-Fisk supper was served at the hospital Friday evening, December 22. On Saturday, December 23rd, another nice evening was planned for the nurses when a festive supper was served, and Santa was present with a gift for each. Carols were sung on Christmas morning throughout the Nurses' Home and Hospital corridors.

# CHAPTER II

## THE FORTIES

The following article was found in the February, 1940, issue of the "Augustana Nurse."

Within the past month, information has been sent you regarding the Augustana Hospital Refunding Program. At our last Alumnae Meeting, Mr. Haverty was with us and explained how this plan would save our Hospital from foreclosure in 1945.

Do we as Augustana Graduates wish to see our Hospital go down defeated? No, never! Do we not retain much of that pride, spirit and enthusiasm which our former nurses had as they labored and struggled to rear the School and Hospital which we are proud to call our own?

Come, come, —let us step forward again. Sacrifice—yes. We must not die, WE MUST LIVE.

Since our membership is so scattered and difficult to reach, we would appreciate if each of you would offer your support without further notification. Write or phone Mr. John Haverty, Room 212, Augustana Hospital, 411 Dickens Ave., Chicago.

In March, 1940, the following Corporate Title was agreed upon, "The Alumnae Association of the Augustana Hospital School of Nursing." Our "History Book" was placed in the Library of Congress and copyrighted. It was decided to send a copy of the book to Their Royal Highnesses, the Crown Prince and Princess of Sweden. It will be recalled that they visited here in 1925, at the time the cornerstone of the new Hospital was laid. Dr. E. H. Ochsner had very kindly placed the History Book in the library of the American College of Surgeons; a copy had also been sent by the Alumnae to Columbia University of New York City; and a copy was also sent to Cumulative Book Index. By September of 1940, the request for a copy of the History Book from the Minnesota Historical Society was

119

not granted because so many requests had been received for free copies of the book.

In March, Mr. Haverty of the Augustana Hospital Refinancing Fund Program asked that nurses who had contributed so far should form a committee to talk over the refinancing plan. The Board of Directors of the Alumnae did not agree, believing that this project should be taken care of by the Hospital Refinancing Committee.

The Private Duty Nurses Section of First District sponsored a Nurses Institute at Mercy and Billings Hospital. Many of our "grads" attended. Registration for six sessions was $1.00.

A tea was given at the Nurses' Residence on March 17th to honor the History Committee composed of Miss Amy Schjolberg, Clarissa Drach, Martha Rohrbeck, Ida Burkhalter and Edna Thornblade. The tables and room were beautifully decorated in spring flowers and each honor guest received a corsage and a small gift. A large group attended.

Capping exercises were held on March 27th for the members of the pre-clinical class. The service was held at 6:30 a.m. The seniors and juniors were already seated when the pre-clinicals marched in to take their places in the front row. Following the hymn "The Lord Is My Shepherd," Miss Haggman gave a very impressive talk. This was followed by the placing of the cap on the head of the nurse and reciting the Pledge of Augustana Nurse in unison.

In becoming an accepted nurse of the Augustana Hospital School of Nursing, I pledge in the presence of God:

That I will always appear on duty in complete uniform as now.

That I will wear my uniform for duty only.

That I will conscientiously carry out the orders of the physician.

That I will respect all rules of the School.

That I will take an intelligent interest in all its activities.

That I will give my loyal support, while a nursing student and after graduation, to all policies adopted.

That I will hold every confidence inviolate and will not gossip.

That I will upon all occasions and by every means at my command, especially by my own personal conduct as a student and a graduate, maintain and endeavor to raise the nursing standards in the professional world.

That I will, immediately upon completion of my course, apply for State registration by examination, become a member of the Alumnae Association and thereby all organizations of which it is a part.

That I will at my earliest opportunity seek membership in the American Red Cross Nursing Service.

Then the hymn, "Take My Life And Let It Be" was sung. In the afternoon, Miss McNall, Miss Thornblade and Miss Klauser entertained at a tea in honor of the newly capped nurses. Miss Viola Lofquist sang two songs and friends and relatives of the nurses crowded around to offer congratulations to this group who in their new uniforms felt a newly acquired prestige.

The student uniform consisted of a striped shirtwaist, short-sleeved style dress with a detachable collar and cuffs. The apron was white and was a wrap-around style with a separate bib. During the probation period the students wore white "scrub dresses."

An article entitled "Aggressive Unionism" (reprinted from The Modern Hospital, Vol. 50, No. 5, May, 1938) appeared in the March issue of The Nurse. (Radical groups were giving some thought to forming unions for nurses). It read in part:

Nurses are organizing not for the purpose of improving themselves professionally or of rendering better service to patients but to gain shorter hours, higher pay and more satisfactory working conditions. Better let it be said that minority groups in this fine profession is thus following the example of labor unions. None will deny the splendid contribution that nurses individually and collectively have made to the welfare, happiness, comfort and humanities of this and other generations. To organize group effort for elevating scientific and professional aims is splendid. More power and influence for good to the American Nurses' Association and National League of Nursing Education and their many fine state organizations. Never from the platform of the national conventions of such groups does one hear a selfish, egocentric or arrogant voice. Instead there is much discussion of the most effective methods for providing better nursing.

But, alas! On the fringes of this fine professional group one observes small, excited emotional gatherings discussing wages, hours and hospitals. Here and there a listener might catch incendiary suggestions as to votes, parties, national or local elections, or the building up or the tearing down of political influence. Some believe that such groups are wholly unrepresentative of the nursing profession and that they consist of the agitator type.

Ethical nurses do not hold such persons in high repute. It is probable that the professional organizer finds the idle incompetent nurse easy to persuade. Such slogans as "eight hours, eight dollars and eight months work" find easy lodgement in their shallow minds. It is likely that the nurse with union tendencies will either gravitate to her own level or else repent and seek reinstatement by her more ethical colleagues. [18]

Finland had been attacked in December 1939, by Russia and the following was from a letter received from Marit Moe '31, who had gone to her home country, Norway.

> "I worked with the boat up till Christmas and then joined the Norwegian Red Cross ambulance going here. We are divided in three places and I happen to come along to the front Casarebt, where we are 2 doctors, 1 student and 3 nurses. The work is plentyful. One of the other nurses and I are in the operating room and one in X-ray. We work mostly at night as all the wounded is being transferred after dark and in the day time we try to sleep some between the airplane alarms. That is when the Russian bombers come. I can not describe the feeling it gives when they are right over us and the bombs are falling. Neither can I describe what we see every day and the harm they are doing. It is such a beautiful place here— lakes and small hills covered with woods and the most marvelous weather. Clear, blue sky and sunshine and moonlight. Cold—40⁰ C. and more sometimes but we are well supported with woolen clothes and furs of all kinds.
>
> "It is such a nice feeling to be in a place where you feel you are of use. It is not always so.
>
> "It is hard to tell now when I will be back in U.S.A. but I should like to come back to Chicago some day to visit. Give my best regards to everybody.
>
> > Sincerely yours,
> > Merit Moe, '31"

Baccalaureate Services were held at the Gethsemane Lutheran Church, Oakdale and Lamon Avenues, at 11:00 a.m. Sunday, April 21st. The supervisors of the Hospital entertained the Seniors on Tuesday Evening, April 23rd, at an informal party in the lounge and the Juniors entertained the Seniors at a dinner on Friday Evening, April 26th, at the Webster Hotel. Graduation Exercises were held at the Trinity Lutheran Church, Barry and Seminary Avenues, at 8:00 p.m. on Tuesday Evening, April 30th. Speakers for the evening were Dr. N. M. Percy representing the staff and Rev. T. L. Rydebeck as guest speaker.

---

18. Reprinted from The Modern Hospital, Vol. 50, No. 5, May, 1938.

Dr. Percy gave an inspiring speech which contained the following:

> You have been taught by experience, as well as by training, to recognize those major and minor emotional disturbances that may attend sickness, and equally have you learned, perhaps many times from bitter experience, the effect on the patient's family and friends of the emotional disturbances which so often accompany the unusual events inseparable from illness.
>
> As the various classes have gone forth from Augustana Hospital training School in this nearly half a century, they have left their mark in the betterment and uplifting of the social conditions of their communities. I know you young women will do the same. I take this opportunity to congratulate you on your entrance into one of the most noble and unselfish of the professions. I congratulate you, not alone on becoming a part of the great organization of nursing, but also on the opportunity that is given you to take part in social progress.

A Reception in the Nurses' Residence to the families and friends of the Graduation Class followed the exercises.

In June of 1940, two $50.00 scholarships were offered by the Alumnae Association to its members.

REPORT OF EDUCATIONAL
SCHOLARSHIP FUND COMMITTEE

The Educational Scholarship Fund Committee of the Alumnae Association of the Augustana Hospital School of Nursing submits the following report.

1. That $5,000 of the accumulated scholarship fund shall be invested in Augustana Hospital First Mortgage Bonds at not less than 3% or more than 5% interest per annum.

2. The income, from the investment together with the annual contribution of the senior class of the Augustana Hospital School of Nursing is to be used as a scholarship award, the amount of which shall not exceed $250.00. The award shall be made at the beginning of each school year.

3. According to need, the recipient of the scholarship award may apply for a loan, the amount of which shall not exceed $250.00. The loan fund shall be established from the remainder of the existing scholarship fund and maintained by the general fund of the Alumnae Association of the Augustana Hospital School of Nursing. No interest shall be paid on this loan and it shall be re-payable within three years from date of loan.

4. The applicant must be a resident member of the Alumnae Association of the Augustana Hospital School of Nursing and in good standing.

5. The Scholarship Award shall be given to the applicant who in the judgment of the Educational Scholarship Fund Committee has outstanding rank in scholarship and shows most promise of future usefulness.

6. The applicant must be enrolled in the department of nursing of an accredited college or university, to whom the award shall be made payable.

7. Should the recipient of the award retire from active nursing within one year following the completion of the school year she shall be obligated to return at least $100.00 of the amount awarded within one year of her retirement.

In the June Alumnae Meeting, a motion was made to recommend to the Board of Directors of the Hospital that only 8-hour duty be permitted at the Hospital. After the summer vacation the Board of Directors of the Hospital considered this matter but refused to restrict the Hospital to hiring only 8-hour duty nurses.

The members of First District of I.N.A. were urging the nurses to subscribe for an insurance policy covering accident and health and hospital. The Continental Casualty had been chosen because of its fine reputation and financial backing.

Two students assisted in the Red Cross Drive for funds. Four students assisted in soliciting funds for Adult Charities on May 6th. It was interesting to learn that the boxes held by our nurses contained the largest amount of any boxes in the city.

On July 3rd, two of our staff physicians, Dr. Natalie Ashmenckas and Dr. Oscar Nadeau were wed. The happy couple were presented with a coffee set by the graduates of the hospital. The honeymooners made a trip from Connecticut to Chicago on the "Nanda" (boat).

The Alumnae Association had plans to raffle a 1941 Ford Standard car. The raffle was to be held on December 14th at 8:30 p.m. It was asked that each nurse sell two books of raffle tickets priced at 10 cents each. In December, it was reported that a profit of $1,882.00 was made on the raffle, and a Mr. William Hennick of Aurora, Illinois was the winner. This project was undertaken to enable the Alumnae Association to purchase one or more Augustana Hospital Bonds.

A tea sponsored by the Chicago Lutheran Nurses Guild was held at the Nurses' Residence on October 18th from 4:30 to 6:00 p.m. and all Lutheran nurses attending the Illinois State

Nurses' Association convention were invited. Illinois State Nurses' Association convention was held at the Palmer House from October 17 to 19th. Discussion was held about educating the public to 8-hour duty and to the term "graduate registered nurse." Lack of cooperation and apparent inertia and failure to attend meetings were listed as being detrimental to the private duty group.

A concert was given on November 11th at the Messiah Lutheran Church by the Nurses Chorus under the direction of Mr. Harry T. Carlson. In spite of inclement weather, many turned out to be entertained by this group. A Red Cross pageant was given as part of the entertainment, directed by Miss Saenger and Miss Chamberlain. The program closed impressively with the sounding of taps. The proceeds amounted to $200.00 and this was turned over to the Hospital.

In December, the editor of the Augustana Nurse reported that she was mailing 528 copies of the Nurse each month. Fifty two members were taken in during the year.

The annual Alumnae Association Christmas party was held in the Recreation Room on December 11th. Edna Thornblade presided and opened the meeting with the reading of the Christmas Story. A lovely supper was served during which time the members were entertained by the student orchestra. Santa Claus had left a gift at each place and the tables were beautifully decorated. The Heinz Soup Company assisted in the planning of the meal and the Alumnae Association realized $16.40 from the project. A representative of the Heinz Company served cream of mushroom soup as the second course and for each signature that evening the Alumnae received ten cents. In addition each guest received a gift can of soup. About 150 nurses attended this party and the collection to benefit the sick nurses was $68.50. Following the supper the guests were entertained in the lounge by the Thalian Drama Club who presented tableaux of the Christmas Story accompanied by beautiful singing coming from behind the scenes. (Student Octet.)

The following article was written by a student and printed in the January '41, Augustana Nurse.

### AUGUSTANA CHRISTMAS

Perhaps one of the nicest memories that we students will carry with us when we venture away from Augustana's doors is the one which we shall have when we recall Christmas and all the activities which it occasions. The hustle of last-minute, hurried Christmas shopping seems to lend an undercurrent of excitement, and looking forward to the annual festivities which will take place furnishes the keynote of that undefinable "something" known as "Christmas Spirit."

The Alumnae Party, on December 10, ushered in the holiday season and was attended by many graduates. And it gave us who were "on the outside looking in" a little thrill of pleasure to think that someday we would be meeting our classmates and celebrating Christmas under similar conditions. From all reports, the dinner in the recreation room of the Nurses' Residence was something to remember, and the Christmas tableaux presented by the Thalian Drama Club were apparently enjoyed.

The "Hanging of the Greens," on December 19, was the next event. Graduates and students, their friends and relatives were invited to take part in the decoration of the lounge. Fir branches were placed around the room, the Christmas tree was trimmed, and the assembled company, including the gentlemen, were admitted to the "inner sanctum" of the entire Nurses' Residence to see the room decorations. Judging from the remarks of many of the guests, our efforts to make our rooms express the spirit of Christmas were well worthwhile.

The Smorgasbord Supper, on December 20, was perhaps the highlight of the season's festivities. The candle-lighted dining room with its beautifully decorated tables, bearing tasty Swedish delicacies, was something never to be forgotten. And for those of us who sampled everything, lest we be deprived of knowing just what "this" was made of or how "that" would taste, even the "overstuffed" feeling with which we left the dining room was not unpleasant.

The January issue of The Nurse printed the following poem sent by a former patient:

> To all the nurses who took care of me
> After my apen-dec-to-my
> From the 20th at midnite to New Years Day
> I've had a swell time and want to say
> "Thanks"—on my 12th P.O. day
>
> For:
>
> Pinning and straightening my belly bands
> For bathing me—my face and hands
> For bringing my trays—water and sippers
> For putting on my dust mop slippers
> Answering my lights—watering my plants

Putting on my bed jackets and pajama pants
Changing my sheets, making my bed
For rubbing my back so it wouldn't get red
For taking my temperature and counting my pulse
For bringing me orange juice and chocolate milks
Getting my Tribune every day
Buying stamps to send my letters away
For a Merry Christmas and a Happy New Year
I want to say thanks for my nice visit here.

—Ann Nichols

Following are two other articles of interest from the January Augustana Nurse:

The beautiful rosewood case electric victrola given to us some years ago by Dr. and Mrs. Percy has been rebuilt with new motor, reproducer, amplifier and power speaker. We are glad to have this machine which will fill a need in the Residence.

Recently the Nurses' Chorus made two recordings, "Sanctus" by Bach and "The St. James Air." Records may be purchased at the Residence for $1.10 each.

Although we were not yet at war, many nurses were joining the Army Nurse Corps. Our February meeting afforded us the opportunity of becoming acquainted with Miss Pearl C. Fisher, the Assistant Superintendent Army Nurse Corps, Sixth Corps Area, Chicago. She outlined for us a picture of a Red Cross Nurse's life in the Army Nurse Corps, from the viewpoints of duty, social activity and a religious and Christian aspect. The Army wants its nurses from the ranks of the Red Cross Nursing Service.

Another speaker of our program was Miss Charlotte Landt, Recording Secretary of the Illinois State Nurses' Association. She had recently been designated as Special Agent by the United States Public Health Service to assume charge of the national nursing inventory in our state. She urged 100% cooperation and asked that we return our questionnaires at once. She stated that "in answering these questions you are not in any way obligated to participate in military activity, but you will aid in a great nursing need should an emergency arise. Our civilian population must also be cared for. As nurses, we have one of the greatest opportunities to serve—let that desire of service to others— never die within us."

The following statistics (see Table 2.1) are for your aid in completing this above-mentioned Questionnaire.

Table 2.1
Bed Capacity Statistics

| Year | Bed Capacity | Average Daily Census |
|------|------|------|
| 1894–1903 | 125 | 90 |
| 1903–1919 | 200 | 150 |
| 1919–1922 | 280 | 260 |
| 1922–1925 | 285 | 200 |
| 1925 | " | 205 |
| 1926 | 375 | 223 |
| 1927 | " | 286 |
| 1928 | " | 261 |
| 1929 | 300 | 268 |
| 1930 | " | 240 |
| 1931 | " | 185 |
| 1932 | " | 180 |
| 1933 | " | 144 |
| 1934 | " | 147 |
| 1935 | " | 142 |
| 1936 | " | 160 |
| 1937 | " | 179 |
| 1938 | " | 180 |
| 1939 | " | 180 |
| 1940 | " | 220 |

"WHO SHOULD RESPOND?"

The Red Cross Nursing Service does not assume the responsibility for saying to a nurse that she should or should not respond to the present call for nurses in the Army Nurse Corps, but it has the great responsibility for giving a true picture of the need so that nurses can, themselves, decide this important question.

We can remind nurses of these points which may help them to decide whether they should respond:

1. That at this time the need is for a large number of nurses for bedside care in Army hospitals.

2. That although nurses in all different types of positions are needed where they are now serving there are some positions from which nurses can much more easily and safely be spared than from others.

3. That although the care of the civilian population is unquestionably of equal importance with the care of the military forces, military forces at the present time lack 4,000 nurses necessary to safeguard their health conditions.

4. That conditions of service in the Army compare favorably with conditions of service in civilian hospitals.

5. That all in all, the need for nursing care in any such emergency is a professional responsibility which must be met by the professional nurses of the country. No other group can meet this need. From this arises our moral obligation to be enrolled in the Red Cross Nursing Service if eligible, as it is through this channel that nurses can be available for such an emergency need. Mary Beard, Director, American Red Cross Nursing Service.

### "PATRIOTISM IS NOT ENOUGH"

In May 1915, in the city of Brussels, Belgium an English woman Edith Cavell who in pity had in her capacity as a nurse, aided wounded prisoners to escape over the border into Holland, was executed by a German firing squad. Her last words were: "Patriotism is not enough. I must have no hatred or bitterness toward anyone."

It was said that though she had asked the privilege of not having her eyes bandaged, her captors were obliged to bandage them, as the firing squad could not bear the look of pity and mercy in her eyes. She could pity those who were about to shoot her. Today, throughout the world, nurses remember the name of Edith Cavell, but how many remember the name of the powerful military governor who ordered her execution? He is forgotten, and he who is forgotten is dead. Edith Cavell will never die, because she is remembered as one who was worthy of her calling and faithful even unto death.

In May, 1917, in New York City, an American woman, Anna Caroline Maxwell, was preparing a group of nurses, most of them graduates of her own school, to go to France to serve their country as nurses in a war hospital. She said many things, but among them she said: "If you have any wounded Germans to care for, I expect you to do it just as well as if they were British, or French, or American." While the nurses assembled applauded her words, and were glad she spoke them, there was no need to have said those words. Those present were all nurses, and filled with the spirit of compassion for humanity, friend and foe alike, and they fulfilled their trust. What is more, when, during their first year abroad, in the service of the British army, they met men from many lands, of many nationalities, including Germans, it was not difficult to care for them all alike, for they were alike, all equally bewildered by the behavior of their different countries, and not quite sure why they had been asked to kill each other.

Today our country is faced with a more serious crisis than we faced in 1917. The half-hearted, blundering efforts of our country, and of every other country, to secure the promised peace and to "make the word safe for democracy," have broken down completely. Nothing is any longer safe. Power-mad dictators have launched a ruthless, cruelly unjust war of conquest and of vengeance. Several perfectly innocent, prosperous, self-respecting, peace-loving small nations have gone down in the wave of ruthlessness that has swept over them. The France that many Americans learned to love and respect twenty years ago is at present bound in chains, partly of its own forging. England is fighting for her very life, is being terribly wounded, her civilians killed by hundreds, and what the end will be we cannot yet foresee.

Opinions may differ as to the part our own country played twenty years ago. Some of us think that the war should have been finished then, in order to prevent future war, and secure peace and justice. Many more Americans believe that if the United States had been differently led, or had been more mature, and had accepted the responsibility of joining the League of Nations, it might have done much more to secure world peace. But we cannot go backward. We must go forward.

In the opinion of many Americans, the present leader of the United States is sincere and earnest in his wish to help secure world peace, as quickly as possible. The question of how that can be done is the awful responsibility of the President and the Congress of the United States. Upon the decisions they make now, even today, rests the entire future of the country, and of the world. It becomes clear that the center of world power and, more important, of world responsibility, is gradually shifting, more and more, onto our shoulders.

For that reason it becomes very important that Americans, more particular young Americans, the young men who, in the event of war, will be called upon to fight, and the young women who as nurses will be called upon to serve in the armies of the United States — that these young people should form a clear conception of what they want to do and of what they want their country to do and to mean to the world. As a young, strong, powerful nation, with great national resources, the task of rebuilding the war-torn world across the sea will devolve very largely upon us.

As nurses, we can do much to help steer a good course in these troubled waters. It behooves us to spread the doctrine, not of so-called "patriotism" — a once good word which has been so misused to fan the flames of hate, of nationalism, of sectionalism in times past that it no longer serves as the right motive for fighting even a just war, if there can be a just war. Idealism, love of humanity, compassion, that high vision which came to Edith Cavell in her last moment of life, are a much worthier banner for nurses to enlist under. We could not do better than to use her words as our slogan if we are again called into battle for freedom and for peace and for world brotherhood.[19]

The School of Nursing pointed to some changes in uniform at this time. This was the first time that students were allowed to wear white shoes and hose. The seniors wore their "whites" on March 31st at the capping for the Class of 1943, and the

---

19. Taken from the American Journal of Nursing, Vol. 41, No. 3.

other students changed on May 1st, changing a very old custom at Augustana. The student uniform was also new. The straps of the bib which formerly crossed in the back and extended to the waist now were to reach the shoulder and buttoned there. A red lined hood had been added to the cape. The hood was detachable and useful in bad weather.

The Junior Class presented a bazaar on April 25th in the Recreation Room of the Nurses' Residence, which was continuous from 2:00 p.m. until 10:00 p.m. The proceeds of this event were used to entertain the Senior Class at the Annual Junior-Senior Banquet which was held in May. The students were hard at work, each one making an individual article to be sold at the bazaar. There were refreshments and admission tickets were being sold for five cents. This fee also entitled one to a chance on the door prize.

Baccalaureate services for the Graduation class of 1941 were held at the Concordia Lutheran Church on Sunday, May 18th at 10:45 p.m. Graduation exercises were held on Sunday, May 20th at the Bethlehem Lutheran Church at South Wells and 58th Street. The event was at 8:00 p.m. and 41 seniors marched in to the hymn "Rejoice Ye Pure In Heart" after which Rev. Sandstedt gave the invocation. The nurses' chorus under the direction of Harry T. Carlson sang several selections. Greetings were extended by Mr. E. R. Jacobson, President of the Board. The address of the evening was given by Dr. Oscar Benson, President of the Illinois Conference of the Synod.

As Chief of the Surgical Staff of the hospital, Dr. N. M. Percy gave a very timely and appropriate greeting to the graduates of 1941 which is applicable to all nurses. He encouraged tact, one of the most important qualities of a nurse. The practice of "talking shop" is very harmful and should be eliminated. Nurses should not feel that graduation ends their study in the profession, but should continue learning by reading current journals. This practice gives the doctor more confidence in the nurse.

Dr. Percy discouraged the use of cigarettes among nurses and cautioned them against over-exercise. A good form of exercise is the popular sitting-up exercises and walking. He maintained, however, that walking should include window shopping, which should be kept as such and warned the nurses against the very poor policy of getting themselves in debt by charge accounts and installment-plan purchasing. These are very great temptations to the nurse who is beginning to earn money for the first time in her life perhaps, and too frequently causes plenty of worry. A reception followed the graduation in the newly decorated Lila Pickhardt Memorial Lounge.

On Hospital Day, May 11th, the "Lamp Light Eternal," a marionette show, written by Darlene Kirkland, a Preclinical student, was presented by the Preclinicals of the School of Nursing and the student chorus under Harry T. Carlson sang at the Olivet Lutheran Church.

Private duty nursing was being discouraged because of the shortage of help in hospitals and group nursing was being encouraged. Changes in wages of the private duty nurse were announced.

$6.00 - 8 hour duty with one meal or fifty cents.

$8.00 - 8 hour duty with two patients.

$9.00 - 8 hour duty with three patients.

$7.00 - 10 hour duty with two meals or one dollar.

$8.00 - 12 hour duty with three meals or $1.50.

$9.00 - 20 hour resident service with three meals or equivalent.

Mental or alcoholic, etc.:

$7.00 - 8 hour duty.

$8.50 - 10 hour duty.

$10.00 - 12 hour duty.

$11.00 - 20 hour duty.

The wages were to go into effect on September 22nd, 1941.

The Edgar Bergan Foundation presented scholarship assistance to some of our needy students. Mr. Bergan with "Charlie" made an effort to meet these students individually and was a guest at the residence on several occasions.

The following article was reprinted from the Journal of the American Medical Association:

Eighty-eight schools of nursing were selected by the U.S. Public Health Service, October 10, to receive federal aid in training additional student nurses. Sixty-seven schools in thirty-two states will offer refresher courses to three thousand graduate nurses, and twenty-six schools will enroll five hundred graduate nurses for postgraduate study. A total of $1,200,000 is available for the program, which includes field training centers for public health nursing.

The student-nurse training program will increase enrollment by two thousand young women in this country, Hawaii and Puerto Rico. Surgeon General Parran has estimated a need for fifty thousand student nurses this year, and the federal program will bring the total to about forty-two thousand. The average yearly enrollment is slightly under forty thousand. It is hoped that schools able to increase their enrollment without federal aid will meet the deficiency.

The federal grants will be made at the end of each quarter of the school year except in cases in which tuition is required in advance. The eighty-eight schools of nursing were selected from a list of three hundred applications. The $1,200,000 was made available by the Federal Security Agency Appropriation Act to help meet a national shortage of nurses created by increased demands of the armed services and defense industries. The money will be spent as follows (all figures are approximate): for student training $900,000, for postgraduate courses $125,000, for public health training $50,000 and for refresher courses $125,000.[20]

The Illinois State Nurses' Association Convention was held October 23–25 in Urbana, Illinois. The meetings were held in the Auditorium of the University campus and the following were delegates from the Alumnae Association: Agnes Hanson, Sylvia Kercher and Lillian Ostrand. The reports were given at the November meeting and following are the highlights of the report.

State problems: Most prominent was the lack of general duty nurses. The solution everywhere was better pay and more pleasant living quarters. There were at the present time 6,000 Red Cross nurses on duty but a total of 13,000 were needed. The Illinois League luncheon was well attended with Miss Anne Goodrich, Dean Emeritus of the Yale School of Nursing speaking on the problems. She

---

20. Taken from the Journal of the American Medical Association, October 18, 1941.

stressed more education for nurses and lamented the fact that nursing was the only profession that had not established a place in education. She said, "Good education means good care for patients." At the private duty section meeting the State President of the group, Miss Harden, opened her talk by saying, "You private duty nurses are in disgrace. You are the largest, yet the weakest." She also stressed the lack of Private Duty nurses on the various boards. "We should not expect any better conditions for our branch until we get out to vote for someone who is interested in our problems." Lectures on sulfanilamide and diabetes were given later by two doctors.

Admiral Isorakus Yamamoto who was the commander of the Japanese Navy attacked Pearl Harbor on December 7, 1941. An emergency session of congress was called to Washington, D.C. and war was declared on Japan and Germany a couple of days later.

The nurses were enrolling for service with the armed forces and excitement was running high. The office of the Nurses' Residence brought out the flag used during the first World War to indicate the number of nurses from our hospital who were members of the armed forces. It was a large white flag and each nurse was indicated by a red star with a total of 72 stars of which one was white. Miss Saenger had ordered a new flag to be used during World War II.

On February 11th, 22 new students entered training. Classes in first aid were begun with Dr. Carl T. Stephan as the Certified American Red Cross Instructor. There was an enrollment of 121 students the first night. They were mostly students and graduates from our school—however, some of the neighborhood women and men enrolled.

Governor Dwight Green spoke at the Chicago Sunday Evening Club in Orchestra Hall on February 8th. His topic for the evening was "Defense of God vs. Godless Forces." Upon hearing his speech, Miss H. Evelyn Johnson, Editor of the Augustana Nurse for 1942 wrote to him about the many nurses from our school who were serving with the armed forces. [Approximately 170 Augustana nurses served in the military during World War II.] She received the following reply:

Dear Miss Johnson:

Thank you for your letter of February 10th which lists the work of some of Augustana Hospital graduates' work in the service of their country. I am sure that all of us are proud of this contribution.

We are engaged in a war to preserve our American way of life. Either we and our allies win completely or the brute forces that are representative of hate, greed and intolerance will dominate the world. Let us make no mistake about that. It is a death struggle between two systems of living.

I am sure that all of us are proud of the sacrifices and heroic efforts the nursing profession is making to give our armed forces victory. In the front lines and on the home front, they have answered the call of their country. They are truly the soldiers of mercy.

Sincerely yours,
Dwight H. Green, Governor

Following is another interesting article received at Augustana. Phil Ault, United Press Correspondent in far-off Iceland wrote his parents who lived in LaGrange the following:

"Recently I played a role in an interesting reunion, involving a Dr. Boice of Augustana Hospital in Chicago, now with the medical corps in Iceland and a Norwegian nurse up here from England. The nurse remarked that she had trained at Augustana before returning to Norway. (Marit Moe,'31.) I told him of her and they got together recently. They had known each other at Augustana. She had returned to Norway and they had naturally lost all contact. After the German invasion of Norway she made an 8 hour trip on skis across the border to Sweden, reached Stockholm, then traveled to Moscow, south to Odessa, through Turkey by rail, across the Mediterranean to Port Said, Egypt; from there to Lisbon to London and finally to Iceland. Now they live a short distance apart. This proves something about the old 'small world' saying, doesn't it?"

The following three articles were taken from the January 2, 1942, New York Times.

OVER 6,000 NURSES JOIN ARMY FOR ACTIVE DUTY IN YEAR
Major Julia Flikke, Veteran of World War, Heads Corps
By Jessie Fant Evans

Wherever the Army sends its troops, Army nurses go along to take care of the soldiers.

Army nurses today are on "around the clock duty" in every Army Hospital base, including those in Alaska, Hawaii, the Philippines, Puerto Rico, the Panama Canal Zone and Iceland. In Iceland, they are cheerfully evolving all sorts of substitutes for accustomed procedures and refusing to be dismayed by the rapidly approaching prospect of 23 hours of darkness out of every 24.

A little over a year ago there were 700 Army nurses. Now, there are 6,877. Before this fiscal year is over it is expected 8,237 will be enrolled. Each is a volunteer, drawn from the Red Cross list of Army and Navy Reserves.

The Army is proud of the fact that it has never had to draft a nurse. During the last World War, 21,480 volunteer, registered nurses served our armed forces. Over 10,000 of this number were with our troops on foreign soil under incredibly difficult conditions in most instances.

### Cupid Often Reduces Ranks

Army nurses must be graduates of class A nursing schools. They must also be in top-notch condition, without physical impairment of any kind. Provision is made for age and disability. Retirement on 75 percent of their pay is possible at the age of 50, after 25 years of service. They volunteer for one year, with the pledge that except for "cogent" reasons, their service if satisfactory, shall be of three years' duration.

Marriage is accepted as a "cogent" reason, despite the fact that Dan Cupid sometimes reduces the nurses' ranks with the virulence of an epidemic. The service is philosophical, however, with regard to authorized defections on the theory that establishment of happy American homes is an asset in building good citizenship and loyalty to country.

The Army's nursing corps functions under the surgeon general. Its immediate supervision is vested in Maj. Julia O. Flikke, R.N., whose office is on the fourth floor of the Social Security Building at Fourth and Independence Avenue S.W. She is the second woman to administer the details of this highly-important Army job of caring for men who require hospitalization. Her immediate predecessor and the first woman to have this position, was Maj. Julia C. Stimson, retired.

### Four Aides Rank as Captains

Under Maj. Flikke, at her headquarters office here, are four assistants with the rank of captain. Assistant superintendents of nursing on field duty, one for every corps headquarters area, hold similar rank. Each and every Army ward nurse is a second lieutenant. All chief nurses are first lieutenants.

There is nothing of the harassed feminine executive about Maj. Flikke. She is serene and apparently unhurried. She has a sympathetic approach to, and an infinite understanding of human frailties and needs in sickness and in health.

Carefully catalogued desk files provide her with statistics or information which may be quickly needed. A combined career of nursing care and hospital administration has given her perspective and the power to administer details without being submerged by them. But she has that "human touch" which has kept her essentially feminine and "motherly" in the finest sense of the word.

Of Norwegian parents who came to this country and settled in Wisconsin where they became American citizens, she entered a nursing school as a young widow. She chose this career because she wished to pay in service to others the debt of gratitude she felt she owed individual members of the nursing profession who for 10 years assisted her with the care of an invalid husband and mother.

Coping with the rapid expansion of an Army nursing setup on a war basis is not a new experience for her. She is a nursing veteran of the last World War. From her post as assistant superintendent of the Augustana Hospital in Chicago, she went overseas with the Red Cross unit organized by the internationally known Swiss physician, Dr. A. J. Ochsner. As chief of nurses at Base Hospital No. 11 she served abroad until July, 1919. Her foreign service with the Army nursing corps has included duty in the Philippines and China. She moved to her present assignment after 12 years continuous duty as chief of the nursing staff at Walter Reed Hospital.

### Likes Smart New Uniform

With her office assistants and members of the corps, wherever they are on duty, she is enthusiastic about the changes in service uniforms which have just been authorized for Army nurses, the first since immediately after the World War. Gone are the olive drab ones, almost universally unbecoming to women.

The smartly-tailored, dark blue new uniforms are intriguing with their color contrasts of brass buttons, braid, other insignia and maroon piping of the Medical Corps.

The skirt of fashionable length is of medium colored blue covert cloth. With it is worn a choice of a white or periwinkle blue blouse, a regulation officer's black tie, a trim jacket of darker blue, black oxford shoes, gray suede gloves and an overseas cap. The jacket has brass buttons down the front. On the lapels are the letters, U.S. and on the maroon-colored piped blue shoulder bar is the insignia, which indicates the official rank of the nurse. The insignia on the jaunty blue, maroon-piped overseas cap is the caduceus.

The darker blue overcoats for field uniforms are water repellant with removable, sharply contrasting maroon colored zippered-in linings.

Extremely attractive, too, are the dark blue capes with their vivid maroon lining. These are worn over the white indoor uniforms, with white shoes and white caps.

An outfitting of six white indoor uniforms with its complement of caps and shoes is issued to all Army nurses, as are the capes and overcoats. Thus far, the out-of-door uniforms for field duty are being issued only to nurses on foreign duty.

In the March 1943, "Augustana Nurse," we had an article quoted from the Journal of Nursing stating that Colonel Julia Flikke retired as Superintendent of the Army Nurse Corps. Her 25 years experience in the Corps. comprised service in France, at many Army posts in the continental U.S.A., in the Philippines and in China. She was the first woman in the United States Army Nurse Corps. to attain the rank of Colonel.

### RUSH TO ENROLL NURSES GROWS
#### Rapid Increase in Enlistment Sequel to the Attack on Pearl Harbor
#### 1,237 JOINED IN DECEMBER

Response to the Campaign for Volunteers Cheers Official of the Red Cross

Japan's first blast at Pearl Harbor on Dec. 7 started a rush of American nurses to register for service, even as their brothers and cousins stormed recruiting offices and as leaders in their field had predicted would happen. Confirmation of a rapid rise in enrollments in the First Reserves of the Red Cross was obtained yesterday from headquarters in Washington, where Miss Gertrude Banfield, assistant to Miss Mary Beard, director of the Red Cross Nursing Service, was on duty for the day.

Appointments to the Army and Navy Nurse Corps are made only from the ranks of the First Reserves of the Red Cross. Enrollment in this class is only open to American citizens, unmarried, between the ages of 22 and 40, and who have completed their training as professional nurses.

"Up to the outbreak of war," Miss Banfield said, "the largest number of nurses enrolling in the First Reserves in any one month was recorded in April of 1941 and numbered 1,615." An intensive drive was put on at that time for volunteers who would sign up for emergency service. In November, the monthly total had dropped to 441. But the December figures shot up promptly after Pearl Harbor, and had reached 1,237 at last report.

At the War Department, where the office of Major Julia O. Flikke, director of the Army Nurse Corps, was also open and functioning yesterday, an assistant declared that no further figures will be released on the size of the corps or the appointments made to it, since these now become military secrets, of interest to the enemy.

The last-mentioned quota of the first reserves of the Red Cross was 50,000, according to Miss Banfield, who added that current records show the enrollment of more than 25,500, including those in service in the Army and Navy Corps.

Nowhere was it said or indicated that many more nurses are not wanted or needed. Indications were that the recruiting would be continued at full speed ahead.

—N.Y. Times, Jan. 2, 1942

STATE IS URGED TO POSTPONE STATE NURSES' PRACTICES ACT
Mrs. Detmold Backs Move In Legislature—Sees Delay Needed as War
Measure To Help Enlist More for Service

Mrs. Mabel Detmold, chairman of the legislative committee of the New York State Nurses' Association, yesterday expressed her complete accord with the proposal made in Albany Saturday by Miss Jane Todd, member of the Assembly, seeking delay in execution of the State Nurses Practices Act.

"When we drafted the law," she said, "we had no idea that we would actually be in the war. Now I feel it should be postponed, not only for one year, as suggested, but for the duration.

"With the law postponed, we will probably canvass the possibilities of bringing others into service. Many nurses who have already left active practice will probably return as a result of this, as the act definitely hampered their coming back into service. They knew that unless their applications for certificates were in by July 1 their licenses would be suspended as of today.

"By postponing the act, which would permit only persons holding State nursing licenses to practice in the State, we will have accomplished one more step in relieving the drastic shortage of trained nurses."

A delay would mark the third for the act. Twice before it was postponed because of small appropriations and because difficulty in checking credentials retarded the process of clearing applications.

—N.Y. Times, Jan. 2, 1942 [21]

The "Augustana Nurse" continued to run the request for empty cold cream jars and bottles of various sizes to be used by the pharmacy. They were difficult to obtain during the war and all jars were being saved along with the tin cans and other articles with metal parts.

Everywhere one could see the "V" for Victory sign and even in the "Augustana Nurse," bond ads and "V" for Victory ads were noted on many pages.

The following item appeared in the "Augustana Nurse" of May 1942:

We hear a great deal about not wasting paper. It seems that printing paper comes in blocks of a certain size. Every time our "Augustana Nurse" was printed, the block had to be cut down, thus wasting a very great deal of paper. So we decided to try an experiment with the larger size, for a time at least.

All meetings of the Alumnae now opened with the saluting of the flag. It was voted by the Alumnae Association to invest all interest from holdings in U.S. War Savings Bonds. The war continued and the "Augustana Nurse" was filled with names of nurses who were in service and also the names of staff doctors and former doctors from our hospital. D. Marguerite Craig '33, entered the service before Pearl Harbor [and spent 20 years in the Army Nurse Corps]. She along with Bert Anderson Henkle '34, and Edna Thornblade '32, were among the first nurses to be called into service overseas; their assignment was India. Many of our nurses were teaching home nursing courses

---

21. The "Augustana Nurse," March 1942.

and otherwise helping out on the war effort. The students had a victory garden on the lot next to the Residence and the hospital. As the students entered training they were required to turn their ration books over to the Hospital. It was difficult to buy soap to wash stockings and very difficult to buy stockings. Another hardship was trying to get passage on a train to go home and then trying to get a seat on the train. Dr. and Mrs. Percy gave their Doberman-Pincher "Percy's Prince Peter" to the U.S. Army to be used as a guard dog for the duration.

The National Biennial Convention of the American Nurses Association was held in Chicago. The theme of the convention was "Nursing at the Nation's Service." Speakers included Dr. Thomas Parran—Surgeon General of the United States and Miss I. Stewart, President of the League of Nursing Education. Augustana Nurses were very active in helping to make the convention a success. Our student chorus sang at the opening joint session of the convention at the Coliseum. Dressed in complete uniform and marching in perfect order it made a truly beautiful picture and it seemed the chorus sang as it had never sung before. The student luncheon was held in the Gold Room of the Congress Hotel. Guests honored at the luncheon included Col. Julia Flikke. A hobby exhibit was held at the Congress Hotel and many of our students and our nurses took part.

Eight members of the class of 1945 published a mimeographed booklet covering the student activities and exhibits at the convention. There were panel discussions on Student Publications and Student Government. An address on Infantile Paralysis was given by Sister Kenny of Australia and she also showed her movies of her treatment procedures. Honorary membership in the A.N.A. was granted to her.

Some topics discussed at the convention were nurse's aides and voluntary workers, socialized medicine and group nursing. Among the discussions, it was mentioned that all states below the Mason-Dixon line do not accept the colored nurse into their state associations. Therefore the colored nurse in those states was not eligible in the American Nurses Association. A committee to discuss the situation and find a solution before this 1942 Convention closed was appointed and met. A delegate from each state below the line was present. The committee reported no solution to the problem had been decided upon and that they hoped to have something definite by the next convention in 1944.

[In 1947 the National Association of Colored Graduate Nurses met with the American Nurses Association to discuss merging. In 1948, A.N.A. inaugurated individual membership. In 1949, a panel of nurse leaders from the South met again. At the 1950 Convention of A.N.A. it was voted to have them become members. In 1951, the National Association of Colored Graduate Nurses dissolved its organization.]

The American Nurses' Association resolution was to go on record as follows: We will meet the need in this war completely unified to help any situation. The Nursing Council sent a telegram to the President of the United States asking for a four million dollar appropriation fund to carry on our war program.

The book, "The Doctors Mayo," was published about this time and there was mention of the early associations of the Mayos with Dr. A.J. Oschner. It was also mentioned that their pathologist, Dr. Wilson, worked out the method of sanctioning, staining and examining under the microscope fresh tissue while the patient was still on the operating table so it could be determined whether it was malignant or not, a method which became widely used in all first-rate hospitals.

Mrs. Louise Westerberg-Annen '39, Instructor, whose junior class in History of Nursing produced a puppet show, was congratulated on having assembled and arranged four miniature puppet stages showing the important periods in Florence Nightingale's life. In addition, this group had also prepared and given a play on the life of Florence Nightingale; a copy of the script was given as favors at the student luncheon. Adjacent to the puppet show exhibit was another set up by the preclinical class ('45), who dressed dolls representing the makers of nursing history from the time of Phoebe to and including Colonel Julia O. Flikke. This project was under the direction of Miss Hallie Amling '39, Instructor, as part of the History of Nursing class activities.

The Augustana Hospital School of Nursing Student Chorus sang two numbers on October 10th over station WLS—the program was called "Angels of Mercy." It was a regular home front program and the theme was on the service given by nurse's aides and nurses. Dr. Preston Bradley was the speaker and his topic was about Clara Barton and the Red Cross.

The American Red Cross sent out an urgent appeal for more nurses to volunteer to teach home nursing. Government statistics state that of the large number of men who failed to pass their physical for the draft, the largest percent were rejected because of cardiovascular disorders, nervous and mental, venereal and TB (in order of rejections). These failures were laid to the type of teaching done in the home, school and medical profession. In the home it was laid to neglect and ignorance, the school attempted to teach but the pupils did not learn, and the medical profession was not as active as it should have been in detecting and teaching.

When the office of Civilian Defense was created, the doctors in Chicago became very active in preparing to meet any emergency. Guided by the national organization, a definite program was arranged with competent officers in charge. They had organizations within institutions, public offices and gathering places and in the residential sections, each block had its own set of officers—block captains, etc. At the Augustana Hospital, Dr. Rudolph Oden was asked to serve as Chief of the Defense unit. There were two separate units each composed of several doctors, one of whom served as Captain, two nurses and one orderly. Each unit was equipped with an emergency supply kit with everything in duplicate as specified by the National Committee. In case of emergency and if our unit was called, they would go at once to the scene of the accident, render proper first aid to the injured and send the lesser casualties home and direct the Red Cross or ambulances to transport the more serious cases to the hospital where a casualty station with 30 cots was prepared to care for the victims. The entire hospital staff—personnel was then subject to call to help render such service as was necessary to care for the seriously injured. A list of graduate nurses who had signified their willingness to assist in this work had been supplied by Miss Haggman, Director of Nurses.

At a U.S. Public Health Meeting held in Rockford in October, the wartime measures were discussed regarding public health nursing in the state. Because of the critical shortage of Certified Public Health Nurses the case load on the individual was very heavy. In 1942, public health nursing was considered equivalent to service to the Armed Forces. Constant study was required by the public health nurse in order to teach the latest trends. Dr. David Slight, Professor of Psychiatry of the University of Chicago was a luncheon speaker and his topic was "Mental and Social Effects of War." He stated, "This, a total war, presents a picture of economic, psychological and social changes due to increased demands for action and service. Delinquency is already apparent. One can expect neuroses to come out of the vicissitudes of war service."

The League of Nursing Education luncheon brought out the shortage of nurses in civilian hospitals and suggested that:

1. Return all inactive nurses to active duty.
2. Increase enrollment in schools of nursing.
3. Accelerate nursing curricula.
4. Prepare more instructors.
5. Make more use of personnel.

The annual alumnae party was held at the Nurses' Home on December 15th. Students' voices blended in harmony as they opened the party with their carols and Miss Saenger led in saying a prayer of thanksgiving.

On December 22, the annual Christmas Smorgasbord was served at 5:00 p.m. for the Hospital family—students, internes and help. The dining hall was decorated with lovely Christmas trees and Mr. Erickson gave the thanks for the food. Included on the menu: brown beans, meat balls, "hard tack," "sylta," pickled herring. lut-fisk, rice pudding, with each person in the room hoping to find the almond in his or her dish. Dainty Christmas cookies, nuts and coffee completed the meal. The Northland Trio, wearing their Swedish costumes, sang in their usual fine manner.

The students' Christmas party was held in the Recreation Room of the Nurses' Residence on the 22nd also. The room was beautifully trimmed with paper Santas, greens and candles. All boutonnieres and favors as well as the decorations were made by the students. A pageant called "One Holy Night" under the direction of Miss Marguerite McNall was presented. Solos, trios and instrumental numbers were also presented and the party came to a close with the appearance of Santa Claus with gifts for all.

The Children's Memorial Hospital wrote to the members of the Alumnae Association telling them that they had many vacancies and encouraging nurses "who are interested in the nursing of children to make a start there now in order to advance to positions of more responsibility."

Letters began to come in from the girls in the Army Nurse Corps and Navy Nurse Corps thanking the Alumnae Association for the gifts of subscriptions to Reader's Digest and American Magazine.

A beautifully embroidered luncheon cloth was sent to the Nurses' Home by the nurses stationed in India. New membership cards were issued to Alumnae members which stated whether or not a member was entitled to hospitalization at a discount. It had previously been arranged with the Superintendent of the Hospital that nurses who had been members for at least three years or since graduation if the nurse was a new graduate, to be eligible for discount. Because the front office of the Hospital had no way of knowing who were or were not members, the membership cards were printed and discount cards given to those eligible for discount, and "courtesy" membership cards to the others. The card was white and the Augustana pin was printed in the center in a pale blue ink.

Over a long period of years capping had been a tradition in our schools of nursing throughout the country. To get one's cap was a symbol of acceptance to the school and it signified one was further entrusted with the duties and responsibilities of a nurse. Tuesday, March 16, 1943,—a class of forty young women were capped. The exercises were held in the lounge in the presence of parents, friends and hospital personnel. Speakers were Miss Haggman, Mr. Erickson and Rev. Christianson of Nebo Church.

First District, Illinois State Nurses Association offered six scholarships of $125.00 each. There were two for each branch of nursing—Public Health, Institutional and Private Duty.

A concert sponsored by the Lila Pickhardt Memorial Fund Committee was held on Sunday, April 4th, at the Ebenezer Lutheran Church. The Nurses Chorus under the direction of Mr. Harry T. Carlson, sang several groups of songs. Coffee was served in the Parish House following the concert. Tickets were sold for 55 cents each. Receipts were $407.00.

In the drive for 65,000 student nurses to fill the vacancies left by the graduate nurses leaving to serve with the Armed Forces, the Office of War Information had window displays in the different large State Street stores. Our Alumnae Association took the responsibility of "manning" a booth at Marshall Fields.

Miss Eula Butzerin, Chairman of the Local Committee of the Council for War Service issued an appeal to all nurses asking that "every nurse find a nurse"—meaning that we should all encourage our inactive nurse friends to come to the front to assist in any way they can during the emergency. At this time there were about 33,000 nurses serving with the Armed Forces.

A group of Nurses' Aides were taking preliminary courses at the Hospital under the supervision of Mrs. Levin, a Cook County graduate.

The Central Council for Nursing Education meeting was held at the Palmer House on April 19th and the meeting was devoted to Student Personnel Problems in War Time. She spoke on the ability of nurses to think accurately on problems. She said we should know a lot about ourselves before we should try to direct and judge others.

The summer of 1943 was a busy time—the students at the Nurses' Residence acquired a Persian cat as a pet. They called him "Bounce" because he jumped so much. In spring of 1944, he jumped over the fence and was run over by a car.

A capping service was held in the lounge on August 11th, at which time 27 students were given their caps. Pastor Christianson, Hospital Chaplain talked, as did Mr. E.I. Erickson who spoke on the Cadet Corps program in the school. A reception was held following the exercises for the friends and families of the students.

On Sunday, August 15th, a flag dedication was held for the block victory square in front of the Hospital. The Nurses Chorus sang a group of patriotic songs. The dedicatory address was given by Father Martin Lawrence of St. Michaels Catholic Church. Representatives of the American Legion, the block captains, and a Drum and Bugle Corps were present. A recording of the ceremony was made and a record was given to the Hospital. Because of the Cadet Nurse Corps, student nurse enrollment increased. On September 7th, 50 students entered the School of Nursing.

The following appeared in the Illinois Conference Messenger: "Mr. and Mrs. C.E. Balliett of Chicago have recently given Augustana Hospital the sum of $550.00 to establish a loan fund for deserving students. Loans are to be repaid after the student has finished nurses' training. The Committee on Nursing will act as trustee and pass on applications. Miss Balliett (Clarice Mae) died after an auto accident and the fund was to be called in her memory, the Clarice Mae Balliett Memorial Fund."

Some improvements were made in the Nurses Residence. Forty new double-deck beds were installed. Mrs. N.M. Percy presented to the School of Nursing bookplates for the library. The bookplate selection was made by a competitive effort on the part of the students with artistic leaning, the only specifications being that the school pin be incorporated in the design. An artist from Kroch's Book Store and Mrs. Percy selected one presented by Bernice Flom '44 who received a monetary prize for her efforts.

On November 30, word spread of the death of Mrs. Beda Munson Lundgren '01 after an illness of many months' duration. She was a charter member of the Alumnae Association, the first Augustana nurse to enroll in the American Red Cross and one of the founders of the "Augustana Nurse" and had helped to build and maintain the high standards and traditions of Augustana. In 1906 she was appointed chief surgical nurse. Her eagerness and enthusiasm for her work caused her to visit hospitals in Chicago and in the East learning new methods to improve her own technique and to enable her to teach students. She continued scrubbing in surgery for Dr. A. Oschner until 1912 when she married Dr. Albert Lundgren. Mrs. Lundgren was very active in the Hospital Auxiliary and in the Alumnae Association. She had been the Chairman of the Committee to furnish the lounge in 1925 and again was on the Committee in 1941 when the lounge was refurnished.

Notice came to us that after January 1, 1944, the Red Cross would not enroll nurses over 45 years of age, thus enabling them to concentrate their efforts on the nurses eligible for military service.

The class of 1918 presented a mirror for the corridor on the first floor of the Home. A beautiful colored portrait of Lila

Pickhardt was placed in the lounge. This was made possible by the presenting of cash donations by older graduates who knew Lila Pickhardt.

In response to numerous requests for information concerning the dues of the nurses who were serving in the Armed Forces, the following was published in the "Augustana Nurse":

Alumnae: Nurses who are in the Armed Forces are to pay dues. They will be carried as members for the duration but they are expected to pay-up when they return. They would not be required to pay a reinstatement fee.

First District—INA: No special ruling had been made but nurses were encouraged to maintain their membership.

ANA: felt that all nurses serving in the Armed Forces should consider themselves actively engaged in the practice of nursing and should pay full dues.

American Red Cross: The American Red Cross waived the rule that required all nurses joining the Armed Forces to be members of the American Nurses Association.

The Tribune carried pictures of Augustana nurses twice during one week. Three students' pictures appeared in the Inquiring Reporter's column and the following Sunday a picture appeared taken of a group of the nurses who had attended the Theatre of the Air performance which was dedicated to the Cadet Nurse Corps. After the broadcast portion of the program our student chorus of 75 voices sang several songs. Miss Victoria Carlsson '08, who held a Phd degree in Health was employed as Professor of Health at the Women's College of the University of North Carolina.

The January issue of the "EMBLEM," the magazine published by the Chicago Chapter of the American Red Cross carried a picture of Lt. Vera Gustafson '39 modeling the new trim olive drab uniform of the Army Nurse Corp.

Volunteer Nurses' Aides had been assigned to Augustana Hospital earlier in 1943 and had been a factor in maintaining nursing standards during the emergency. The graduate nurses greatly reduced in number had been able to carry on with the help of these trained volunteers who performed many of the routine duties under the direction of nurses. The Chicago

Chapter of the American Red Cross recruited and trained the women for service in civilian hospitals. The 85 hour course was divided into two units—the first 40 hours being spent in a classroom (lectures, demonstrations and practice) and the second half of the course was spent in hospital wards where the recruits under the direct supervision of the instructor had actual experience in caring for patients. The hospital also had difficulty securing interns and instead of the usual 10, they had only 4 in 1943.

On June 15, 1943, the Bolton Act was passed which formulated the U.S. Cadet Nurse Corps. It went into effect on July 1, 1943. The main purpose of the plan was to ensure ample nursing service for the duration. The potential student entered training with all expenses paid by the government. She was also supplied with an outdoor Cadet uniform and a monthly stipend. Students already enrolled could join the Cadet Corps and receive the stipend and uniforms. The student received $15.00 a month for the preclinical period. Then for the next 21 months she was paid $20.00 a month and for the last six months received not less than $30.00 monthly. The last 6 months the student could be sent to Federal, Military or other civilian hospitals, wherever her services were most needed. Their choice of service was indicated on the forms which they were required to fill out.

On March 1, 1944, we had 154 nurses enrolled under this plan at Augustana. Capping exercises were held in the lounge on March 14 at 2:30 p.m. for 41 students. Of this group, 35 were Cadets. A total of 226 students received their training through the Cadet Nurse Corps.

The second annual spring concert sponsored by the Lila Pickhardt Memorial Fund Committee was held on Sunday, April 16, 1944, at the Ebenezer Church. This concert was given every year to raise funds to be used in the maintaining and refurbishing of the Lounge in the Nurses Residence. On April 23, Baccalaureate services were held at Messiah Church with

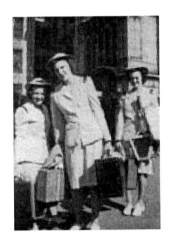

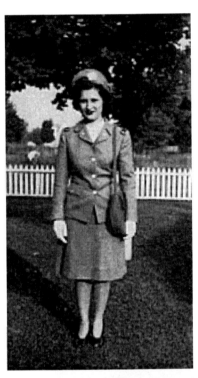

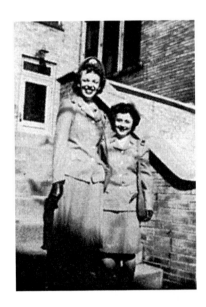

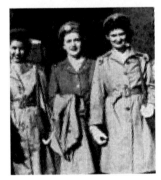

Cadet Nurses, Circa 1943

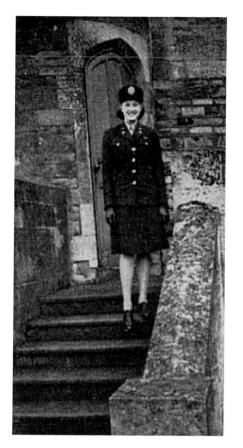

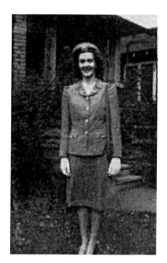

Cadet Nurse

U.S. Army Nurse

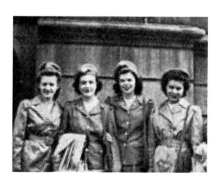

Cadet Nurse

Pastor Sjostrand giving the sermon. The graduation ceremonies were held at Bethlehem Lutheran Church located at 58th and Wells Street on the south side. Talks were given by Mr. E.I. Erickson, Dr. Percy, Mr. Jacobson and Rev. H.E. Sandstedt. Miss Mable Haggman assisted by Mrs. Thyra Lindstrand awarded the pins to the nurses. The Nurses Chorus sang and Mrs. Rudolph Oden offered vocal selections.

Miss Mary E. Falk ("Peg" Bleeker '32), Assistant Executive Secretary of the Illinois State Nurses Association was appointed special agent in Illinois for the Nurse Education Division of the U.S. Public Health Service. First District was offering four scholarships for the year to graduate nurses, two each for institutional and private duty.

On May 4, the Chicago Herald American carried a picture of four of our Cadet students taken in the pool at the Nurses Home. Those shown were Virginia Nyce, Harriet Johnson, Eloise Schmitz and Marjorie Huseby.

The following article appeared in the May 1944, issue of the "Augustana Nurse":

CADET NURSE CORPS

The members of the U.S. Cadet Nurse Corps gathered in the lounge of the Nurses Residence on Saturday, May 13, at 3:30 p.m., to join with Miss Haggman, Director of Nursing and Miss Marguerite McNall, Educational Director of the School, in the induction broadcast. This program was carried out on the air (NBC) with the following participating from Washington, D.C.: Congresswoman Bolton, Mrs. Eleanor Roosevelt, Helen Hayes, Lucille Petry, who was Division Director of Nurse Education of the Federal Security Agency, U.S. Public Health Service, and Surgeon General Thomas Parron, U.S. Public Health Service. Dr. Parron administered the Cadet Pledge.

Of the 144 Cadets, more than 100 were in the Lounge, which we thought was a very good showing in spite of many away on vacation and a few attending the special induction program at WMAQ Radio Station in the Merchandise Mart building. We were all much impressed with the content of the program and felt it a real privilege to be a part of this effort.

Monday, May 10, 1944, was another highlight as far as I was concerned, for it was on this day that I was privileged to model the U.S. Cadet Nurse Uniform for a group of 800 women having tea at Marshall Field's. This gathering was sponsored by the Woman's Symphony Orchestra of Chicago, to help raise funds in order to maintain the orchestra during the war.

The afternoon consisted of a style show and music by a group of musicians from the Woman's Symphony Orchestra. This was all very lovely. A light luncheon was served. During the intermission I was introduced by Mrs. Stanley, President of the Woman's Symphony Orchestra. I drew the stubs for prizes out of a hat box, making two women extremely happy and the other 798 a little bit disappointed. First prize was choice of any dress and hat from Field's 28 Room; second prize, a lovely white hat.

I was then given the opportunity to explain a little about the Cadet Corp—how, when and why it was organized, and the benefits and satisfaction one has from being a cadet nurse, knowing we are helping to serve our country.

After the intermission was over, the style show proceeded and my job was done. It made me very pleased and proud when several ladies came to me and said how attractive they think our cadet uniform is, and how thankful and proud we should be to know we are doing something as worthwhile as nursing is. I want to say here that all the nursing students of your and our Augustana Hospital truly are happy in this great work.

V.A.N.—A Cadet Nurse of 1946<br>(Virginia Nyce)

The cadet uniform was a medium gray suit with a straight skirt, worn with a white blouse. It had red epaulets and an insignia on the sleeve picturing a Maltese Cross, representing the beatitudes from the Sermon on the Mount, and the words "Cadet Nurse." The summer uniform was cotton as was the beret, and the winter uniform and hat were wool. Both had pewter buttons and were worn with dark hose and black shoes in the winter and white in the summer. A long winter coat, a raincoat and shoulder bag were also part of the uniform. When on duty, the cadet wore the regular student uniform for bedside nursing.

Following is a letter received in 1987, also from a '46 graduate:

I have always been very happy and proud to say that I graduated from Augustana. Even as recently as last Saturday I said, "I'd go back into training at Augie tomorrow if I could." Even while in training I felt that we were getting excellent training in that we were given valuable opportunities not only in actual nursing procedures but also responsibility. This was very evident when we affiliated at Children's Memorial; and when a procedure was ordered by a Dr., a student from another school responded that she didn't know how, and the Dr. said "Ask a girl from Augustana—she'll know."

I have often said that I never worked so hard in my life either before or after training, but it has certainly made a better person as a result.

Because money was always in short supply, I was thankful to be a member of the Nurses Cadet Corp.—if for no other reason than to ride the CTA free of charge; a reduction in the price of our train fare on the CNW allowing me to get home twice a year; and also to board the train with the Service Men to eliminate standing in line, especially at Christmas; and then to know that I'd have a seat on the train once I got on.

As student nurses we were able to purchase white nylons and would then dye them in order to have colored nylons for street wear.

I have to this day no desire to have frozen green peas for Sunday dinner since I had them 52 Sundays a year for about 3 years.

Miss Haggman certainly kept us all in line with her reminders both verbally and written. Fortunately I never did get sent back to the Residence before reporting on duty because my shoes and/or shoe laces weren't clean but know of girls that were.

She arrived early in Chapel each morning to mentally take roll as to who was not in attendance in Chapel, but would come to breakfast (15 minutes maximum) and report to the floor at 7 a.m.

Having to report to her office following a tour of night shift was always a "nerve wracking" experience. It seemed unnecessary in that she had the schedule on her desk, but it did afford her an opportunity to either praise or criticize us for something or everything. My most humiliating incident involved my reporting to her following a month of mid-nights on 5th floor (which for all of us was 12-7 a.m. 7 nights a week with the 1 hour off adding up to 7 hrs. which then was considered our day off for the week!!). She asked when was the last time I had seen the mantle clock on the marble top piece of furniture (similar to a dining room buffet) in Room #528. I didn't know that I was also being held responsible for the room and its furnishings in addition to the patient and his/her care. The clock had disappeared and later it was learned that Mrs. Lindstrand had had it sent out for repairs. Yet when it was returned safely, I got no apology from Miss Haggman.

In one of her sessions on etiquette and moral values, we were told to never sit on a boy's lap without first placing a telephone directory—"and I don't mean a small town directory—I mean the Chicago directory" on his lap.

It is and was only by the Grace of God that I can say I am a graduate nurse of Augustana. On one of my tours of mid-nights, my room-mates (I had 3 as we had a suite of rooms) and I decided to go on an all day boat cruise to Benton Harbor, Michigan. We waited for a day when 2 had the same day off and the third requested the day off. They signed out for late leaves in case we didn't return by 10:30 p.m. I couldn't sign out at all as my late leave would have meant 12 o'clock noon so I just left. Since I could not then appear in the office to sign in, I quickly took to the stairs while the 3 went into the office to sign in at 10:15 p.m. As I'm dashing up unnoticed by Miss Sanger, I met another student who informed me that one of her class-mates was expelled from training that day because she was not in the residence after 10:30 a.m. during a room check. I knew that my day was coming!!!! I did nothing but report for work at mid-night and back to my room as soon after 7 a.m. as I could so as not to encounter either Miss Haggman or Miss Sanger. You see—while out on the boat cruise, I got very sun burned and to explain it would be disastrous. I had 4–5 nights yet to work before having to report to Miss Haggman that my schedule of mid-nights was complete. I was then scheduled for my vacation. When she told me to enjoy my vacation and that she'd be eager for my return, I said "Thank you, Lord" as I happily walked out of her office.

Another episode in her office came following my room-mates and my return from a few days at home during Christmas. She'd been hesitant about allowing us to go home but finally agreed. On our return we went to her office to thank her and to let her know how grateful we were and also our families' appreciation to her had been, when she tells us in all sincerity—"And we got along very well without you!" Don't think that that didn't deflate our ego!!!! I can still see the snow flakes fluttering down as she said that. Then there was Miss Sanger. My room-mate, her sister (who was in the class ahead) and her room-mate and I decided that we all wanted to live together after our first year in a suite of rooms. We'd already checked out the rooms in the Residence and knew that 415–417 were vacant. We approached Miss Sanger who said that there weren't any adjoining rooms. When we informed her of 415 and 417, her reply was that those rooms were infested with bedbugs. We quickly replied, "Oh we don't care!!!!" To us that was very highly unlikely as surely the place would have been fumigated if there were bugs of any kind. We moved in and are nicely settled with our 4 beds (cots) and a dresser in 417; and 415 with a dresser, 2 desks, a cupboard (containing a 2 burner hot plate, pots, pans and dishes) and an easy chair that we'd purchased at a fire sale when Miss Sanger comes along and informs us that we cannot live like that because it's too difficult for the cleaning lady to clean. We kindly told her that we'd clean our own rooms. She agreed saying that the first time she found our rooms unkept and/or dirty, we'd have to break up our arrangement. I venture to say that we had the cleanest, neatest rooms at 427 W. Dickens as we were never reprimanded or told to break up house-keeping.

The best years of my life were my days in training—believe me. There was just one time that I was about to call it quits, but not having money for a train ticket home, I soon dismissed the thought and have been forever grateful. I've done various kinds of nursing since I finished training and have thoroughly enjoyed each kind, but can honestly say that my best days were spent doing bedside nursing as a student.

As always,
Ruth Martinson Potter '46

On June 11, the nurses who served in Unit number eleven of World War I held a reunion for the first time in 26 years. The party was held at the Nurses Home with the Augustana Nurses serving as hostesses. There were 17 nurses present and messages had been received from those unable to attend. Since the war, many of our girls had remained in Government service and the list included: Col. Flikke, Esther Julian who had served as chief nurse at Hines and at present was at Veterans Hospital at American Lake, Washington, Laura Erickson of the

Veterans Hospital of Augusta, Georgia, and Lillian Olson who served as First Aid Nurse at the Chicago Post Office.

The Alumnae Association was doing its share to purchase War and Government Bonds. In June the treasurer was authorized to withdraw $2,000.00 from the Scholarship Fund and $2,500.00 from the Sick Benefit Fund for the purchase of Government Bonds. Whenever the membership felt they could, they would move to purchase war bonds of smaller denominations—$25.00, $50.00 or $100.00.

About this time many promotions were coming through for our nurses serving with the armed forces and a map had been placed in the mail or office room of the Nurses Home with colored pins indicating spots where our nurses were stationed.

The following is an article from the Chicago Daily News:

> Two Chicago nurses, oblivious of a battle raging 200 yards away, today were calmly caring for the wounded Americans in a hospital on Leyte, according to an AP story.
>
> Rose Chapman of Mount Sinai and Olga Kmet ['39] of Augustana landed on the island yesterday with the first group of American nurses to return to the Philippines. Less than two hours after their ship arrived they went on duty in the wards of the hospital to relieve the exhausted corpsmen.
>
> Bitter fighting swept in and around the courtyard of the old Catholic church which serves as the hospital. But nothing stopped the women from giving the wounded men their first feminine care. Nor did the Filipinos fail to attend daily masss at the altar.
>
> The nurses were looking forward to being with the American forces when they rescued the 66 nurses captured at Bataan and Corregidor. Those women are now working in a concentration camp in Manila.[22]

On Sunday, October 29, 1944, Granger Westberg was installed as Chaplain of the hospital. The service was held at Messiah Lutheran Church. Rev. P.O. Bersell, President of the Augustana Synod and of the National Lutheran Council delivered the main address and Rev. Oscar Benson, President of the Illinois Council, assisted by clergy of the Hospital Board conducted the rites of installation. The Nurses Chorus sang

---

22. Chicago Daily News, November 2, 1944.

under the direction of Harry T. Carlson. Refreshments were served to about 400 persons in the Parish House.

The 43rd annual convention of the Illinois State Nurses Association was held at the Palmer House on November 9, 1944. The talks seemed to dwell on postwar nursing. Emphasis was laid on the group's responsibility to postwar planning. Naturally all speakers admitted that "specific plans" still remained vague, but that we must look to the nurses who will return as "changed" personalities. Miss Isabel Stewart of the Division of Nursing Education of Teachers College of New York City was the speaker at the Illinois State League of Nursing Education.

An appeal was received for 26 nurses to volunteer for duty at the Gardiner General Hospital, Chicago, and 42 for Vaughn Hospital, Hines, Illinois. The Office of Indian Service also had vacancies for nurses in the Indian reservations located in practically every state west of the Mississippi. The wounded were coming back in such numbers that a serious situation had been created in the hospitals, made worse by the lack of civilian nurses. Nurses volunteering to assist in the army hospitals made application directly to the hospital and those interested in serving in the Indian Service could apply directly to Civil Service in the new Post Office Building.

The Alumnae Christmas Party was held on Wednesday, December 13, with a program in the recreation room of the Nurses Home. Rev. Granger Westberg, Hospital Chaplain, read the Christmas story and the student octet sang several songs. The Drama Club presented a two act play called "The Bird's Christmas Carol." Many of the nurses serving with the armed forces sent messages and several were able to attend the party. Two tea tables had been set up in the lounge and refreshments were served following the program.

General Dwight Eisenhower was very much in the news and the Augustana nurses were thrilled to read of the baptism of Linda Elsa, daughter of Elsie Koski Stack '29 in Washington, D.C. with Mrs. Eisenhower serving as Godmother.

On February 6, 1945, a group of 52 students enrolled to pursue the course of nursing. In accordance with the latest request from the Red Cross Recruitment Office the entire 1944 graduating class had registered with the American Red Cross. A class of thirty-three were capped on April 4th. The capping exercises were held in the Lounge with Chaplain G. Westberg giving an appropriate talk to the class and relatives. Miss Haggman assisted by Mrs. Lindstrand placed the caps upon their heads.

April 1945, was designated by an Act of Congress as the Cancer Control Month. A group of students attended a clinic of the American Cancer Society held at Hines Hospital.

The following is a summary of a lecture given at another clinic sponsored by the Chicago Surgical Society.

### TOLL OF WOUNDS IN ABDOMEN CUT 50% BY SURGERY

#### Vaughn Hospital Medic Tells of Strides

Skilled surgery has resulted in a 50 percent mortality reduction from abdominal wounds in World War II as compared with World War I, Maj. George B. Sanders, assistant chief of medical service at the Vaughn General Hospital, told a clinic at the hospital yesterday.

Blood plasma and the new "miracle" drugs, penicillin and sulfa, were given secondary rating as "useful adjuncts" by Maj. Sanders.

Mortality in wounds of the colon, once 60 percent, has been reduced to 30 percent, it was brought out.

Members of the Chicago Surgical Society, who hold meetings in 10 different hospitals yearly, participated in the clinic.

#### Use of Colostomy Told

Colostomy—the surgical procedure associated with the repair of wounds of the bowel—has proved to be one of the most effective methods of treating abdominal wounds, he continued. While colostomy was known before World War II it was not utilized much, Maj. Sanders said, but since the war great strides have been made in its use.

The colostomy treatment, he explained, consists of making a temporary opening in the abdominal wall thru which contents of the colon are detoured temporarily to put the injured part at rest and to prevent peritonitis.

#### Cites Improvement Factors

Highly improved surgical skill in the Army Medical Corps, Maj. Sanders said, is the result of two factors: 1—Adaptation of the residential (hospital) system among civilian doctors for the last 20 years, which has produced highly trained surgeons. 2—Lessons learned in World War II as the result of careful observation, new technological advances in evacuating the wounded, well equipped and well staffed hospitals near the fronts, and intelligent use of such aids as penicillin, plasma, whole blood and sulfa drugs.

To illustrate some of the principles which were discussed several soldier patients were presented at the clinic. One of these was a Major of the Medical Corp, a Chicago resident, who was thrown from a jeep on the western front. The head and neck of his right hip joint were shattered and fragments were destroyed beyond repair.

This subject was discussed by Lt. Col. Thomas Horwitz, chief of the orthopedic section, who described the operation in which the fragments were removed and the ballsocket action restored with a vitalium (metal) cup. The doctor who suffered the injury five months ago, walked before the doctors with the aid of a cane and without pain.

### Treat 4,000 Since August

Of the 1,900 battle casualties now enrolled in Vaughn Hospital, 1,350 are on surgical treatment and 75 percent of them are orthopedic problems, Col. Horwitz said. Over 4,000 patients have been treated in the hospital since it was opened last August.

Dr. Lester Dragstedt, president of the society and professor of expert surgery at Chicago University, said the hospital has a fine staff and is performing marvelous service. He too credited the special surgical training of young men in hospitals as residence doctors for the advancement in surgical skills.

In 1945, the hospital made the last payment of the outstanding debt, described by Illinois Conference reports as "the most gratifying single event in the history of the hospital."

The debt was incurred when the depression brought an end to the expansion, the optimism, and the lofty plans launched in the 1920s. The East Wing, which brought such pride to the institution in 1926, proved to be a major concern in the 1930s, as it seemed almost impossible to redeem the bonds which had provided money for the East Wing construction.

The Illinois Conference records are a testimony to the hospital's search for survival:

"Bonds issued began to mature and the earnings were not sufficient to redeem them. The corporation answered by authorizing the board to inaugurate a campaign for $500,000 in the fall of 1930 (among Lutheran churches) but when the financial depression began to develop, it became evident that a general drive would not give the desired results. The board decided to issue a series of Junior bonds to redeem bonds that mature in the near future." (1930)

"The board surely regrets that for the first time it has to report a net loss. It has done everything in its power to prevent it." (1931)

"The emergency appeal (to Lutheran churches) has passed the $100,000 mark."
(1932)

"Efforts have been made to reduce the number of student nurses to the least possible number. The average number last year was 110 compared with 136 the previous year. A substantial saving in expenses has been made by this reduction."
(1932)

"Twice the employees have received a wage cut of 10 percent. Many employees have been dropped." (1932)

"The work of refinancing the debt has proceeded during the year, and we are glad to report it has been very near to a successful completion." (1935)


Augustana Hospital was saved, thanks to a sale of bonds, a fund raising campaign, cost-cutting measures and debt refinancing.

On April 29, graduation exercises were held at the Irving Park Lutheran Church with Dr. Joshua Oden officiating. Mr. Jacobson of the Hospital Board spoke and Dr. Carl Hedberg gave a short and friendly greeting from the medical staff. Chaplain Granger Westberg gave the address "Stability in Chaos" and the Nurses Chorus sang two groups of songs. Of the 56 nurses graduating, six were related to former Augustana graduates.

The Alumnae Banquet was held at the Swedish Club on May 5. There were 240 at the annual dinner and music was furnished by the student nurses. Greetings were read from nurses in the service. Augustana conferred an honorary membership on Augusta Johnson '05 for her 40 continuous years of membership. This marked the 50th graduating class from our School of Nursing. One member of the first class was present (of the six still living at that time)—Josephine Oberg Lofgren 1896.

[Mrs. Lofgren died at her home on June 14, 1946. She was the widow of north side physician, Dr. Carl A. Lofgren who died in 1936. Mrs. Lofgren was a native of Stockholm, Sweden and came to Chicago at the age of 16. She served as an army nurse at Matanzas, Cuba during the Spanish American War. Military services were held by Columbia Camp number Two, Spanish War Veterans.]

Our student chorus took part in a Hospital Day Program in

the John B. Murphy Hall of the American College of Surgeons Building in Chicago. A group of Augustana Student Nurses helped in the bond drive at the Bond Platform which had been erected at State and Madison Streets (between where Mandels was and Carsons). They rendered a program of patriotic songs. Appeals were being published by all the papers and the "Nurse" for more nurses to serve in civilian hospitals. It encouraged nurses to serve full or part time in the hospital nearest them. On February 23, 1945, the American flag was raised on Iwo Jima. On May 8, 1945, Germany surrendered (VE day) and on September 2, 1945, the Japanese surrendered (VJ day).

The "Angels of Mercy" were the Army and Navy nurses of World War II: a small force of 7,719 when war began in 1941, but by war's end, their numbers had increased to 44,802 in the Army and 8,896 in the Navy.

They were trained in their profession, but they had no shock- or battle-trauma medical training and little or no military training. They were issued combat uniforms in men's sizes and, in many areas, began their work with leftover WWI medical supplies.

Wherever there were American Troops, the nurses trailed within sight, sound and smell of the battle. They were at field hospitals and division-level clearing stations. They served on hospital ships, hospital trains and in evacuation and general hospitals. They flew on planes that sometimes carried cargo and combat troops one way and wounded on the return flight. Working hours were as long as the lines of the wounded on stretchers or operating-room tables.

Sixteen of the 201 Army nurses who died during the war were killed by enemy action. They fell at Anzio, in Belgium, and aboard the hospital ship "Comfort" in the Pacific. Named in their honor were five hospital ships, a camp in North Africa and one general hospital.

For the 29 nurses at the Pearl Harbor Navy hospital that day in December 1941, the glamour of Hawaiian duty ended with the first wave of Japanese planes. Within an hour, they had set up receiving stations that functioned "like a human conveyor belt" to classify the hundreds of casualties for additional treatment. Their efforts were, perhaps, the first application of the triage concept in medical care. In any event, the recovery room techniques the Army and Navy nurses developed would become a standard in post-surgical care.[23]

Before it was finally over, 57 nations fought in World War II. About 70 million people served in their country's military; 17 million of them were killed. At least another 20 million civilians—perhaps many millions more—died as a result of the fighting.

---

23. The American Legion Magazine, September 1995.

There were more than 8 million displaced persons in Europe alone when the hostilities ceased. Almost as many Japanese, Chinese and other Asians had to be repatriated. Hundreds of thousands of people were missing and never accounted for.

World War II confirmed the value of air power and high-tech military equipment. It also provided the impetus that split the atom and developed the nuclear bomb. The existence of the bomb—exceedingly more powerful and unimaginably more deadly now than when it was dropped on Hiroshima to end the war—may, ironically be humanity's best protection against World War III.

World War II not only left bereaved and dispersed families and ruined cities, it did damage to the human psyche that has not yet completely healed. Few people would have believed any human beings to be capable of the holocaust until inescapable proof was made public after the Nazis' defeat. And no one can understand modern Israel and the unresolvable tensions of the Middle East without a knowledge of the gas ovens.

World War II changed lives and nations and expectations and history more than any other similar time span ever. Never was there so much horror and death on the face of the Earth—or so much courage and effort aimed at stopping what was seen to be intolerable evil.[24]

The September "Augustana Nurse" records the honoring of Mrs. Julia Flikke by Wittenberg College, Springfield, Ohio. She was awarded a Doctor of Science degree at the Centennial Commencement at the college on June 12. The citation was given her with the words: "By reason of her notable service she fully deserves the high place of honor accorded her among American Women." Both Dr. Rees E. Tulloss, President of Wittenberg and Dr. Franklin Clark Fry, President of the United Lutheran Church of America were high in praise of Mrs. Flikke.[25] She also authored a book, "Nurses in Action," the story of the Army Nurse Corp.

The October issue of the "Augustana Nurse" carried an article from the Illinois Hospital Association on Miss Amelia Dahlgren '03. She had served as an administrative person in the medical field for 42 years—the last 30 being spent as superintendent of the Lutheran Hospital of Moline. She started

---

24. Chicago Tribune, August 3, 1989.
25. Copied from Luther Place Church Paper of Washington, D.C.

by serving as acting Superintendent of Nurses at the Blessing Hospital of Quincy, then maternity supervisor at Presbyterian Hospital of Chicago. Next she was Superintendent of Nurses of Englewood Hospital of Chicago and in 1916 went to Moline. She was recognized as one of the forward looking hospital administrators in Illinois. She had served the Illinois Hospital Association in various capacities. She became a member of the American College of Hospital Administrators in 1938. Besides being a member of the above-mentioned organization, she was also a member of the Illinois Hospital Association, American Protestant Hospital Association, American Nurses Association and the League of Nursing Education.

First District, Illinois State Nurses Association sent the following announcement concerning the fees of private duty nurses:

$8.00 for 8 hour duty.

$10.00 for two patient 8 hour duty.

$11.00 for 20 hour duty in homes and hotels.

For alcoholism, drug addiction, attempted suicide, manic depressive psychoses, violent mental patient in restraints, diphtheria, epidemic cerebrospinal meningitis, poliomyelitis (acute anterior), scarlet fever, TB and typhoid fever, the fee will be $9.00 for 8 hour duty.

Three delegates were sent to the one day meeting of the Illinois State Nurses Association held in Peoria on October 20, 1945. The House of Delegates without interrogation or debate unanimously approved the following recommendations:

The Illinois State Nurses Association authorize its Board of Directors:

1. To institute standards of personnel policies and practices for nurses.

2. To serve as sole representative for its membership in per sonnel policies and practices.

3. To act as a mediator when desirable in cases where differences occur with employers.

4. To increase dues of $2.00 to finance the various projects which were discussed at the meeting.

5. To set up a Committee on Professional Counseling and Placement Service whereby the nurses could obtain new positions without a placement fee.

An approval of these new practice acts required a favorable vote from 51 percent of the membership.

The National Nurses Association in Europe sent in a request to the American nurses to help in their clothing shortage. They asked for uniforms in good condition; caps which were washable, shoes in good condition; stockings with the size indicated; capes, clean, wearable and with hooks and eyes, watches in good repair, scissors, fountain pens and pencils. All articles were to be sent prepaid to the Chairman of the American Nurses Association Committee for Uniforms for Nurses in War Areas.

On the evening of December 12, about 200 graduates gathered at the Nurses Home to hold their Christmas party. A technicolor movie "It Came Upon the Midnight Clear" was projected on the screen and the group joined in singing the song. Rev. Granger Westberg read the Christmas story and led in prayer. The students presented the play, "Pop Reads the Christmas Carol." During the social hour, music was furnished by two student pianists.

On the 21st, the students had their Christmas party with the freshmen and preclinicals acting as hostesses. The play "Pop Reads the Christmas Carol" provided the entertainment along with piano and marimba music, vocal selections and carol singing. The party followed the sumptuous smorgasbord supper in the candlelit dining room of the Hospital.

On the 22nd, the Nurses Home had an "Open House." For two hours the building was buzzing with visitors—including many men who took advantage of the opportunity to visit "No Man's Land"—the rooms in the Nurses Residence. The rooms had been decorated and refreshments were offered in many of the rooms. At nine o'clock the play was given and enjoyed by all.

On Christmas Eve a carol service was held in the Hospital Chapel—at 2:00 p.m. and the chapel overflowed with patients and hospital family. The chapel had been decorated with pine boughs and candles.

The following morning Miss Haggman and a group of students arose at 5:00 a.m. and caroled at the hospital bringing joy to the patients. The Lounge of the Home was decorated with a fine tree, plants and greens. A scene of the Nativity had been made by two students and placed in the alcove of the fireplace.

In January, eight students sang before the women's group of the Chicago Rotary Club.

The Alumnae decided to furnish the Alumnae room and the front office of the Nurses' Home and to pay for it from the general treasury. All during the war the Alumnae meetings were opened by repeating in unison "The Pledge Of Allegiance" to the flag. The Alumnae Association was taking a month of each year to serve in the workroom of the hospital pulling gauze. This was under the wing of the Auxiliary but the nurses were doing their month and enjoying it.

The February meeting of the Alumnae had as its program a movie "Winter Carnival." The newly enrolled preclinical students were guests. A class of 24 had entered training on February 6th.

The students were taking orders for the year book which they were publishing. The price of $2.50. The students rented the film "Happy Landing" and showed it to students and graduates off duty to raise funds for the year book. In April, the seniors appealed to the Alumnae for financial aid on this project and were given $25.00. They then presented a skit entitled "The Follies" which was enjoyed by the members attending the Alumnae meeting.

Lt. Col. Oscar Nadeau of the Medical Corps of the U.S. Army was cited and received the Legion of Merit award. He organized the surgical service at Fletcher General Hospital in Cambridge, Ohio and served with distinction as its chief from

May 1943, to October 1945. He brought to this assignment broad surgical knowledge and experience, enthusiastic interest in his work and unselfish devotion to duty, inspiring those with whom he served to utmost endeavor. He personally performed many delicate operations on the severely wounded. He guided and instructed members of his staff with successful performances on the part of these officers. Col. Nadeau's professional capacity and administrative ability were evidenced by the efficiency and high standards with which the surgical section functioned even when peak numbers of the sick and wounded were hospitalized. From the date of activation to the cessation of hostilities, there were no surgical deaths recorded at this hospital, an achievement symbolizing the skill, resourcefulness and high level of care and treatment Col. Nadeau provided for the patients of Fletcher.

Dr. and Mrs. Percy presented the residents of the Nurses' Home with a fine ultra violet lamp. It was expected that it would bring much comfort and relief to many of the sufferers from head colds.

On April 7th, the Lila Pickhardt Memorial Fund Committee sponsored a benefit concert at the Trinity Parish House, 1034 Barry Avenue. The 80 voice student chorus sang under the direction of Mr. Harry Carlson. Mr. Robert Quick, concert-master of the WGN Philharmonic Orchestra accompanied the chorus and Mr. Ralph Niehaus, the tenor soloist.

Louise Bylander of the class of 1896 passed away at the home of her sister in Andover, Illinois on May 11, 1946. Miss Bylander was the first probationer to enter Augustana and graduated with the first class. After graduation she had worked as a private duty nurse, completed a course in Swedish massage and followed that profession until 1918. She then devoted her time to making a home for other Augustana nurses.

The Stolley-Anderson post of the American Legion had installation of officers at the Knickerbocker Hotel on May 5th with six officers of Post 1022 being put into office. The post was composed of nurses, physiotherapists and dieticians of

World War II. The post was named in honor of Donna Stolley, graduate of Cook County Hospital who died in Chicago while on terminal leave and Miss Helen B. Anderson '44, Augustana graduate who was killed in a plane crash on Okinawa on September 29, 1945.

Dr. Anders Frick died on May 9, 1946, at the Hospital after a long illness. He had come to Chicago in 1896 from Malmo, Sweden where he was born on January 12, 1868. He was graduated from the Karolinska Medikokirugiska of Stockholm in 1896. He started to practice shortly after coming to this country in a section of the north side of Chicago that was thickly populated with people of Swedish extraction. He served as assistant professor of clinical medicine at the University of Illinois College of Medicine; associate professor of medical therapeutics at the Rush Medical College from 1901 to 1905. He was a Fellow of the American College of Physicians, was made Knight of the Swedish Royal Order of the North Star by King Gustaf of Sweden; chairman of the medical advisory board number 38 during World War I; in 1913 attending physician at the Cook County Hospital; in 1903 appointed to be attending physician in the medical department of Augustana Hospital.

In 1925, Dr. Frick became chief of staff following the death of Dr. A.J. Oschsner and remained in this capacity until his retirement in 1938. At about this time he developed Parkinson's disease which progressed gradually and from which he died at the age of 78 years. He was a member of the Swedish Association of Physicians and belonged to the Swedish and Lake Shore Clubs of Chicago. Dr. Frick became a Fellow of the Institute of Medicine the year it was founded (1915) and became Emeritus in 1938. He was a member of the original committee on necropsies in the hospitals of Chicago and served as a member for ten years. During this time and as a result of the committee's efforts, the percentage of autopsies was definitely stepped up in the Chicago area.

Dr. Frick was a fine, upright, gentlemanly type of doctor of the older school. He was an excellent teacher and trained many young men in the general medical field. His death was a loss to his patients and to Augustana Hospital.

The annual Homecoming Tea was held at the Nurses' Residence on Saturday, May 25. Two hundred and twenty-five graduates came to renew old friendships. The railroad strike was on and many nurses who had planned to come by train had to cancel plans to attend. The banquet was held in the evening and 261 attended the affair which was held at the Swedish Club. For the first time the members of the Board of Directors and officers were all seated at the Speaker's table. Col. Julia O. Flikke who had retired from military service gave a short greeting to the members. Miss Haggman addressed the seniors and Miss Saenger gave a word of greeting. Miss Ida Ehman, Director of the School of Nursing from 1922 to 1927 gave a greeting. Miss Elsa Odman who had served in World War I greeted the World War II nurses. Life membership cards were presented this day to members who had maintained continuous membership for 40 years.

Miss Amy Chamberlain returned from California to take the position of Matron at the Nurses' Home held formerly by Miss Saenger.

Psychiatric affiliation with the Veterans Administration Hospital, Downey, Illinois, or Visiting Nurses Affiliation (8 weeks) was introduced into the curriculum, although the Visiting Nurse Association could handle only 12 students per year. [In 1948, the psychiatric affiliation of 12 weeks at Veterans Administration Hospital was incorporated into the curriculum for all Augustana students and was used continuously through 1969.]

Dr. Emmy Carlsson Evald, noted Lutheran woman leader died in New York on December 9. Funeral services were held at the Immanuel Lutheran Church in Chicago. Dr. Evald was among the nation's most notable woman leaders. It was she who nominated Susan B. Anthony to head the woman's suffrage movement which culminated in the constitutional amendment granting women the franchise and for this she was made a Dame in the Royal Order of Vasa by the King of Sweden in 1922. In 1927, Dr. Evald went to China for the dedication of the Emmy Evald High School founded in her honor. The degree of Doctor of Human Letters was conferred on her by Upsala College. She was an ardent worker in behalf of the Augustana Hospital and was a member of the Hospital Auxiliary.

The annual Christmas party was held at the Nurses' Residence on December 11, with approximately 200 guests. Rev. Granger Westberg, the Hospital Chaplain read the Christmas story and led in prayer. A sextet of students sang carols and a play "The Christmas That Bounced" was given by the student drama club. Following the program, the guests gathered in the lounge which had been decorated in the Holiday motif and refreshments were served.

Miss Martha Rorhbeck '15 passed away at the hospital on December 13, 1946. She served overseas in World War I and became supervisor in surgery at Augustana in September 1926, and held that position until she was hospitalized. She was a very active and faithful member of the Alumnae, having assisted in the writing of the first History Book and in serving on various committees. She was Past Commander of Jane Delano Post of American Legion #185 and members of the Post acted as pall bearers at her funeral. The Jane Delano Post through its Commander Cecilia Hillstrom '16 presented the Alumnae with a check for $25.00 in memory of Martha Rorhbeck. The Association purchased a clock which was placed over the door of the Lila Pickhardt Lounge.

The following resolutions were adopted by the Alumnae Association on the death of Martha Rorhbeck. They read in part: "be it resolved that a tribute be recorded to her excellent service as a nurse; to her service to her country in World War I; to her service as Surgical Supervisor; to her constant membership in the Alumnae Association . . . ." The Alumnae voted to place the name of Martha Rorhbeck on the In Memoriam Plaque in the lobby of the Hospital.

The Augustana Nurses Chorus rendered a Christmas program at the Concordia Lutheran Church on the 15th of December. The title of the program was "A Christmas Song Service and Pageant," written and directed by Marguerite McNall, Director of Nursing Education at the Hospital. Harry T. Carlson played the organ and directed the chorus. The narrators for the pageant were Rev. Granger Westberg and Miss Kvidahl. Visiting artists in the form of a quartette assisted in the program. An offering was received that was to be used toward the expense of building new offices for the Hospital Chaplains.

The president of the Senior Class appeared at the meeting and invited the Alumnae members to attend the Senior Follies Minstrel Show held at the Home on March 13, 1947. The funds collected were to be used to defray expenses incurred in publishing the annual, called the Augie Log.

At this time, First District and Augustana Hospital had the policy that all Augustana Nurses doing Private Duty Nursing must be a member of the Alumnae Association of the Augustana Hospital School of Nursing and a member of the First District Private Duty Registry.

The eight hour duty charge to the patient was $9.50. The patient was charged 50 cents for the nurse's meal. This made a total of $10.00 to the patient.

The Private Duty Nurses in First District of Illinois Nurses Association were privileged to charge more for their services after July 1, 1946, as follows:

$10.00 for 8 hour duty.
$12.00 for 12 hour duty.
$13.00 for 20 hour duty.

March 11, 1947, at 2:00 p.m., 37 preclinical students were capped in the Lounge of the Nurses' Residence. Miss Haggman introduced the members of the faculty. Dr. Joshua Oden addressed the group using two words as his text, "THINK AND

THANK." Mr. Erickson extended a word of greeting on behalf of the Hospital Staff. Following the ceremony, friends and relatives of the newly capped students enjoyed a social hour.

May 10th was the date of the annual Alumnae tea and banquet. 180 graduates and children attended the tea. The banquet was held in the Grand Ballroom of the Hamilton Hotel (Dearborn and Madison) at 7:30 p.m. The senior class of 1947 was honored and out of a class of 69, 59 attended. A total of 269 graduates attended the banquet.

The class of 1922 had collected funds from their class and presented to the Alumnae Association a life size reproduction bust of Florence Nightingale finished in oxidized bronze. The original was made by the late Sir John Steell, the eminent English sculptor in 1862 when Miss Nightingale was at the height of her career.

Mrs. Dag Anderson Olsen '22 was unable to attend the Banquet Reunion but she wrote a letter describing the experiences and hardships under the rule of the Japanese in Manchuria and later the Russian Communists. (Their school was closed when they would not bow to their god.) She remembered the quote of Dr. Lang when he gave their commencement address. Matt. 28:19 "I am with you always even unto the end of the world." She said that this Bible passage also sustained them. Matt. 5:41, "And whosoever shall compel thee to go one mile, go with him two." She wrote that in Denmark, the Nurses' Association was very active in foreign mission work.

The May 1947, issue carried some material on GI readjustment allowances. It dealt with allowances given those who served with the armed forces. The Illinois Unemployment Agency acted as agent for the Veteran's Administration. The G.I. Bill for education was managed under this agency.

Because many nurses went right into the U.S. Military Service before they could take State Board Exams at the scheduled time, the Illinois Nurse Practice Act was revised. Section 32 would provide Illinois Registration to those who had practiced professional nursing at least 2 years within the period preceding July 1, 1947; and had qualifications which would have enabled such a person at the time of graduation from a school of nursing approved by the Department of Registration and Education to take an exam. Application had to be made to the Department by July 1, 1948.

The following article appeared in the March issue of the Augie Nurse:

### PUBLIC HEALTH NURSE WEEK APRIL 11–17

Know Your Public Health Nurse Day was observed for the first time on January 26, 1945. By 1948, the Day has grown up and become a "Week," from April 11-17. Through radio, press, speakers, film strips, libraries, churches, posters and displays the work done by the public health nurses will be brought to the attention of the people during this week.

How many public health nurses do you know? How many jobs do they do? Public health nurses' activities are extremely varied because they had proved their value in many phases of community health protection.

This branch of the nursing profession is not crowded, however. It is estimated that at least 7,000 more public health nurses are needed immediately. Forty-two million hours of nursing service are given each year but still more are in demand.

In order to provide adequate living quarters for student and staff nurses, the Hospital had purchased the apartment building located at the northeast corner of Hudson and Dickens, directly opposite the Hospital. The building contained six 5-room and six 4-room apartments and with only slight remodeling accommodated from fifty to sixty very comfortably.

It was necessary to await the expiration of the leases of the present occupants at the end of 1948 before the building could be occupied by hospital personnel.

The Board of Directors had been keenly aware of the need for more space during those past several years. The residence had been filled to overflowing and the inconvenience of this arrangement could not continue indefinitely even though it was cheerfully accepted as a War Measure.

Plans for an addition to the hospital were also being prepared which would include a modern maternity division, a chapel, and the enlargement of various supporting departments. At that time, however, there was no definite assurance as to just when this project could be undertaken.

As the new students were admitted, psychometric pre-admission tests became a requirement for prospective students in addition to the other pre-admission tests.

In September, actress, Tallulah Bankhead, appearing in Noel Coward's comedy "Private Lives" was a medical patient at the Hospital, causing quite a flurry.

The committee on Revision of By-Laws had been meeting and presented at the December Alumnae Meeting a set of proposed revisions. The members could gain life membership in the association by the following two methods:

1. After 30 years of membership, a member could become a life member by the payment of fifteen dollars.

2. After 40 years of membership, the organization automatically confers life membership without the payment of fees. Following the business meeting, the Junior B Class of students presented "Thoughts at Christmastide" written by Miss Poole, instructor. The Christmas Story was read by students.

Amy Chamberlain '12 who had retired as the Director of the Nurses' Home was replaced by Agnes Carlson '24.

Augustana was in the news on New Years Day of 1948. The first baby to be born in Chicago for the new year was delivered at Augustana.

The Alumnae Association Membership Committee arranged a "Get Acquainted Tea" for the senior nurses on January 16. 37 seniors attended and were introduced to the Members of the Board of Directors and Membership Committee members.

The Committee on Program was allotted the sum of one hundred fifty dollars for the year. Previously the committee had arranged free programs. However, since the war, and with all performers being in demand it was deemed necessary to allot some money to the committee.

The Educational Scholarship Fund Committee had carefully studied the agreement between the Class of 1928 and the organization and presented the following suggestions to the members at the April meeting: The plan now used by the organization of offering two $50.00 scholarships from the general treasury be discontinued. That one scholarship be offered annually from the Scholarship Fund and that it should amount to $300.00. This scholarship was to be made available to any member of the Alumnae Association who was in good standing and who had not less than one year experience in nursing. The above was passed and for the first time since 1928 the Scholarship Fund was put into use. In May, the senior class presented the Alumnae $75.00 and the Class of '23 (25th anniversary) presented $110.00 to the scholarship fund.

Dr. and Mrs. Percy presented a radio complete with AM and FM and with a record changer to the Nurses' Home. The cabinet was of blond wood to match the furnishings of the lounge. The previous year, Mrs. Percy presented a beautiful oil painting which was hung over a desk in the lounge, and the Class of '21 donated a floor lamp.

The Student Nurses sponsored a May Day Formal at the Knickerbocker Hotel on May 1st. The price was $5.00 a couple.

Pastoral ministry to the sick, with the advantage of all modern resources of medical science and psychiatry, was the subject of a five-week course of study offered clergymen by Augustana Hospital. Chaplain Granger Westberg, assisted by a faculty of 153 conducted the seminar which began June 14. The faculty consisted of doctors, psychiatrists, special workers and clergymen. Special emphasis was placed on the psychosomatic approach in the treatment of the sick. There were three full-time chaplains at Augustana, together with a secretary-librarian. Reading material for patients was prescribed as part of the healing process. The seminar was said to be the only one of its kind to be conducted during the summer of 1948.

The American Nurses Association Biennial Convention was held at Chicago, Illinois, May 31-June 3, 1948.

The Chicago Lutheran Nurses invited all Lutheran nurses attending the ANA Biennial Convention to come to the Lutheran Deaconess Hospital Nurses' Residence, 2236-40 W. Haddon Avenue, for supper, at $1.25 a plate, which was served from 4:30 to 6 p.m. on Monday, May 31. Dr. S.M. Miller, former dean of Lutheran Bible Institute and who was Director of Immanuel Deaconess Institute, Omaha, spoke on: "Working Together With Christ In Nursing." At 6:00 p.m. the hostesses of the evening invited the entire group to go to the chapel to enjoy an hour of devotions, which had, in addition to inspirational messages from Lutheran leaders, information regarding the activities of the National Lutheran Nurses Guild.

The following was the address to the Graduating Class of 1948 by Dr. A.T. Lundgren, given on April 25 at Ebenezer Lutheran Church:

"Mr. Erickson, Miss Haggman and Associates, Class of 1948, and Friends:

We have gathered here today in salutation of your graduation from the School of Nursing and the Commencement of your life's profession.

I am not going to offer any admonitions concerning your professional duties which have been so adequately imparted to you during these past years, by your very efficient instructors in the practical and didactic work which you have now completed. You are now your own didacticians, ever mindful, however, of the instructions received at your Alma Mater.

In contrast, I shall attempt to bring before you briefly, a true picture of the present spiritual, economic, and political aspect of our present day dilemma; the solving of which we must look forward to direct leadership from you, the Youth of America and the coming generations.

We need leadership today, comparable to that of the Christian Martyrs who could enter the Arena with hymns and praise on their lips. Again, our own Martin Luther, struggling with the loyalties of his own convictions could utter those never to be forgotten words as he journeyed to the Diet at Worms. Would that we had had such devotion and leadership during the first post war assembly at San Francisco when we forfeited the Word of God to appease that individual who now seeks to destroy the very fundamentals of our existence.

We are looking to you, the future generations of America, for devoted loyalty, dedicating yourselves to this worthy cause. The spheres of action will vary according to your own inclinations and talents. But the ennobling effect of loyalty to your ideals will impart meaning and dignity to the lives of humblest mortals.

The consciousness of your now being members of that great profession of nursing, impels you not only to the liberation of human suffering, but to the furtherance of a clear vision toward the ideals acceptable to both God and Man.

During these troublesome days, when various ideologies are clamoring for allegiance, may you be ever steadfast to those teachings imparted to you during your formative years, and listen not to false ceremonial conventions. By keeping in mind the supremacy of ethical values over material gains, then can you be loyal to the ideals which give you true happiness.

And now, on behalf of the staff at the Augustana Hospital, I wish to express thanks and appreciation for your loyal and devoted cooperation, and may we in return bequeath the stars of the skies, the red roses by the wall, the bloom of the hawthorn, the sweet strains of music, and aught else your hearts desire.

We wish you God Speed."

[Dr. Albert T. Lundgren died January 23, 1949 at Augustana Hospital, where he was a staff member from 1910. He was a graduate of Rush Medical School, and was a member of the Chicago Crime Commission.]

The Homecoming Tea was held at the Nurses' Residence on the afternoon of May 22 with 220 guests registered. In the evening the banquet was held at the Edgewater Beach Hotel. 289 guests attended the affair.

The resignation of Miss Mabel E. Haggman, as Director of Nurses and Director of the School of Nursing, evoked a desire to express appreciation for the capable and inspiring leadership which she provided under rapidly changing economic conditions. She came to Augustana Hospital in 1927, and the responsibilities of her position called for a high order of understanding, initiative, and hard work, all of which she provided in full measure. Many of these years were difficult because of the depression, and later the war brought even greater but different problems.

Being ever mindful of the fact that the hospital was an institution of the Lutheran church dedicated to the ministry of mercy, Miss Haggman set a high example by word and deed for her associates and for the student body. Personal problems were confided to her as to a mother, and she gave endlessly of her time, wisdom, and experience in their solution. There were few, if any, who from time to time had been associated with the hospital as members of the Medical Staff, the graduates or student nurses, or other personnel who had not been benefited by her assistance and encouragement, particularly when unusual difficulties and trials arose.

As the future history of Augustana Hospital is recorded, the name of Mabel E. Haggman will stand out as one who for over two decades contributed greatly to its progress.

September 13, 1948, brought the news that Dr. John Christenson had passed away at the Hospital. He had been on the staff since 1911. He was born in Sweden and was 76 years of age at the time of death. Graduated from University of Illinois Medical School in 1905, he served as Health Commissioner in Manistee, Michigan until 1911. He was past president of the University of Illinois Alumnae Club, Scandinavian Medical Society of Chicago, Swedish Club of Chicago, Swedish Society Old Peoples Home and American Federation of Lutheran Brotherhoods, and was formerly President of the Board of Augustana College.

In the Fall, Sophie Robertson '25 attended the give-away radio program, "Ladies Be Seated," and was selected the Toni Girl (Toni permanents) of the Day. The prize was a beautiful diamond wrist watch.

The regular business meeting of the Alumnae Association was held on December 8th in the recreation room with the Christmas party following. The organization voted to send $5.00 to the Community Fund and to give the students $15.00 to the Student Government to defray expenses of "Open House" at Christmas. The offering for the sick nurses amounted to $121.10. Following the business meeting, children of Alumnae members presented a program of songs, dances and musical selections.

Martha Salemme (Blomgren '34) had a water color exhibition at the Van Diemen Galleries in New York and received many fine comments.

At the March Alumnae meeting it was voted to direct a communication to the President of the Illinois Conference of the

Augustana Church requesting that a Graduate Registered Nurse of the Augustana Alumnae Association be allowed to represent the group on the Board of Directors of the Augustana Hospital, with the understanding that the member selected was a member of a church of the Illinois Conference, Augustana Synod. This communication was acted upon favorably by the Synod Board and presented at the open meeting of the Synod held in Chicago in April. We were given the opportunity to send a nurse to the meetings (she was not given voting powers). Mrs. Mable Huntley '23 was elected to represent the group.

In the March 1949 Augie Nurse, Karen Shrader '31 placed the following article:

> The Post Office Department requests that we Zone all our mail, particularly the "Augustana Nurse," which is mailed on Permit. New addressograph plates must be made. I have zone numbers for Chicago nurses (Chicago Postal Zone Directory). Out of town nurses living in areas using Postal Zone numbers please send me this necessary information. To complete our records and to make Postal Directory service available, ALL married nurses please send me your husband's first name, and your telephone number. PLEASE DO IT NOW. Thank you. After March 1, the "Augustana Nurse" will be mailed to paid members only.

On April 14, the Lila Pickhardt Committee sponsored a rummage sale at 2318 North Lincoln Avenue. For weeks the store room in the Nurses' Home was the receiving room for boxes of clothing, knickknacks, etc. After the items were moved to the store, the police had to be called to restore peace and quiet after a group of merchants from Maxwell Street tried to walk off with most of the merchandise. The proceeds from the sale were $357.15.

The annual Homecoming Tea was held in the Lounge of the Nurses' Home on May 14 with approximately 280 nurses present. The Annual Dinner was held at the Edgewater Beach Hotel the same evening with Miss A. Elizabeth Galloway and the graduating class as guests. This was the last year that the seniors were invited as guests.

## START ANNEX TO AUGUSTANA HOSPITAL SOON

New Maternity Division to Accommodate 70

Construction will begin soon on the long planned addition to Augustana Hospital, Dickens Ave. and Sedgwick St., it was announced recently by E.I. Erickson, hospital superintendent.

The new building will cost 1 million dollars and will adjoin and harmonize in architectural style with the present buildings. The new structure will consist of a basement and three stories but will be constructed in such a way that other stories can be added. Mr. Erickson said officials hope to raise the structure to eight stories eventually.

Reinforced concrete, brick and stone will be used in the structure. Architects are Schmidt, Garden and Erickson. Hospital consultant for the project is Dr. Herman Smith.

### Increase Maternity Care

Supt. Erickson said plans to meet the increasing needs for patient care include a modern maternity division with accommodations for 70 patients. There will be three labor rooms, three delivery rooms and six nurseries.

A combination chapel and auditorium will seat 300 and will be used for school purposes as well as for general and religious meetings. Sliding doors will separate the room's chapel area from the seating area.

Two new nurses classrooms will be included, bringing hospital classrooms to eight.

An entrance unit will contain admitting offices, out-patient department, increased space for nursing, X-ray, and physiotherapy departments, a library and administrative offices. The building will be heated by the present central heating plant.

### Active in Program

The new building was planned at the time the present structure was erected in 1925.

Officers of the hospital board are E.R. Jacobson, president, the Rev. O.V. Anderson, vice president, E.G. Erickson, secretary, and M.N. Ranseen, treasurer.

The building committee consists of E.G. Erickson, chairman, E.R. Jacobson, Carl Bergendoff, W.A. Goranson, Dr. N.M. Percy, Dr. Rudolph Oden, the Rev. O.V. Anderson, the Rev. J.H. Olson, the Rev. H.W. Linden, the Rev. C.O. Bengtson, the Rev. G.E. Westberg and Supt. Erickson.

The hospital is an institution of the Augustana Evangelical Lutheran church. Hospital service was first provided by it in 1884 in a remodeled residence at Cleveland and Lincoln Aves. This original building was replaced in 1893.

In 1916 the institution acquired its present location which for many years had been the site of a brewery. The seven story nurses residence was completed in 1922 and a few years later the present eight story patient pavilion which contains facilities for 275 patients, was constructed.

When the new building is completed next year and some renovations made in the present structures the hospital will be able to care for about 350 patients, officials said.[26]

At this time the new rates from the First District for the Private Duty Section were put into effect:
$12.50 - 8 hour duty with one patient
$14.50 - 8 hour duty with 2 patients
$14.50 - 12 hour service with one patient
$15.50 - 20 hour duty
$13.50 - 8 hour duty for special group

In September we received an interesting letter from one of our graduates. Doris Bruce '46 who was serving as a medical missionary in Assam, India, arrived at Shillong on May 2 with 3 other missionaries for language study. The trip of 150 miles was made in one day by Jeep. She stated that mountain roads were very poor in places and accommodated only one-way traffic. The girls were taking room and board in an Anglo-Indian home. They had electricity which seemed like a real luxury after the kerosene lamps and candles used at the compound. Miss Bruce found the study of the language very fascinating. She had 3 hours of class each day with a teacher, and many more hours of study. In addition to the work of ministering to patients' physical needs (including lepers) it had been her privilege to help with the services of the colony. She played the folding organ, or marimba, and assisted in teaching hymns which had been translated from Bengali or Hindu. The Messages were often given by Flannelgraph illustration. Miss Bruce joined the Assam Nurses Association and was making arrangements to join the India Association. There was to be a law in India that no nurse could attend deliveries without a midwife certificate, so she was arranging to take the midwifery course as soon as possible.

"New Horizons in Nursing" was the topic of the 48th An

---

26. Chicago Tribune, May 26, 1949.

nual Convention. A summary of reports of delegates to the ISNA Convention at Peoria, October 5–8, 1949, follows:

### PRIVATE DUTY SECTION

Membership in the section seems to remain about the same with no district having a sufficient number of private duty nurses to fill the calls. The District Chairmen stress the need for more educational programs. A plea was made to directors of nursing service to help curtail this practice of working more than one shift in the 24-hour period. Some districts had non-professional registries. Projects and aims ran from putting Personnel Policies into practice, to Institutes, Educational Meetings, increasing membership, influencing non-professional registries to become professional registries, to better program planning, to review of professional ethics to assisting with the national reciprocity movement, to solving the Practical Nurse Problem, to better security for nurses and more educational opportunity. There was general voicing of the public's inability to distinguish between R.N. and P.N. There is a need for educating the public of the difference and rates. As of October 1, 1949, there is a total of 3,413 nurses engaged in the private duty field.

A State Practical Nurses Committee organization has been formed called the S.P.N.C. A motion was made and seconded that a recommendation be made to have a Private Duty Section Council Nurse represented on S.P.N.C.

There was some discussion on the subject of Malpractice Insurance. This is protection for about $10 a year for the self-employed. Metropolitan Life Insurance or Mutual may be referred to in this regard.

Dr. David B. Owen, President of Bradley University, Peoria, lectured on "What is Expected of Nurses and Nursing by General Education?" at a luncheon meeting given by the Public Health and Private Duty Sections combined.

He said: "General Education is similar to liberal education to prepare to lead a richer life and to become a more worthwhile citizen. Liberal Education is pursued as an end in itself (for mere satisfaction). General education might expect of nurses and nursing education the following:

1. Be a good practitioner in the field.
2. Be a well adjusted human being.
3. Good knowledge of science of human relations.
4. Reasonably sound orientation of civilization.
5. Sense of Balance.

(Tolerance here, remembering that when ill the patient is a person out of balance)."

—Ethel Jensen '47

### INDUSTRIAL SECTION

It was resolved that the Illinois State Nurses Association would not endorse socialized medicine. A motion was made, seconded and carried that a copy of this resolution be sent to the Federal Representatives and Senators from the State of Illinois.

It was reported that the Industrial Section now has a membership of 519 members in Illinois.

"Employment Standards for Nurses in Industry" has been revised by the Industrial Nurses section this year and has been approved and printed by the Illinois State Nurses Association. The revised edition is much simpler than the original and copies of this edition have been sent to each member and to management of each industry.

Dr. Harold Vonachen, Med. Director of the Caterpillar Tractor Company of Peoria, addressed the session on "The Nurse and Human Relations in Industry."

He pointed out that Industrial Medicine was recognized by the A.M.A. in Atlantic City. That 25 years ago Industrial Medicine was still in its infancy.

Dr. Vonachen mentioned that the emotional status of an employee was just as important as his physical status. That this factor has become much more noticeable since World War II.

—Dorothy Herbert '40

INSTITUTIONAL SECTION

"Policies for a Better Understanding of the Student Nurse" were summarized from questionnaires sent to students. It can be gratifying to the profession that the students did not ask for anything radical, but wanted education based on sound and democratic principles, an interest in their health and welfare, a professional attitude from the graduates, and counseling which would not be mere reprimanding, but a guide to maturity and good adjustment.

Dr. Seay, Dean of the University of Kentucky, and a representative of the Kellogg Foundation, gave six excellent principles as guides in planning for future education:

1. Have a knowledge of the world and its resources.

2. Consider leadership in the recognized plan for democracy. Rule out the *don't* because it is prohibitive. Emphasize the *do* to bring about participation, collaboration, and free use of abilities. Good leadership finds ways to keep people free to participate and it instills confidence.

3. Give more emphasis to general education. A specialty needs a firm foundation.

4. Use all facts as to supply and demand.

5. In-service Education is a necessity. It is impossible to complete one's education today for life tomorrow.

6. Service will be the reward you will most prize for "He profits most who serves the best." Dr. Seay concluded his remarks with the well known biblical verse: Acts 20:35. "It is more blessed to give than to receive."

The entire convention was stimulating and educational and I am sincerely grateful for being privileged to act as delegate for the Alumnae Association.

—Bertha E. Klauser '34

PUBLIC HEALTH SECTION

The Education Committee planned a program for an institute on the relationship between the public and the public health nurse.

The School Nursing Committee presented a report on vision screening and hearing screening with recommendation that the report be made public, and a training program be held for both teachers and nurses for hearing and vision screening.

The Legislative Committee gave a report on certification. A survey was made on the attitude of various states on certification. Non-certified states were asked why they did not have it. The certified states were asked questions on the qualifications required for certification and what they felt were the weaknesses of the bills. The recommendations of the committee were to:

1. Repeal the law.

2. Arrive at some plan where certifications could be issued without examinations.

3. Change the law.

The committee further stated by way of clarification that certification is mandatory in Illinois for all tax-supported agencies and non-mandatory for any voluntary or private agency.

In the past few years we have been taking a critical look at ourselves as nurses and at the field of nursing, itself.

—Ruth Buntrock '46

The first District announced a change. The dues for 1950 were to be $17.00 for the district plus $3.00 for Alumnae. It was no longer necessary to be a member of the Alumnae Association to be a First District Member.

At the October Alumnae Meeting, members of the senior class sold Christmas cards and fancy wrapping. Miss Galloway resigned as Director of Nurses and Miss Maud Doherty, the new Director of Nurses was our guest along with Miss Olga Solberg, Instructor. Dr. Joshua Oden (Pastor) reviewed the book "Kinfolk" by Pearl Buck. The Alumnae presented him with a copy of the book "Stalin."

On December 14 at 2:00 p.m. the ceremony of the laying of the cornerstone of the new annex to the Hospital was celebrated. Dr. C.O. Bengston, President of the Illinois Conference of the Evangelical Lutheran Church was in attendance. Mr. E.R. Jacobson who was president of the Hospital Board presided. Chaplain Granger Westberg led the responses, the Student Nurses Chorus sang, and Chaplain E.T. Anderson gave the Benediction. About 70 additional beds and facilities for additional Diagnostic Procedures were added. The building was completed in 1951.

A most enjoyable Christmas play, "Thoughts at Christmastide," was presented by the student nurses for the Alumnae Christmas party, held on December 14 in the Recreation Room of the Nurses' Residence. The play was written by Francis Poole, and the play chairman was Joan Kirk.

# CHAPTER III

## THE FIFTIES

Alumnae dues payable to January 31, 1950 were $3.00 and meetings were held in the lounge at the Nurses' Residence. The February meeting of the Alumnae Association, however, was held in the Recreation Room of the Nurses' Residence because students of the class of 1951 presented a comedy skit, "Augie Potpourri." The President thanked the class for its program and gave them a donation of $10.00.

The Korean War erupted on June 25, 1950, when the North Korean Army, organized, trained and equipped by the Soviet Union, invaded the Republic of South Korea. China also fought on the side of North Korea. Three days later, President Harry S. Truman ordered U.S. forces to defend South Korea.

Encouraged by the prompt action of the United States, the United Nations condemned the act of aggression. For the first time in its history, the U.N. created a United Nations Command, with the U.S. acting as its executive agent, to repel the attack of North Korea from Communist domination. General Douglas MacArthur was named commander in chief of the United Nations forces. In addition to the United States and South Korea, twenty other nations provided military contingents which served under the United Nations banner. Forty-one countries sent military equipment or food and other supplies. The U.N. sent more than 90% of troops, military equipment and supplies.

The fighting raged on for more than three years, as the U.N. forces drove the North Koreans from the Republic of Korea,

185

then stemmed the tide of the Chinese Communist Army attacks.

The active hostilities ended on July 27, 1953 when the U.N. and North Korea signed an Armistice agreement. A permanent peace treaty between the two was never signed, however, U.S. military forces remained in South Korea to discourage resumption of hostilities between the two parts of Korea. About 1,000,000 South Korean civilians were killed and several million made homeless. About 580,000 U.N. and South Korean troops were killed or wounded or were reported missing.[27]

Following are remarks by Secretary of Defense, Frank C. Carlucci on July 27, 1988.

"Today is not too late to counter history's slight of this war and its veterans. The Korean War was the first real test of America's pledge to contain Communism. We met that test, in spite of the remoteness of the challenge and the burden it entailed...

For America, the human legacy of the Korean War is the sterling performance of her uniformed sons and daughters who, uncomplaining, took up arms to defend a nation they never knew and a people they never met...

In a land so remote from America and America's consciousness, heroes came to the fore and the inner strength of our troops showed through. They fought brilliantly and tirelessly and enabled our Nation to achieve its aim, and to prove to ourselves and the world that America comes to the aid of its friends, defends its principles, and never retreats from freedom's fight."

Thirty-two students, class of September, 1952, received their caps in a very impressive Capping Ceremony held at the Grace Lutheran Church on Monday evening, March 13, 1950. The processional was awe-inspiring as each girl, with her big sister, entered the auditorium as Harry T. Carlson officiated at the organ. The Nurses' Chorus made its second appearance of the year under the direction of Mr. Carlson. The selections sung by the chorus were: "Praise We Sing to Thee" by Haydn, "Jesu, Priceless Treasure" by Bach, "The Nightingale" by Tschaikowski and "The Nation's Prayer" by Franck.

---

27. Excerpts taken from the World Book Encyclopedia, 1993 Edition

After receiving their caps from their big sisters, the newly capped students repeated "The Nightingale Pledge." The unlighted lamps held by the girls were lit from the lighted lamps held by the older students and in unison they joined in singing the hymn, "Blest Be The Tie That Binds," depicting a beautiful picture of faith and steadfastness in striving for the goal of the nursing profession, realizing probably for the first time that although they had reached the first milestone of their career, they had only begun their work. The ceremony concluded with the benediction which was pronounced by Rev. Arthur L. Mahr, pastor of Grace Church.

The April Alumnae Rummage Sale held in the Nurses' Residence realized receipts of $218.26, benefitting the Lila Pickhardt Memorial Fund. The Alumnae Association unanimously voted to donate $1000 for a stained glass window in the new Chapel as a memorial to the nurses. (The window is now in the Lutheran General Hospital chapel and was dedicated in a special service 12/19/91.)

The 55th annual graduation exercises were held at the Irving Park Lutheran Church, Sunday, April 23, 1950. The invocation was given by Rev. Granger Westberg, Chaplain. The Augustana Student Nurses Chorus sang several choral selections, and greetings were given by the Board of Directors and the Medical Staff. The address was delivered by Rev. Joshua Oden, D.D. Miss Maud Doherty, Director of Nurses led the Florence Nightingale Pledge, followed by the presentation of diplomas and the school pins. The benediction was pronounced by Rev. E. E. T. Anderson, Associate Chaplain.

The Alumnae banquet was held at the Edgewater Beach Hotel on April 22 at 7:30 p.m. with 250 in attendance. This was held following the afternoon tea held at the Nurses' Residence from two to five p.m. where 276 were present. Tickets were $4.50 for members and $5.50 for non-members. The class of '25 gave a liberal check at the banquet for completion of the silver service.

Our delegates to the 37th American Nurses Association Biennial Convention (May 7 to 12, 1950, San Francisco, California) presented excellent and comprehensive reports of the convention at the June meeting. A resume of the house of delegates business meetings follows:

The American Nurses' Association, largest organization of registered nurses in the nation, with 171,000 members, blazed trails into new territory at its 16th biennial convention. For the first time in history, it voted to admit inactive nurses as associate members, and adopted a code of professional ethics for nurses. It aligned itself in favor of merging the six national nursing organizations into two, to meet the nation's nursing needs; one a strictly professional association, the other, joining nurses and lay people. Delegates instructed ANA officers to take steps to provide personal liability (malpractice) insurance for nurses on a nationwide basis.

A 5-year series of studies of the nursing function was decreed by the 1,500 delegates who indicated their willingness to meet financial assessments to pay for the studies.

A request by the American Medical Association for adoption of a resolution condemning compulsory health insurance was tabled by the convention. Nurses indicated a desire to remain free to provide nursing service in any plan the American people adopt.

Other action included ordering final liquidation of a nurses' relief fund established in the early days of the Association which was founded in 1896; directing discontinuance of studies of the so-called Lenox Hill Retirement Plan but continuance of studies of other plans; adopting a "platform" to guide the nursing profession during the coming two years.

After twenty-five years of preparation, the following code for professional nurses was adopted:

1. The fundamental responsibility of the nurse is to conserve life and promote health.
2. The professional nurse must not only be adequately prepared to practice,

but can maintain professional status only by continued reading, study, observation, and investigation.

3. When a patient requires continuous nursing service, the nurse must remain with the patient until assured that adequate relief is available.

4. The religious beliefs of a patient must be respected.

5. Professional nurses hold in confidence all personal information entrusted to them.

6. A nurse recommends or gives medical treatment without medical orders only in emergencies and reports such action to a physician at the earliest possible moment.

7. The nurse is obligated to carry out the physician's orders intelligently, to avoid misunderstanding or inaccuracies by verifying orders and to refuse to participate in unethical practices.

8. The nurse sustains confidence in the physician and other members of the health team; incompetency or unethical conduct of associates in the health professions should be exposed, but only to the proper authority.

9. The nurse has an obligation and in return is entitled to just remuneration for services rendered.

10. A nurse accepts only such compensation as the contract, actual or implied, provides. A professional worker does not accept tips or bribes.

11. Professional nurses do not permit their names to be used in connection with testimonials in the advertisement of products.

12. The Golden Rule should guide the nurse in relationships with members of other professions and with nursing associates.

13. The nurse in private life adheres to standards of personal ethics which reflect credit upon the profession.

14. In personal conduct, nurses should not knowingly disregard the accepted patterns of behavior of the community in which they live and work.

15. The nurse as a citizen understands and upholds the laws and as a professional worker is especially concerned with those laws which affect the practice of medicine and nursing.

16. A nurse should participate and share responsibility with other citizens and health professions in promoting efforts to meet the health needs of the public—local, state, national and international.

17. A nurse recognizes and performs the duties of citizenship, such as voting and holding office when eligible; these duties include an appreciation of the social, economic and political factors which develop a desirable pattern of living together in a community.

On Monday, October 9, at 3:30 p.m., on WGN-TV, the public saw and heard the actual procedure in preparing a patient for surgery. Dr. John C. Scully, Dr. Bernard Patrick, members of the surgical staff of Augustana Hospital took part in the demonstration. Ruth Schroeder '41, Jean Olson '48,

Edith Goplin '48, Nelle Vincent, anesthetist and Mildred Wickman '38 participated in preparing the surgical patient. Jean Olson acted as the patient. The "Health Talk" was presented each week by the Educational Committee of the Illinois State Medical Society, in cooperation with WGN-TV.

The Augustana Alumnae Association had a complete revision of By-Laws, deleting the words First District and State Association wherever it appeared. The only reference was that in Article 4 it stated: The President and Vice-President shall be members of First District, Illinois State Nurses' Association. This was due to the fact that at the ISNA meeting in 1949 it had been voted that it would no longer be necessary for members of the ISNA to be members of their Alumnae Associations. Up to this time, the Alumnae Associations in the state had collected the dues for all the nursing organizations. However, now a nurse could go to the district or state and pay dues, work in any hospital without belonging to the Alumnae Associations.

A new American Nurses Committee for Illinois was announced. It was the State Committee on Nursing Resources to meet Civil and Military Nursing Needs to assure maximum preparedness of the nursing profession. Madeline McConnell, Director of Nurses of St. Lukes Hospital, Chicago, was Committee Chairman and Esther H. Nelson '28 served as secretary. Mrs. Nelson had served as Executive Secretary for the Procurement and Assignment Service of the War Manpower Commission for Illinois during World War II.

The Christmas Alumnae meeting was well attended. The program was: An original dramatic presentation "His Birthday" presented by Everett Clark, narrator. Mr. Clark did the speaking parts on the Theatre of the Air productions of WGN on Saturday evenings. He was accompanied by a vocal soloist and pianist. It included singing of hymns by the audience. Dr. and Mrs. Beilin presented a television set for the lounge for the use of the students.

A beautiful and impressive service, held in the new Chapel

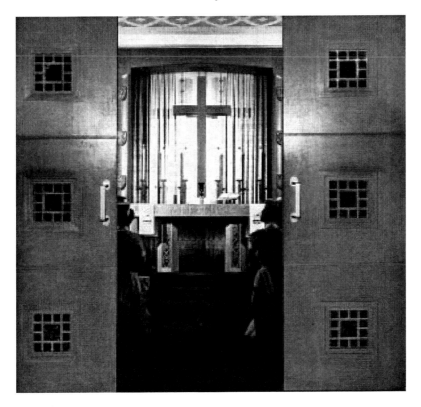

Chapel of the Good Samaritan

for the first time, marked the solemnity of the Capping and Candle-lighting for forty-five nurses, March 1, 1951. Officiating at the service were Chaplain Granger Westberg, Associate Chaplain Sandstedt, and Miss Maud Doherty. The chorus was directed by Mr. Harry T. Carlson. The caps and the lights with which to carry on the lighted lamps were received from the "Big Sister" nurses.

The following information was printed on the back of the program.

## THE CHAPEL OF ST. JOHN — LARGE CHAPEL

Named for the Lutheran Hospital Order of St. John founded in 1852.

Seven pillars on each side—three for Trinity—four for the four corners of the world.

Eight windows in the doors—symbolize Regeneration—eight saved in Noah's Ark in the flood.

Each window has a quotation from the Gospel of St. John.

Altar Rail—symbol of the Fruitful Vine—Isaiah 5:1, John 15:1, Jeremiah 2:21.

Three steps to the Altar—the Trinity.

Reredos—around and behind the Altar—symbols of the four Evangelists—"Gloria in Excelsis Deo"—"Glory to God in the Highest."

The Altar—hand carved of Korino wood from the Belgian Congo in Africa.

The Candles—Christ the Light of the World.

The Cross—The center of our Faith and Message.

## CHAPEL OF THE GOOD SAMARITAN

*(Always open for Meditation, Prayer and Waiting)*

WEST WINDOW—The Good Samaritan.
    —The Healing Ministry of Christ fo the man born blind.

CENTER WINDOW:

*West Panel top*—The Hand of God and the Triangle of Trinity
    Father, Son and Holy Spirit.

*2nd from top* —The dove of the Holy Spirit with its gift of "PAX"—Peace.

*3rd from top* —The Nurses' Capping Service.

*4th from top* —The shield of faith.

*East Panel top* —Eminating from Cross—Red Cross organized in Geneva, Switzerland in 1862 and the National Tuberculosis Association.

*2nd from top* —The Old Testament scroll with the Hebrew "Jehovah,, inscribed, the New Testament with the Maltese Cross on a red cover, and the candle representing Christ in the light of whose life they gain meaning.

*3rd from top* —Christ commissioning the graduate nurse to serve in His name.

*4th from top* —The Healing Power of the Cross.

EAST WINDOW—Light from the Hand of God guiding the work of the surgeon in the operating room.
    —The Nurse assisting the Chaplain in administering Holy Communion.

———

The Pastor faces the *Congregation* as an ambassador of God; he bids to worship, reads the Scripture, pronounces absolution and preaches from the Word of God.

The Pastor faces the *Altar* as he joins with the Congregation in Confession, Prayer and Praise.

———

If out of gratitude to God you wish to leave an offering, receptacles are placed by the doors for your convenience.

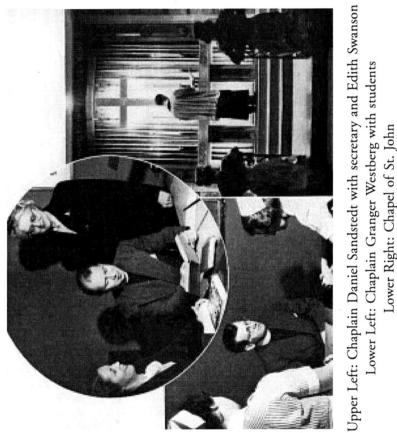

Upper Left: Chaplain Daniel Sandstedt with secretary and Edith Swanson
Lower Left: Chaplain Granger Westberg with students
Lower Right: Chapel of St. John

At the April '51 Alumnae meeting, Mrs. Nelson gave a report on the mass of data collected for the next history book covering 1938 through 1950. The Class of 1951 was honored at this meeting. Each Graduating Senior was presented with a beautifully wrapped Augustana History book together with an orchid as a gift from the organization.

Dr. Alton Ochsner, who was the guest speaker at the Illinois Divisions "Kick-Off" Luncheon on April 3rd, was the former National President of the American Cancer Society, Inc. Dr. Ochsner was a surgical interne under Dr. A. J. Ochsner at Augustana Hospital. He spent 2–1/2 years as a surgical assistant in various hospitals in Europe and was an outstanding surgeon at the Ochsner Clinic and Foundation Hospital in New Orleans, where he was a director of the section on General Surgery. He was also President of the American College of Surgeons at this time.

A concert was sponsored by the Student Chorus under the direction of Mr. Harry T. Carlson. It was given at the John B. Murphy Memorial Auditorium of the American College of Surgeons, located at 40 E. Erie St. on Friday, May 4, 1951. A free will offering benefitted the Student Scholarship Fund. The Student Chorus had in the past year performed an annual concert to benefit the Lila Pickhardt Memorial Fund of the Alumnae Association. As an added feature, the student Folk Dance Team of 24 students (started in 1950) danced. They had just been outfitted with new costumes and they were a smash hit every time they performed.

It was the year of the Alumnae Association's 50th Anniversary. The following very descriptive article was printed in the June issue of the Augustana Nurse.

With almost 400 reservations in for the tea and 261 for the dinner the members of the Social Arrangements Committee worked diligently in order to offer the graduates a lovely 50th anniversary reunion day.

Into the newly decorated and flower bedecked Lila Pickhardt lounge trooped graduates from near and far—young and old. Some were attending their first reunion affair and others their 50th.

Two attractively arranged tea tables had been set—one at each end of the lounge and were presided over by the various members assisted by Agnes Carlson '24 and Miss Maud Doherty. Flower arrangements consisted of pink carnations, a bouquet of roses and daisies on the piano; and the table centerpieces were Styrofoam figures of a nurse complete with cap, set in a container and surrounded by an attractive arrangement of specially dyed blue daisies and yellow carnations. The color scheme represented the Honor Class of 1926 celebrating its 25th anniversary, class colors. Tapers trimmed in gold to indicate our Golden Anniversary were set on either end of the table. The lovely sterling silver trays presented recently to the Alumnae Association by the Class of 1925 were used for the first time to serve the daintily pastel colored iced petit fours. In addition nuts, mints, and Neapolitan ice cream squares were served. Each guest registering was given an attractive lapel badge in white and gold, cut to match the figurines on the tea tables. At 7:30 p.m., the Gold Room of the Belden-Stratford Hotel was crowded to capacity with graduates to celebrate the Golden Anniversary of the Alumnae Association. The seating as in previous years was arranged by classes so that all could visit with classmates.

Following the entrance of the Honored Guests, Mrs. Esther H. Nelson '28, President, gave a short speech of welcome. Following a delicious dinner the program portion of the evening was opened by the Secretary, reading messages from members who were unable to attend.

Genevieve F. Kalthoff, '27 brought greetings to the class of 1926, and reminisced a bit of the "good old days." On behalf of the class, Katherine Johnson Rapp responded, with a brief activity report on each member and reintroduced them all as "they may not be recognized since they had changed their figures in the last 26 years from a straight six to an hour-glass 8." In addition, on behalf of the class, she presented Miss Ehman who had served as Director of Nurses at the time of their training days with a gift, to which Miss Ehman responded and also thanked for the orchid corsage which the class had sent her in time for the tea. Several members of the class then brought in their gift to the Alumnae Association which was a pair of beautiful silver trays, rectangular with handles. The President accepted them on behalf of the Board and also thanked the class of 1925 for their gift of 2 sterling trays in a rose pattern and a donation of $20.00 to the Lila Pickhardt Drive.

Life membership awards were then presented to celebrate 40 years of membership. The Alumnae song, written by Margaret Saenger was then sung. Miss Maud Doherty, Director of Nurses of our Hospital School of Nursing brought greetings to the honored guests and members. A brief moment of silence was observed by the group in memory of the nurses who had died during the year, with the secretary reading their names.

Following the singing of Auld Lang Syne the 50th anniversary festivities came to a close and old friends and class mates separated with high hopes that next year would bring them together again. Incidentally, The Illinois State Nurses' Association also celebrated its 50th Anniversary this year.

Laura Jensen Thompson, '12, who served as a Red Cross nurse in World War I, was the mother of Lt. Jean E. Thompson, Kenosha, Wisconsin, who was one of the flying nurses in the Pacific. Laura wrote that one nurse and two technicians cared for a plane carrying 36 litter patients; a flight with 65 patients had twice that number in attendance.

Some of the duties of a flight nurse were administering oxygen, controlling hemorrhages in high altitudes, giving transfusions, changing dressings, keeping shock patients under sedation, serving meals and feeding the helpless, and trying to bolster the morale of anxious wounded young boys, most of them just out of high school.

The evacuation flights varied from 10 to 15 hours, with 12 hours between flights to re-equip medicine lockers, and have a good night's sleep, except in an emergency, the layover might be only half that time or less.

Dedication of the new wing, lobby, chapel, gift and coffee shop was held on Sunday, September 23, 1951 at 4 p.m. It was attended by doctors, nurses, pastors of the Chicago area and many other guests. An impressive dedication service was conducted by Dr. C. O. Bengtson, president of the Illinois Conference of the Augustana Lutheran Church and Choral numbers were sung by a choir conducted by Mr. Harry T. Carlson. Among the many memorials that were given, the Alumnae window in the Good Samaritan side chapel was dedicated. It had been given this name because the nurses' school pin carried that insignia. This was actually the dedication service signaling the completion of the new construction. "Open House" had been held on May 13th.

The addition provided more beds, modern facilities, and equipment for diagnostic and treatment procedures, as well as the obstetrical department. During this construction, a stream of bad luck left many in the Nurses' Residence wondering if they might have to move out. Prior to Augustana's purchase of the land on Dickens Avenue, a brewery had been located there to take advantage of an artesian well. Early in the construction of the west wing, this well was hit and the entire excavation was flooded. A loud pump kept all awake while it caught up with the well's flow. Meanwhile, a night thunderstorm's lightning hit the roof of the residence and a cornice fell off into the street so that when a fire started on the roof where old rags had been left, the fire engine had to detour around the cornice. If this was not enough, a bulldozer ran out of control a few days later, hitting the residence, shattering a number of windows and cracking the walls. The wing and chapel were completed without further incident. [In 1958, the modern 10-room operating suite and laboratories in the west wing were built.]

Dr. Percy was honored by the board of directors and a number of professional associates who had created a research foundation named for him, the "Nelson M. Percy Research Foundation." The purpose of this foundation was: "To perpetuate the name and memory of one of the masters of American surgery by adding to the sum total of medical knowledge through research and clinical investigations to the end that medical care may be developed to the highest possible level within the Augustana Hospital and the medical and hospital field as a whole."

Mr. E. I. Erickson, Superintendent of the hospital, was elected to serve as President of the American College of Hospital Administrators at its meeting held in St. Louis the second week of September. Mrs. Erickson (Blanche Lauger '22) accompanied him on the trip.

For the first time in the history of Augustana Hospital, a nursing Deaconess, Sister Dorothy Samuelson, had been appointed to our staff. Sister Dorothy was well qualified for her work as clinical supervisor and student counselor. She had her R.N. from the Immanuel Hospital in Omaha, her B.S. degree from the University of Minnesota, and her Deaconess degree from the Immanuel Institute in Omaha. It was interesting to note that Deaconesses gave their services without remuneration. They received only board, room and laundry and necessary expense money.

In 1952, the preclinical period was 25 weeks in length. Remodeling was taking place; clinical space and room for clinical teaching was being provided. Assignments for student practice within each department were made by the clinical instructor. Four clinical instructors had a full time teaching function spent in formal classes, conferences and bedside supervision of the student.

Operating Room—An 8 week operating room experience was now begun in the first year. Students averaged about 50 scrubs (being the instrument nurse during the operation). Sixteen hours of formal class were either given before or concurrently with Operating Room, with 36 hours of clinical instruction.

Obstetrical Nursing—A new unit ranked first in the city by the Department of Health for its excellent set-up and record of patient care. Students had a four week experience. Clinical instruction was planned by three head nurses and the supervisor.

Diet Therapy—The first week the student made menus; the second week she made salads and desserts; the third week she did cooking. One week was spent in taking care of special requests and special feedings. The last weeks were spent in calculating special diets.

Central Supply Service—This service was of 4 weeks duration, and gave the student experience in ordering and maintaining supplies and equipment. There were few disposable items, so the students had to sharpen and wash needles for injections, wash syringes and re-supply the dressing carts with dressings which had been put up in glass jars and sterilized.

Medical Surgical Nursing—There were 270 private and semi private beds. Assignments for student practice were made by clinical instructors.

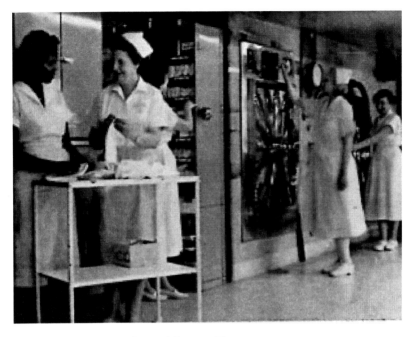

Central Service Department
Edith Pauline Johnson Supervisor (2nd from left)

Visiting Nurse Association—A two month practice was set up with the Visiting Nurse Association to give students practice in giving bedside care in the homes of indigent families.

Pediatric—One hundred twenty hours were given during a thirteen week assignment at Childrens Memorial Hospital. Students walked there daily in good weather and bad. Assignments and instruction included care of infants and older children, recreation and working in the outpatient department.

Psychiatric Nursing—Students had 13 weeks affiliation at a Veterans Hospital. Students had 125 hours of instruction in which lectures, discussions, demonstrations and conferences were provided for, during the weeks of observation and supervised practice in selected clinical areas.

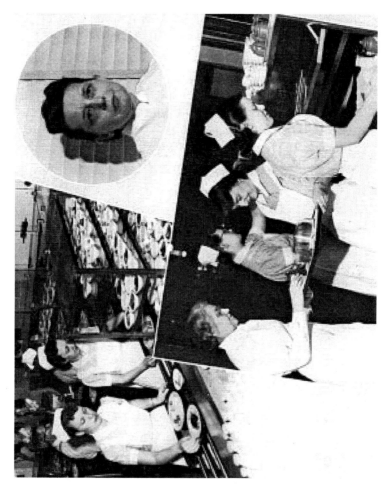

Hospital Cafeteria and Diet Kitchen, Mrs. Jones, Dietician (upper right)

The second Monday of every month at 7:30 p.m. a school for brides and grooms—a clinic on marriage, was being held at our Hospital. A large picture appeared in the Herald-American showing Rev. Sandstedt speaking to a group of about 60 persons in the Hospital Classroom. He stated the following:

"Marriage is a matter of adjustment, both physical and mental. But the carrying on of little niceties and courtesies of courtship mean much.

"Married people should live their lives with understanding, kindness and patience. They should answer their children's questions freely and fully, without any feeling of shame.

"In marriage, both parents should share in teaching the children moral values and in setting the precepts for right living.

"Marriage is an adjustment between individuals which should be sustained. Because of maladjustments, sometimes because of rushing into wedlock and sometimes because of lack of knowledge of their physical and emotional selves, marriage sometimes goes on the rocks."

Mrs. Edith B. Swanson '20 recently spent a week touring the Upper Peninsula of Michigan, to recruit prospective students for Augustana Hospital. She did this annually until 1963.

The Illinois State Nurses Association marking the start of its second one-half century of service held its Fifty-first Annual Convention at the Abraham Lincoln Hotel, Springfield, Illinois with approximately six hundred delegates representing eleven districts in the state and acting upon one of the most important programs ever put before the House of Delegates.

A summary of the meeting was printed in the November, 1952, Augustana Nurse and excerpts follow:

Mrs. L. B. Patterson, First Vice President of the A.N.A. states: "To meet this problem of the present shortage of nurses and the shortage that can be seen in the future, requires the improvement of working conditions for general duty nurses in hospitals, salaries of these nurses have not kept pace with the cost of living and the work week should be shortened to forty hours. The profession, for these and a variety of other reasons is not attracting high school girls to nursing careers. The whole aspect of Nurses Training is changing. The nurse is now the head of a team that includes nurse aides, practical nurses and auxiliary workers and must be trained for supervisory training for the nurses who direct them.

In Summary: the problem will require all of the efforts of Nursing Schools to recruit trainees. It will require an increased public interest in the Nursing profession, the kind that could bring influence to aid nurses to receive better salaries, and more attractive living and working conditions. Scholarships and other inducements to study nursing could be provided by groups or individuals in a position to do this."

Alumnae President Esther Nelson '28 reported that on Saturday, May 10, 1952 all nurses residing in First District would be asked to register. Hospitals, First District Headquarters and locally designated stations would serve as registration spots. Registration included all active and inactive graduate professional nurses and active and inactive practical nurses. This registration was necessary at this time in order to:

1. Ascertain the nurse strength of this area
2. To obtain Civil Defense rosters for each city
3. To enlist volunteers for American Red Cross Major Civilian Disasters.

They were asked questions; such as their name, marital status, School of Nursing, year of graduation; interest in taking a refresher course, if inactive; interest in taking a brush-up in Home Nursing and First Aid. If interested in working, which type of work did they prefer, etc.

These were critical times. It behooved all nurses to cooperate on nursing projects, sponsored by nursing organizations in order that they might, as individuals, be prepared to help themselves, families and communities in the event of an emergency.

The Alumnae sent $150.00 to "Week of Free Care." The president informed us that this particular fund was maintained by 1st District for the benefit of nurses in need of medical care because of tuberculosis.

An appeal was made through the Augustana Nurse for donations for the Lila Pickhardt Fund. The Alumnae maintained the room and in January alone, 102 donated and in February, an additional 126 donated. On January 18, 1953 the senior students held a Silver Tea in the Lila Pickhardt Lounge of the

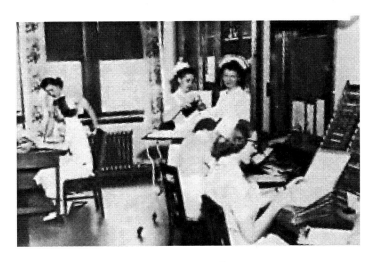

Nurses at Work
Nurse Station

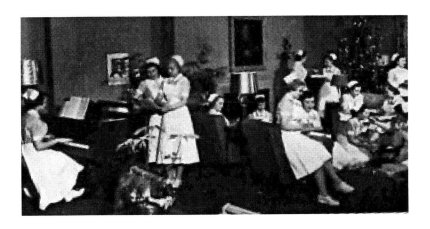

Nurses at Play
Lila Pickhardt Lounge

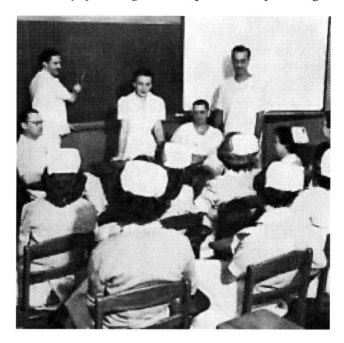

Classroom

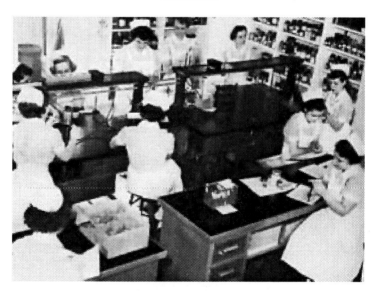

Laboratory Classroom (see page 72)

Nurses' Residence, from 2 to 5 p.m. The proceeds of this Tea were used toward the printing of the Augilog.

The National League for Nursing advised us that, as a result of the inspection which was conducted early in May, 1952, our School had been approved for the year 1953. As with all approval programs, this was made on an annual basis and could be withdrawn from a school which ceased to maintain standards acceptable to the approving body. Therefore, our aim was to put forth every reasonable effort to retain this recognition. It was a notable achievement and was in keeping with the traditions and uniformly high standing of the Hospital and the School.

It was fifteen years since the League embarked on a program of accreditation. World War II interrupted its progress. Thereafter, the program was reactivated, and all schools were invited to fill in a questionnaire giving pertinent data with respect to their programs. On the basis of the returns from this questionnaire, the schools were, after careful study, divided into three groups. Twenty-five percent were placed in Group One, which indicated that they most nearly, or completely, met the standards recommended by the League. Fifty percent of all schools were placed in Group Two; and the remaining twenty-five percent, consisting of schools which had failed to reply or had submitted incomplete data, were listed in Group Three. Our School was placed in Group Two. This step was not intended as a method for determining approval, but was to provide data on which to build a good program. Since there were several hundred schools in Group Two, it was evident that it would be a physical impossibility to inspect them individually except over a period of several years. It was, therefore, decided that the schools in this group could apply for temporary accreditation for a five-year period, or until such time as the school was ready for an inspection. We applied and received this temporary approval of accreditation early in 1952.

We took just pride in this accomplishment and expressed sincere thanks to Miss Maud Doherty, our Director of Nursing, for her leadership and persistent efforts in the development of the program. Appreciation was also due to those who had been charged with details of the School's educational program, including the members of the faculty, and for the cooperation that had been received from our Medical Staff. At the same time, the cooperation of the Assistant Directors and the nursing supervisors in providing patient care and supervising the work of the students in the various stages of their development had been equally important; and their loyal services were also appreciated.[28]

In 1952, the Illinois State Board examinations became a part of the machine graded National State Board Test Pool.

Esther Nelson, President of the Alumnae Association, welcomed all the seniors and invited them to join the Alumnae. At this time there were over 850 members. Each senior was then presented with a history book of the Augustana Hospital School of Nursing.

The Class of 1917 presented a beautifully bound book "Book of Remembrance," to the Chapel. In this book were to be inscribed the various gifts to the Chapel and those who had given them.

The Alumnae Association was pleased that "FIRST" the official publication of First District, Illinois State Nurses Association carried the following: "Augustana has an interesting Alumnae Publication. Published monthly, ten issues, the 'Augustana Nurse' is sent to members of Augustana Hospital Alumnae Association, and additional copies sent to the Students library, to hospital administrators and to First District."

The first symposium on Cancer for nurses was held at the University of Illinois School of Nursing from February 18-20th. Fifty instructors in medical and surgical nursing were guests. Miss Bertha Klauser represented Augustana. At the March

---

28. The "Augustana Nurse" January 1953.

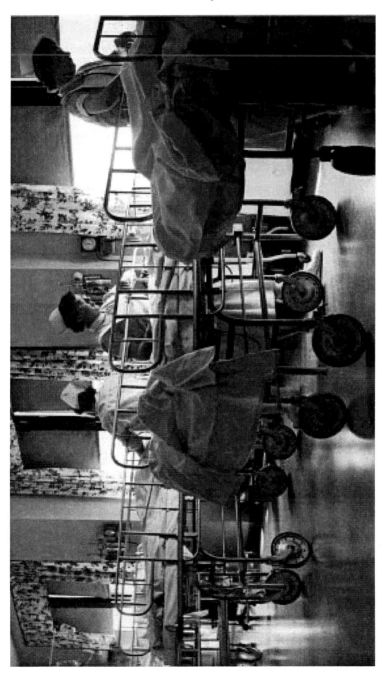

Recovery Room Early 1950s

Alumnae meeting she distributed a 5-page mimeographed report which she had prepared for the hospital staff nurses. It was an excellent report and those attending the meeting were fortunate to secure this latest information on cancer.

The Junior class of student nurses entertained the seniors at a banquet on March 26 at the Svithiod Club on Wrightwood Avenue.

On April 16, 1953, in the Haber Corporation fire on North and Clybourn Avenues in Chicago when 35 persons lost their lives, many severely burned patients were rushed to Augustana Hospital. Local papers had high praise for the way in which these emergencies were handled. The Daily News mentioned among other things that "Augustana Hospital's newly opened post-operative recovery room was pressed into service to handle victims from the Haber Corporation blaze. The room was quickly converted into an emergency ward with 12 physicians and 24 nurses on hand to treat the flow of injured."

On May 7th Dr. Alfred Murray showed his movie on "Hawaii" in the hospital chapel. The students sponsored the showing of the very beautiful color film, shown with a musical background. The free will offering was placed into the Augilog Fund. Dr. Murray had received much recognition for his work, having been cited by MGM studios for his excellence in motion picture photography.

The American Goiter Association held its annual meeting at the Drake Hotel on May 7–9, 1953. At that convention an award was presented which read: "To all to whom these presents shall come, Greetings: Be it known that by unanimous vote of the membership of the American Goiter Association, this Certificate of Meritorious Service is presented to Nelson M. Percy, M.D. These letters bring testimony of his untiring interest and devotion to this Association." This award was given annually. It was presented to Dr. Frank Lahey of Boston and our own Dr. Percy.

Dr. John Weston Nuzum, 62, a surgeon at Augustana Hospital for the last 30 years died at the hospital on Sunday, June 14, 1953. Dr. Nuzum received his medical degree from Rush Medical College in 1915 and served from 1918 to 1923 as pathologist and chief of the laboratory at Cook County Hospital and associate professor of pathology at the University of Illinois Medical School. In 1917 he was credited with perfecting an anti-polio serum which was used with some success. He maintained offices at 2051 Sedgewick from 1923 to 1953.

# OPENING NIGHT
# ICE FOLLIES
## JOHNSON AND SHIPSTEAD

### OCTOBER 22, 1953
### 8:30 P. M.

ARENA — 630 North McClurg Court — CHICAGO

Tickets from: $2.00 to $3.80

The Augustana Hospital Auxiliary is sponsoring this opening night performance. Let's all save this evening—bring the family —make up a party of friends—tell everyone you see. Ticket booth at arena will be open for sale of tickets to this event the end of August or first of September. For answers to questions you may have you may write to Auxiliary President Linnea G. Engberg, 508 Lemont Street, Lemont, Illinois.

We were proud that our relatively small and unknown Auxiliary was chosen to sponsor the opening night, inasmuch as that year, several larger and very important groups were intensely interested. For years it had been the big Fall attraction of the Service Clubs and Infant Welfare Societies. This was the first big project sponsored by the Auxiliary.

The Sunday Chicago American carried a group picture of members of the Ice Follies Benefit Committee—they looked happy over the fact that the tickets had all been sold weeks in advance and that this would be a successful venture. Many dinner parties were given before the performance. The hospital family turned out en masse, as well as members of the Alumnae and Auxiliary, with their families. For days after the event the papers carried pictures of "first nighters," and the Alumnae Association congratulated the Auxiliary on the "bang-up" job that was done to bring Augustana Hospital into public notice, as well as to raise this wonderful sum of money for the Free Bed Fund. The final proceeds made by the Auxiliary were $9,583.51.

On Tuesday, August 25th, the First District invited its members to the first annual picnic which was held on the 55th Street Promontory and the Lake. Approximately 700 nurses attended the affair, and the ten from Augustana had such a good time. Supper was served from 5:00 p.m. on and there was entertainment, games, dancing and fellowship. The food had all been donated and was delicious.

In the Chicago Medical Society Bulletin of Sept. 26th, we noted an article prepared by Dr. Earl Garside, Secretary of the Chicago Surgical Society. It informed us of the 1954 Nelson M. Percy Award of $500 for Surgical Research. The contestants had to reside in Cook County and must have been preparing for a surgical career. This was another "first" and we at Augustana were proud. It was hoped that this would continue to be made an annual award. Dr. Percy presented the award to someone recommended by the Award Committee.

At the September Alumnae meeting, a talk was given to the nurses by Dr. Milles, Chief Pathologist. Highlights of the talk follow:

Accurate diagnosis is the keystone of effective treatment. Laboratory diagnosis has advanced far more rapidly during the past ten years than in any previous decade in medical history. The laboratory sciences have developed new tests, on the one hand, and new instruments for performing the tests more accurately and more rapidly, on the other.

The laboratory of the Augustana Hospital has met the increased needs of its staff for laboratory services by more than fourfold expansion of its physical plant and personnel, and by departmentalizing for more efficient operation.

A brief survey of the several departments, their personnel and their work load will serve to illustrate the growing place of clinical pathology in the whole structure of medical practice.

Surgical Pathology: 3000 tissues from surgery and 170 autopsies processed a year. A single room and the services of one and one-half technicians. Every tissue removed in surgery must be sent to the laboratory, where the decision relative to its being sectioned rests with the pathologist. Quick frozen sections can be prepared and a report returned to the surgeon in eight to ten minutes.

Chemistry: 18,000 tests. A single larger room (formerly the sewing room) and the services of three technicians. The modern photoelectric colorimeters and flame photolometer permit accurate and economical results with the vastly increased demands on this department.

Bacteriology: 4,652 examinations yearly. One room and one technician. The demand for accurate estimation of the effectiveness of the available antibiotics have increased the responsibilities and the work load in this department.

Serology and Blood Bank: 14,393 tests and 1,312 donors yearly. Two rooms and two full time and a part time technician. The growing use of whole blood transfusions has been a large factor in the improved results in major surgery.

Hematology: 13,534 tests. Dr. Limarzi, who is a specialist in the field of hematology, is directly in charge of this department. It utilizes the services of three full time technicians.

It must be evident that those whose contact with the practice of medicine antedates the last war that progress has been rapid and both instruments of precision and trained personnel have greatly facilitated the application of the advances which have depended largely upon fundamental work done in the various sciences.

An entirely new department has been added under the direction of Drs. Lindon Seed and Bertha Jaffee. This is the radioactive laboratory wherein the newly developed field of radioactive isotopes in their application to medicine is being applied. The use of radioactive iodine in the diagnosis and treatment of hyperthyroidism and cancer of the thyroid are becoming widespread, and the use of radioactive phosphorus in the treatment of polycythemia is standard therapy today.

Financial support from the Nelson M. Percy Foundation has permitted carrying on of experimental studies, both in application of radioactive isotopes in the treatment of cancer and in other departments within the hospital so that Augustana Hospital is now taking its rightful place not only as a general hospital but as an institution of higher learning.

We were informed of the death of Johanna Nelson Hanson on September 30, 1953. According to the History of the Alumnae Association, Mrs. Hanson was a Charter member of the organization (see pp. 23, 25 and 28).

The annual Halloween Party was held in the recreation room October 30th. This should arouse a few memories—rubber gloves filled with water, blind musicians, bazaars, a room full of gals dancing with each other . . ..

The students sponsored a spaghetti dinner in November with the proceeds going to the Student Scholarship Fund to help with miscellaneous expenses for needy students. The student nurses had been a particularly busy group those days. They held a bake sale, and on November 5th the seniors of the September division sponsored an authentic Italian spaghetti dinner in the recreation room of the home—$1.25 a plate. The girls served from 5 to 7 p.m. with one of the mothers serving as chief cook.

On December 4th the Christian Nurses' Fellowship sponsored an evening program in the hospital chapel. A missionary from the American Missions to Lepers showed color slides.

"Calling American Nurses to Action," was the theme of the 1954 A.N.A. Convention held in Chicago, April 25–30.

The opening program meeting was held at the Coliseum, on South Wabash Avenue, Monday evening April 26. Frances L.A.Powell, President of the Illinois State Nurses Association, welcomed the convention attendants and invited them to "make this week the opportunity of a lifetime." Between 8 and 9 thousand nurses attended this convention and 26 countries were represented on the platform at the opening session of the House of Delegates.

An estimated minimum of 50,000 nurses in addition to the more than 334,000 registered professional nurses actively employed today, were needed to fill budgeted positions open and waiting to be filled.

Meeting in joint convention with A.N.A. for the first time

were 2,000 student nurses representing the new National Student Nurse Association organized in June 1953.

The First District urged that every nurse have an annual chest x-ray as a health measure for the nurse and for the patient. An x-ray unit was set up in the City Hall, 121 North LaSalle Street, Monday through Friday, 9:00 a.m. to 4:00 p.m. where you could get a free x-ray.

The Chicago Daily News, printed the following article on Monday, April 26, 1954.

TELLS NURSES TO KEEP UP WITH WORLD

"A nurse should know more than how to handle a patient — she should know about world affairs too."

That is what Mrs. Elizabeth K. Porter, of Cleveland, president of the American Nurses Association, told 7,000 nurses here Monday. She was the keynote speaker at a week-long convention of the association which opened general sessions at the Coliseum.

She said keeping abreast of world affairs is "the first challenge to nurses in 1954."

"It is impossible to carry well our share of the responsibility for adequate service in hospitals and homes — unless we understand conditions responsible for man's present ills and his impaired health," she declared.

The Association has two broad purposes, she said; To promote the continuous improvement of nursing service, and to promote the welfare and protection of nurses.

THE AMERICAN NURSES' ASSOCIATION has reiterated these ethical standards in regard to radio and TV advertising:

—A nurse's name can't be used in the endorsement of a product.

—A registered nurse in uniform, even though unidentified, cannot appear in an ad or commercial, if this would imply professional endorsement.

—Since nurses understand that only a physician may prescribe treatment and medication, special care must be taken in commercials advertising pharmaceutical or therapeutic products.

In 1954, two year Associate Degree Programs were established in the United States (mainly in conjunction with Junior Colleges).

A tuberculosis affiliation was established with the Chicago Municipal Tuberculosis Sanatorium for the Augustana students, and continued until 1962. The previous year, 1953, the students had an affiliation at the Lake County Tuberculosis Sanatorium in Waukegan, Illinois. Students moved into the residences of the facility of affiliation excepting the Visiting Nurse Association.

The floors at the Hospital were renumbered. The ground floor was now one, and we had a total of nine floors. The Hospital Auxiliary refurnished the 5th floor which had been known as 4th.

The September 1955, Junior Class was very busy during the winter. They sponsored a dance for student nurses early in January. Students from a number of neighboring colleges and universities were invited guests. This class also sponsored the monthly Friday night movies and slides in the Chapel. These movies and slides were taken and were presented by various members of the hospital family.

The annual Junior-Senior banquet was held in an impressive dining room at the Palmer House. The Junior classes did a splendid bit of arranging for this banquet and were very gracious hostesses to the senior classes and other guests.

Mrs. Edith Bergeson Swanson, '20, Student Counselor, accompanied by Mrs. Bernadine Rehn Johnson, '29, went on a student recruitment tour of many points South and West in Illinois. During this tour they talked to 40 high school students who were interested in the profession of nursing. Information regarding admission to the school of nursing was presented to all. They were on tour for two weeks and contacted Alumnae members who resided in or near towns they visited. The tuition for the 3 year program from 1955 to 1957, was $250.00, in 1958, it was $325.00 and in 1959-1960, it was $500.00.

The Annual Home Coming Tea was held in the Lila Pickhardt Lounge in the Nurses' Residence on the afternoon of June 5, 1954. The Banquet was held in the evening at the Lake Shore Athletic Club. Tickets for Alumnae members were $5.25 each. Cost of ticket for a non-member was $6.25.

The following very interesting letter was received by the Alumnae Association:

c/o Topline, P.O.B. 1348
Beirut, Lebanon
Nov. 22, 1954

Dear Alumnae Members:

In spite of the mailing address, I live over 400 miles by air (550 by car) Southeast of Beirut, in the Northern part of Saudi Arabia. The Trans-Arabian Pipeline Co. has a few pumping stations along the pipeline, which extends from the Persian Gulf area to the terminal at the historic city of Sidon, Lebanon. The other pumping stations have small hospitals staffed by male nurses and a doctor for each station, but Badanah recently opened a new complete hospital which will have four doctors and male and female nurses. I am the only American on the staff at present and the only single American woman who has worked in Arabia for Topline.

In Badanah there are ten American families and about six bachelors, most of whom work part of the time at other stations. With the exception of five Dutchmen and three Indians, all other expatriates are from Arab countries, chiefly Lebanon, Syria and Jordan. Saudi Arabs fill the jobs requiring little or no training.

Because there is water at Badanah for their camels, as many as 25,000 Bedouins camp here during summer months. Bedouin women in Saudi Arabia usually have some tattooing on their faces and sometimes on their neck, hands and feet, and frequently wear a nose ring through one nostril. Many of them have beautiful eyes until they are ruined by trachoma which is very prevalent. Bedouin men wear their hair long and often in several braids.

The first two weeks of December I hope to visit Jerusalem and environs, Istanbul and Athens. I want to be back in the desert before the rush of Christmas travelers begins.

Several weeks ago I spent a most interesting day in Damascus, where I saw craftsmen make beautiful brocades; furniture and boxes inlaid with wood, mother-of-pearl, and ivory; the popular Arab coffee pots and other metal items; rugs, etc. Although the newer parts of the city are very modern, some of the streets in which I walked probably have changed little in general appearance since that fateful day when, following his conversion, Paul of Tarsus was led into the city.

Sincere wishes to all Alumnae members for a Merry Christmas and a Happy 1955.

> Cordially,
> Berniece Hess, Class of 1947

The Christmas season came early to those who attended the annual Alumnae party on December 1st. A good number of Alumnae members and nurses on the staff at Augustana attended the program which was presented in the hospital chapel. Reverend Sandstedt, Chaplain of Augustana Hospital, was introduced and called upon to render the invocation and to read the Christmas Story from the Bible. The Northland Trio, com-

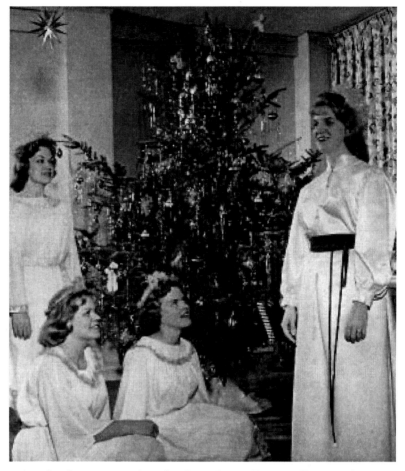

Students presenting the Santa Lucia Pagent, Circa 1960

prised of Lillian Carlson, Gerda Carlson and Magda Erickson, assisted by Mrs. Effie Freedlund were introduced by our President, Karen Shrader. They presented a program in three parts as follows:

Part I—Christmas Chorals. These were rendered beautifully and sincerely. The messages of these songs brought one the feeling of meditation, serenity and joy.

Part II—Mrs. Freedlund narrated a Christmas story based on excerpts from everyday happenings. They were short stories with impressive messages. After each message the Trio sang a Christmas Carol to express the meaning.

Part III—CHRISTMAS IN SWEDEN. This was the highlight of the program. The Trio wore authentic Swedish costumes to portray the holiday customs. Mrs. Freedlund told the story of Santa Lucia, the Queen of Light, and the meaning of that important event in their festivities. The lights were dimmed and Queen Lucia, wearing a crown glowing with candle light, came in with all her grace and beauty. (The role of Queen played by a student nurse.) The Trio then sang many Swedish Christmas songs. They also portrayed the custom of Lighting the Candles in the House, and sang the traditional song. Many other customs associated with Christmas were described. The front of the Chapel was decorated with many types of candle holders from small to large and from regular shapes to those shaped like Christmas trees.

After the Benediction, the nurses adjourned to the Lila Pickhardt Lounge where the Social Committee welcomed them. The Lounge was decorated with pine boughs and attractive ornaments which were made by graduates from the Class of 1928. Two long tables were attractively set for buffet lunch consisting of rolls, ham slices, pickles, potato chips, beautiful gelatin molds in Christmas colors, dainty delicious cakes and salted nuts. The attractive ornaments, made by Miss Sandra Fleming '28 and her classmates '28, were sold during the evening to add more money to the Sick Nurses Benefit Fund. The Christmas party of 1954 was acclaimed one of the best given by the Alumnae Association.

Jennie A. Larson wrote, "I thought you might be interested in knowing that one of the Augustana Nurses in the 1914 class has written music and words of a religious song. Mrs. Clara Lawson Carlson is the composer of 'On The Cross,' published by Fiesta Music Inc." This song was performed at our April

Alumnae Meeting in the chapel by students Carolyn Gonsallus '57 and Jill Anderson '57 accompanied on the piano by Marilyn (Mimi) Johnson '57.

Harold Henning became the instructor for the Swedish Folk Dancing class in 1954. Authentic Swedish costumes were obtained and performances were given at the Museum of Science and Industry, the International Trade Fair and the Lake View Citizens Club. The Student Nurses' Chorus and the Swedish Folk Dancing Class gave a benefit performance on April 28th at the Swithoid Club for $1.25 per ticket.

A special benefit to Alumnae members, who were patients at the hospital, was receiving 50% off the hospital bill after payment by their insurance. Other benefits were receiving the monthly newsletter, voting privileges at the monthly meetings, and the opportunity to apply for a scholarship.

A class of 69 pre-clinical students entered the School of Nursing on Monday, August 29, 1955: 21 from Michigan—17 of these were from the Upper Peninsula, 8 from Wisconsin, 5 from Indiana, 31 from Illinois—12 of these were from Chicago, 1 from Virginia, 1 from New Mexico, 1 from California and 1 from Pennsylvania.

Margaret Samuelson Tessberg '27 was employed at St. Mary's Hospital in Wausau, Wisconsin in the Isolation Ward. Early in 1956 she was caring for two children in iron lungs. Although Dr. Jonas Salk developed a polio vaccine in the late forties, in 1950, there were still 35,000 cases reported nationwide. [In 1949, Dr. Salk became the first man to use dead viruses to immunize against polio. By 1954, he was so sure of its safety that he tested the vaccine on himself and his family. It was approved for use in 1955. Dr. Albert Sabin's live-virus vaccine was approved in 1961. Because it could be taken orally and didn't require booster shots, the Sabin form became the polio vaccine of choice. In the early 1990's there were less than 90 new cases reported.]

The Alumnae Association voted to sponsor a needy student

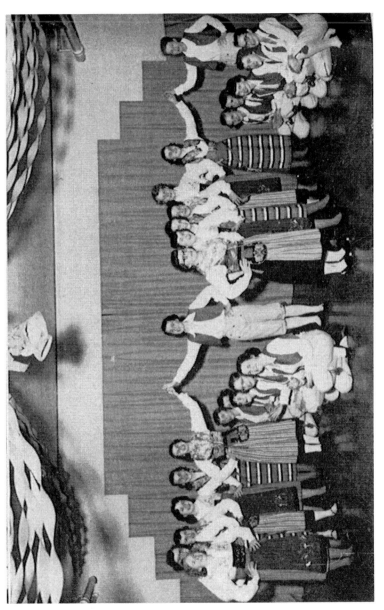

Swedish Folk Dancing Class in 1952

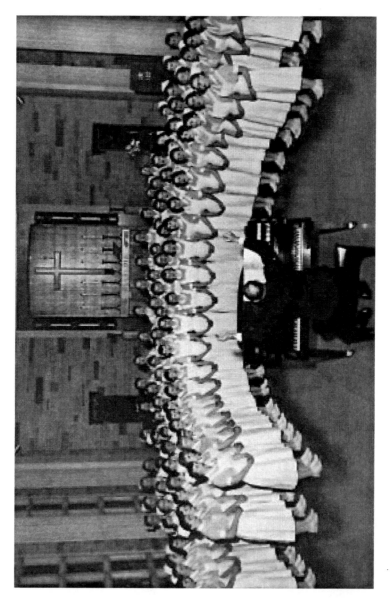

The Nurses' Chorus in 1955 Conductor Harry T. Carlson

nurse by paying her tuition of $250.00 and her Public Health affiliation in her senior year. They also voted to give the student nurses $50.00 for the year book and the school $75.00 for new books for the library.

The American Nurses' Association's 40th Convention was held May 14-18, 1956 in Chicago. The Augustana Student Nurses Chorus sang at the opening meeting.

Miss Bertha Klauser reported on the special committee appointed to set up a program for a reorientation course planned with the hope that Augustana nurses interested in returning to nursing would avail themselves of this type of refresher course.

Because of the growing concern over the current shortage of nurses, a desire to assist in giving good nursing care, and also to make more nurses available, a request was made at its April meeting that our association study hidden resources.

At a meeting attended by representatives from the hospital board of directors, the medical staff, and the alumnae association, a committee was authorized to formulate plans for a refresher course, tentatively June 25-June 29. The purpose of this course at Augustana Hospital was to re-orientate inactive nurses with the hope that they would be interested in returning to full or part-time service; and further, to answer a request of many of our nurses for such a program. The content of this course was tentatively designed to include basic techniques, drug therapy, changing trends in treatment, pre- and post-operative care, parenteral and oxygen therapy and gastric decompression.

A most outstanding event in the Hospital Auxiliary history was that of their fiftieth anniversary celebration on the evening of May 25, 1956. The program was held in the Hospital Chapel with three student nurses contributing the musical numbers. Representatives of the Hospital, Medical Staff, Board of Directors, Illinois Conference and the Alumnae Association gave greetings and the former Chaplain, Dr. Granger Westberg gave the address "Recapturing the Spirit of the Pioneers."

A social coffee hour for the three hundred or more members

and friends was held in the Lila Pickhardt Lounge. Several beautiful bouquets of yellow roses, carnations, and gladioli were in evidence of congratulations from florists through the committee on arrangements. It was indeed a memorable evening. Those of the Alumnae Association present at the program were very proud of their president who gave the greeting from the Alumnae Association.

> The members of the Alumnae Association extend Greetings and Best Wishes to you on the 50th Anniversary of the Augustana Hospital Auxiliary.
>
> We are happy to have this opportunity to congratulate you and to express our thanks to you, as individuals, for your loyal and faithful service to Augustana Hospital. We are aware of your accomplishments—we too benefit by your many contributions.
>
> Our thoughts go back to Thursday afternoon coffee service in the lobby. It made Thursday a special day at Augustana. Everyone loved the custom. The dream of a Coffee Shop became a reality, thanks to far-sighted, interested Auxiliary members.
>
> One cannot measure success in dollars alone. No price tag can be attached to the faithful, unselfish services of a group such as yours. We are most fortunate that through the years the Hospital Auxiliary has been blessed with loyal members, who in turn donated their time and tireless efforts so that hundreds might benefit daily. We are thinking now of all the washed gauze you have made into dressings—the many pleasant hours spent together in the work room doing a very important and necessary task—one that could not have been done without you. Those of you who have worn dressings know the comfort of washed gauze. Never underestimate the importance of that project, unglamorous as it may sound.
>
> We, as Augustana nurses are most grateful to you all for the many ways in which you have helped us by helping the hospital serve the patient. The Hospital Auxiliary is truly Augustana's friend and benefactor. You fill in the gaps, take up the slack, add the frills, and provide the social contacts which are a very necessary and important part of every successful organization. The warm touch, the extra comforts, the many, many things you do reflect thoughtfulness and consideration.
>
> Your progress in the past few years has been amazing. Your courageous undertakings—your faith in what you could do, have been rewarded by success and accomplishment. There is a special happiness and deep satisfaction, an inner joy, shared only by those endowed with a spirit of service. The gift of giving of one's self is in itself rewarding. May you feel richly rewarded. Happy Birthday, Congratulations. Thank you, and best wishes."
>
> Karen Shrader, '31 President

The Manager of the coffee shop was Florence Strom Stange, '26, who was an Alumnae and Auxiliary member. The

Auxiliary's 50th anniversary was celebrated at the Ice Follies on October 16, and the Alumnae Association donated $100.00 to the 50th Anniversary Free Care Fund.

The '26 sewing club living in Chicago donated to the Augustana Gift Shop over $2,000.00 in hand-made articles since they started this club in 1954.

The following was copied from the July 11, 1956, St. Charles newspaper.

Three new community grade schools have been named after well-loved and respected St. Charles ladies who gave years to the education and care of children. The nurse—Amelia T. Anderson, who after finishing a nursing course at Augustana Hospital in 1901, was a home nurse until shortly after World War I when she became school nurse and city and township nurse, serving in these capacities until 1941.

She is best remembered for her work during the depression of the 1930's. Without regard for her own personal comfort, she collected food, money and clothing for the children of poor families, and saw that they got proper medical and dental care.

She was one of the founders of the St. Charles Welfare Association which was organized during the depression for the general welfare of school children. It was through this group and Miss Anderson that school milk and dental care was started.

Her unselfish devotion during these years is still talked of in St. Charles by the many people who benefited.

Miss Anderson resides in the little red house at the corner of S. Sixth Ave. and Adams.

Augustana was very happy that Miss Anderson was honored in such a wonderful, glorious way. Those who had the privilege of meeting her could readily understand the esteem and devotion of the people of St. Charles in naming her for this public recognition.

Mrs. Lillian Johnson Bandt, '20 of Iron Mountain, Michigan was named "Michigan Nurse of the Year" at the Michigan State Nurses' Convention in Lansing. She had been in public health work for 25 years.

The citation for Mrs. Bandt said:

"During her long career in private and public health work, she has displayed singular ability and a deep understanding of human nature. Her eagerness to help is true to this tradition of her profession and her sympathetic approach to her work with both children and adults is sincere and warm hearted. She is the 'Florence Nightingale' of her community. With patience and skill that enables her to meet problems with calm judgment and assurance, she brings hope, help and encouragement to those in greatest need."

Miss Maud Doherty, Director of Nursing and Nursing Education since 1949, retired as of November 15, 1956. Miss Doherty came to us in August 1949, from the University of Akron. She had a long and successful career as an administrator and nursing educator. During her service at Augustana Hospital, full accreditation was accorded to the School of Nursing by the National League for Nursing. This was a tribute to her leadership and purposeful efforts. A farewell reception was given in her honor at the Nurses' Residence on Sunday afternoon, November 11.

Miss Mary Frey, R.N., M.A., entered upon her duties as Director of Nursing and Nursing Education on November 16, 1956. Miss Frey was a native Illinoisan. She was a graduate of the School of Nursing at the Mennonite Hospital, La Junta, Colorado, and received her Bachelor's degree at Goshen College, Goshen, Indiana. Her Master's degree was earned at the University of Colorado. She also pursued postgraduate studies at The University of Chicago and Columbia University. She had extensive experience both as a Nurse Administrator and in Nursing Education. One of her former positions was that of Director of Nursing and Education at the Methodist Hospital, Peoria, Illinois.

The School of Nursing approved students marrying during the last six months of their training. Some students had married before graduation in prior years without the school's knowledge.

In January, 1957 Miss Stella Dytko reported the Alumnae had 910 members, 55 life members, 33 of which were Honorary members and 22 Paid Life members.

The Alumnae Association organized the first aid booths at the 17th Annual International Lutheran Conference.

The Alumnae Association voted to allot one dollar per capita to the Lila Pickhardt Fund annually from the General Treasury. The Hospital Auxiliary presented a check for $2,500.00 for the new carpeting in the Lounge, as the nurses lounge was totally refurbished.

The following letter was received:

At the meeting of the Board of Directors held May 6, 1957, it was reported that your Association has completely refurnished the Lila Pickhardt Lounge in the Nurses' Residence at a cost of more than six thousand dollars.

This generous contribution to the hospital is greatly appreciated; and by motion, the undersigned was directed to express our sincere thanks for your ongoing support of hospital activities.

> Yours very truly,
> Board of Directors
> Augustana Hospital
> Rev. Philip A. Johnson, Secretary

Dolores Fischer '51, who had been working in Pikeville, Kentucky, in the United Mine Workers Hospital there sent this letter:

I don't know how much you have heard or seen about the floods in this area, but believe me, there is no one who can possibly visualize the devastation that it has caused unless they have actually been here to see it. 90% of the people in this town had their homes flooded, and only those on the hill were safe. The water rose so rapidly that people had no chance to save much. We had almost six feet of water in the first floor of our hospital; we were cut off from phone service, electricity and water. At that time I made rounds and made sure that all the patients were in bed and covered with extra blankets since our heating plant was knocked out also. The rest of the night we worked by flashlight. I must say the patients were really wonderful. They had no idea what was happening to their families or homes, or whether they were safe or not. They remained calm, and during the night the water began to recede. For breakfast our patients had cold cereal and milk, as there was nothing else to serve them. Around noon we started evacuating our patients by boat, discharging those we felt could safely go home on medication, and transferring the others to another hospital. Those of us who came to work on the P.M. shift worked straight through for 24 hours. On Friday after the flood, I was sent to our hospital to help out there, and we thought it would be able to reopen. Our engineer rigged up some pipe to a mountain stream, and a hose at the end, and everyone started washing down the walls and the floors and furniture. We were able to transfer our patients back just seven days after the flood. This whole thing has been a terrific experience, and will be the subject of conversation for many a day yet. In the meantime, the clean up job in town is still going on and we will be digging out for many months to come.

The Committee on By-Laws recommended with the permission from the American Nurses Association that we will include in our By-Laws their Code for Professional Nurses.

### THE CODE FOR PROFESSIONAL NURSES

Professional nurses minister to the sick, assume responsibility for creating a physical, social and spiritual environment which will be conducive to recovery and stress the prevention of illness and promotion of health by teaching and example. They render health service to the individual, the family and the community and coordinate their services with members of other health professions involved in specific situations.

Service to mankind is the primary function of nurses and the reason for the existence of the nursing profession. Need for nursing service is universal. Professional nursing service is therefore unrestricted by considerations of nationality, race, creed or color.

Inherent in the code is the fundamental concept that the nurse subscribes to the democratic values to which our country is committed.

With reference to the following statements, the profession recognizes that a professional code cannot cover in detail all the activities and relationships of nurses, some of which are conditioned by personal philosophies and beliefs.

1. The nurse provides services with respect for human dignity and the uniqueness of the client unrestricted by considerations of social or economic status, personal attributes, or the nature of health problems.

2. The nurse safeguards the client's right to privacy by judiciously protecting information of a confidential nature.

3. The nurse acts to safeguard the client and the public when health care and safety are affected by the incompetent, unethical, or illegal practice of any person.

4. The nurse assumes responsibility and accountability for individual nursing judgments and actions.

5. The nurse maintains competence in nursing.

6. The nurse exercises informed judgment and uses individual competence and qualifications as criteria in seeking consultation, accepting responsibilities, and delegating nursing activities to others.

7. The nurse participates in activities that contribute to the ongoing development of the profession's body of knowledge.

8. The nurse participates in the profession's efforts to implement and improve standards of nursing.

9. The nurse participates in the profession's efforts to establish and maintain conditions of employment conducive to high quality nursing care.

10. The nurse participates in the profession's effort to protect the public from misinformation and misrepresentation and to maintain the integrity of nursing.

Word was received that Miss Margaret Saenger, '10, World War I overseas nurse, died November 7, 1957, in her home.

She had lived in Janesville since retiring from the staff of Augustana Hospital, where she served as supervisor of the nurses residence for many years.

A graduate of Augustana School of Nursing, Miss Saenger was second in command at Base Hospital II, Nantes, France, during World War I and was recalled to Augustana nursing staff during World War II. She was a Red Cross disaster nurse, having nursed during several catastrophes including the Dayton flood. She was a member of Jane A. Delano Post, American Leg-ion in Chicago and of First Congregational Church, Janesville.

The following Resolutions were read at the December 1957, Alumnae meeting.

"With a sense of sadness and loss we note the death of Miss Margaret Saenger, a former Assistant Superintendent of Nurses and Supervisor of the Nurses' Residence.

First, that we acknowledge God's infinite mercy to all who will receive it, even in the passing from this life to the life beyond;

Secondly, that we express our sympathy to her family in their sorrow and pray for them the comfort which only God can give;

Thirdly, that a copy of these resolutions be sent to her immediate family."

WHAT NURSING MEANS TO ME
Nursing . . . a way of serving God
Nursing . . . a way of inner peace
Nursing . . . a way of serving the afflicted
Nursing . . . a way of serving a community

In the parable of the good Samaritan Christ asked, "Which of these three was neighbor unto him that fell among the thieves?" And he said, "He that showed mercy on him." Then Jesus said, "Go, and do thou likewise." I feel that each of us is here for one purpose—to serve God and do His will, and in helping my fellowman by caring for his needs, I feel I am best serving my God.

Nursing also means to me a way of achieving inner peace and happiness. Only by having this peace can I give of myself to others. Many times throughout a day I have become discouraged, tired of criticism and weary of patient's complaints and yet at the end of the day I have joy in knowing I have helped someone—either, physically, mentally, emotionally, or spiritually along life's way.

Yes, nursing is a way of serving afflicted and suffering humanity. Easing the pain, comforting the oppressed, or giving hope to the weary, are just a few of the many ways I can perform my duties as a nurse.

Nursing also means to me a way of serving people of a community. I feel the nurse is the interpreter of the findings of medical science and can act as a "bridge" between the sources of knowledge and the people. Because of this association with these people, she establishes a relationship which offers many opportunities for teaching. The nurse is also a leader and must participate in civic affairs as she performs her role as a citizen of her community and country.

I wish to serve . . . that is what nursing means to me.

Written by Karen Latola Sarasin '58 during her Senior year of training and perhaps reflects how many of us feel.

The Alumnae Association received the following letter in the spring of 1958:

We are interested in knowing if Alumnae nurses who have small children and who are not employed now, might accept employment here if there was a day nursery established close to the hospital.

We have considered from many angles the feasibility of establishing a day nursery in this vicinity. We would endeavor, of course, to meet all the Board of Health requirements and other recommendations for managing a day nursery. This project would be developed for the purpose of bringing nurses back to work who have small children and have no satisfactory provision for their care while they work.

It was suggested that this be brought before the Alumnae Association. We would appreciate your bringing this to the attention of the group for consideration and discussion.

Thank you, and we shall appreciate reply.

Sincerely yours,
(Miss) Mary Frey, R.N.
Director, School of Nursing
and Nursing Service

Miss Frey later reported that a nursery school would not be practical as only three persons replied that they would be able to put in more working time.

Mrs. Swanson reported that the student library needed a book cart and shelves. The Alumnae Association responded with a gift of $75.00 for those items and at Christmas time the Class of 1933 sent $50.00 for a magazine rack for the school.

The following poem was written by a patient for the nurses on the 8th floor at Augustana.

TO WONDERFUL PEOPLE
I've never really thought about
The life among the ill,

The trials and tribulations that
A hospital does fill.
A patient enters on his own
Or flat upon his back;
From that time on the nurse's job
Involves that perfect tact.
No one wants to enter here,
Although they really must,
Rebellion is in each of us;
To the girls, it's so unjust.
We know unpleasant tests are made,
And hear of them outside.
By these and many other things,
We impatiently abide.
We blame our ills on many things;
Inner anger comes to front.
And who is there so patiently,
To get most of the brunt.
We pull the switch and wonder why
A nurse is not at hand,
Forgetting that these lovely girls
Are always in demand.
Their job is one incessant trip
Throughout their hours of work.
Just one shift of this I'm sure
Would send us all berserk.
And yet, we put this all aside
And say "Well, it's their job,"
By saying this we brand ourselves
Pure and selfish snobs.
Each day I spend upon my bed
I marvel at their calm.
Example should be learned from them,
To give a patient balm.
A nurse, a student, or an aide,
To me is heaven sent,
Without them God knows what I'd done
To pass the time I spent.
Their smiles throughout the day and night
Assured me all was fine.
A little word, a thoughtful deed
Showed me their time was mine.
Augustana should be proud
The girls will give their time
To help to heal and soothe the sick
In manner so sublime.
So in passing may I say,
I think you're all just grand.

There is no one who has refused
To lend a helping hand.

Mrs. Larry Goetz

The Alumnae Association was tendered an invitation to the annual Spring Formal held May 16, 1958 at the Graemere Hotel, 3400 W. Washington, by the senior class. The admission price was $4.00 per couple.

Dr. Nelson M. Percy, 82, internationally known Chicago surgeon of 2130 N. Lincoln Park West, died Friday, October 10, at Augustana Hospital. He was chief of staff at Augustana for 21 years until his retirement in 1956. He was graduated from Rush Medical College in 1899, was professor emeritus of clinical surgery at the University of Illinois Medical School and taught there from 1920 until 1940. During World War I, Dr. Percy went overseas as surgical director of Base Hospital No. 11. He was a member of the American College of Surgeons of the Chicago Surgical Association, president of the American Goiter Association in 1937 and in 1953 received a special meritorious award by the association. He was also a member of the Illinois Medical Society, the Chicago Medical Society, the Lake Shore and the University clubs. In 1951, the directors of Augustana Hospital organized the Nelson M. Percy Research Foundation in his honor. The Alumnae Association voted to become life members in the Percy Foundation for a donation of $250.00.

The following ad appeared in the Augustana Nurse (Oct. '58).

HELP WANTED

At long last a Volunteer Program is about to come into being at Augustana Hospital. Volunteer workers are needed desperately for non-nursing duties. Would you or one of your friends wish to spend some of your leisure moments extending care and courtesy and doing the small things that busy nurses just do not have the time to do for the patients at Augustana Hospital? For full details contact the Volunteer Director, Mrs. Florence Stange, at DI 8-1000 or write to: Volunteer Director, c/o Augustana Hospital, 409 West Dickens Avenue, Chicago 14.

Of the 56 graduating seniors, class of 1958, 51% accepted employment as General Staff Nurses at their Alma Mater and 50 of them joined the Alumnae Association.

In January, the Chicago Hospital Council sponsored a student nurse uniform fashion show at the annual meeting held at the Congress Hotel. Over thirty schools of nursing of the Chicago area participated, including Augustana. Each school was asked to have a student model the original uniform of their school and the present day uniform. A freshman student, Judith Enoksen, using pictures of the class of 1896 made the uniform and modeled it. The dainty and beautiful cap was made by Mrs. Edith Swanson, '20.

Mary Frey, Director of Nursing, sent the following report to the Alumnae Association. In July, the students were placed on a 40-hour week (class and practice). Many improvements were made in the school. Books and charts were updated and classrooms were added. A new Bell-Howell silent-sound movie projector was purchased to replace the old one. The school library consisting of five rooms on the first floor of the nurse's residence was upgraded. As of December 31st we had 1,558 books and instructional materials in the library. Of the 248 persons employed in the Nursing Department on December 31st, 117 were graduate and/or registered nurses, of which 59% were Augustana graduates.

In the past year we opened negotiations with the American Nurses' Association for graduate nurses on a visitor's exchange basis. Two nurses from the Philippine Islands each accepted a six months' assignment here, one in Obstetrics and Gynecology and the other in Surgery. At that time we had graduate nurses on our staff from England, Sweden, Germany, Norway, Philippine Islands, Chile, Argentina and China.

On Sunday afternoon, March 8, 1959 at 3:00 o'clock a short service of dedication for the new surgery was held in the Chapel of St. John at Augustana Hospital. The service was attended by a large congregation of hospital personnel, staff doctors and their families and Augustana friends. The service, led by Augustana's Chaplain, Daniel Sandstedt, included a Dedicatory Address by Dr. O. V. Anderson, President of the Central Conference of the Augustana Lutheran Church and greetings from Mr. E. G. Erickson, President of the Hospital Board, Dr. C. A. Hedberg, Chief of Staff, Mr. M. H. Hough, Administrator, and Dr. A. Howard Weeg, President of the Illinois Synod of the United Lutheran Church. A lovely solo was offered by Suzanne Nuske S.N. and Benediction was offered by Augustana's Assistant Chaplain, John Benson. After the service all visitors were welcomed to inspect the new addition.

In the early 50's, the Chicago Fresh Air Hospital for tubercular patients found that due to new techniques their facilities were no longer needed in Chicago. The Board of Directors of that hospital elected to give all of their assets, including a good deal of real estate, to a cause that would be perpetuated through the years. In December of 1955 these assets were turned over to Augustana Hospital. After a mortgage was paid the real estate was sold for $785,000.00, almost the exact cost of the new addition.

The new addition consisted of two floors; Four West housed the Surgical Department and Five West housed the X-Ray and Pathology Departments, the Laboratory, a Cardiac Catheterization Station and a Respiratory Testing Center. All of the units were designed with the advanced techniques of brain, bone and lung surgery and especially heart surgery in mind. Both floors were air-conditioned and sound-proofed.

The Surgical Department included ten operating rooms, all tiled in pastel green. The rooms were equipped with modern lighting, built-in x-ray projectors, piped-in oxygen and suction plus other modern equipment too numerous to mention. A special Cystoscopic room included its own drainage system and another room had its own x-ray unit. Automatic instrument sterilizers and cabinet warmers for saline, blankets, etc. were also provided. Another innovation was a new transformer located in the basement for use in case of power failure.

The staff doctors claimed that Augustana now had the most modern Surgical Department in Chicago. (They should know since they helped design it.) The first surgery in the new operating room, a Caesarian Section, was performed on April 22, 1959, by Dr. William Browne.

During the first quarter century of the hospital's existence, 27,484 patients were cared for; in the second quarter century 115,182 patients were cared for; and in the third quarter century 202,910 patients were cared for. A grand total of 345,576 patients who received more than 3,750,000 days of hospital care, for an average stay of 11 days.

In 1959, more than 25,000 persons made use of the hospital's services in the course of the year. Of this total, more than 10,000 persons were admitted for regular hospitalization; the balance consisted of patients who came to the hospital for various kinds of laboratory examination, X-ray examination and treatment, physiotherapy, first aid, etc. There were, for example, 16,840 such patient visits in 1958.

The School of Nursing graduated its first class of 8 in 1896. The class of 1959 numbered 57, bringing the number of Augustana graduates to a total of 2,203. The school was fully accredited. Over 200 medical technicians and 300 clergymen were also trained at Augustana.

Patients of all races and national origins, whether rich or poor, received care. For those who could pay nothing, or only in part, the hospital rendered free service to a total of $3,000,000.00. This was made possible in part by gifts, legacies and fundraising efforts totaling approximately $2,000,000.00. Last year's benefit provided 750 days of free care at Augustana.

The Nightingale Service for the freshmen class was held March 15 in the Hospital Chapel. There was a very large crowd, with both the Chapel and classroom being filled. Two alumnae nurses who were mothers of two members of the class, were able to be there. This service climaxed successful performance by the freshmen students of their first six months in the School of Nursing. One of the highlights of the service, as in previous years, was the Nightingale Pledge, sung to the tune of a Scottish chant. It was not a capping service, as the students now received their cap in the beginning of their first year when they received their uniform. Our new "Need No Starch Cap" was now available for $2.50.

The Convention of the National League for Nursing, was held in Philadelphia May 11th through the 15th. A junior student, Donna Jones of Preston, Iowa, attended, representing the Student Association and a senior student, Marjorie Johnson of Dixon, Illinois, attended as an officer of the State Student Nurse Association. The Director of Nursing also attended.

On May 18, 1959 two members of the freshman class from Augustana were elected to office in the First District of the Student Nurse Association of Illinois. Miss Karilyn Sterrenberg was elected Vice President and Miss Ruth Tronet Treasurer.

The Nursing student's Chorus gave two public performances. They sang for the All Chicago Luther Youth Lenten Vesper Service at the Rockefeller Chapel and at the Civic Opera House for the Women of Chicago, under the direction of the Salvation Army.

Miss Siri Persson, '28, membership chairman, reported that the entire class of 1959 joined the Alumnae Association. This was the year of the sixty-fifth anniversary of Augustana Hospital School of Nursing. At the founding of the hospital, February 28, 1882, a Charter was issued authorizing the hospital, "to train well qualified nurses." The School of Nursing endeavored to meet this call and challenge since its inception in 1894.

The first class, consisting of eight student nurses enrolled early in the fall of 1894. The course was two years in length, including one month of probation. Requirements at this time were meager, for there were no "standard-setting" bodies either on a state or national level. Training schools then in existence conducted nursing programs in keeping with the needs of the hospitals with which they were identified. Doctors were the first teachers of nurses as well as our first writers of textbooks for nurses. Much emphasis was given to learning from the doctors and from working with and observing older nurses. Interest in the education of the nurse was characteristic of the medical staff of Augustana Hospital throughout the history of the school.

Augustana nurses have been known to serve on many fronts of disaster and war, including the Spanish-American War, the flood of Dayton, Ohio, the San Francisco earthquake, the Eastland Disaster on the Chicago River, and later in World Wars I and II. A number also responded to the call of the mission field. [Our Graduates also served in Korea, Viet Nam and Desert Storm.]

The School of Nursing believed its function was to serve God where He presented himself for man's service—a specific form of that service being to care for the sick and disabled. The faculty accepted this challenge and endeavored to operate a curriculum open to change and new knowledge, challenging the student to achieve satisfaction professionally and personally. The aim of the School of Nursing was to select young women with an aptitude for nursing, and provide such an environment and experience as would help them develop their potentials for professional nursing.

The School offered both the diploma and degree programs. The basic three year diploma program included instruction and practice in medical and surgical nursing, and obstetrics in the home school. Pediatrics, psychiatry and tuberculosis nursing were acquired through affiliation. In 1958, psychiatric experience became a requirement of all schools of nursing in the United States. At this time, Augustana students affiliated with the Veterans Administration Hospital, Downey, Illinois. Affiliation with the Chicago Visiting Nurse Association was offered as an elective. In 1959, a tuition charge of $50 per student was made by Childrens' Memorial Hospital. Board, room and laundry continued to be provided by C.M.H. Expenses to the students for the three years at Augustana were, first year $323.00, second year $92.00 and the third year $85.00.

The degree program was in affiliation with Augustana College located in Rock Island, Illinois. The program was four and one half years, consisting of two academic years, one summer of college work, and two and one half years at the hospital where practice was obtained in the clinical areas. Upon completion of the program the student was awarded the Diploma in Nursing and the Bachelor of Science degree. The first students in the newly arranged program enrolled in the fall of 1959.

On September 3, 1958, eighty-eight students enrolled, which was the largest single class ever to enroll in the history of the school. The School of Nursing had steadily moved forward over the years, and much credit goes to the early leaders of nursing, the doctors, the administrative body and the devoted church leaders.

On September 9, 1959 we enrolled 84 students in the School of Nursing, the second largest class in history. A few figures revealed some interesting things about the class. They came from six states: Illinois, Michigan, Minnesota, Indiana, Iowa and Wisconsin. Fifty-one or 60% were from Illinois, with twenty-seven from Chicago, Michigan was second having twenty-one. Of the group, four were born outside the United States: representative of Cuba, Germany, Latvia and Nigeria, West Africa. Twelve had some college preparation ranging from one course to two years. Thirty-two students, or 38% of the class were recipients of scholarships of amounts ranging from $100.00 to $500.00. Ten of the group received $100.00 each from the $1,000.00 given by the Women's Auxiliary of Augustana Hospital and five were granted $100.00 each from a scholarship fund created by the Board of Directors of the Hospital. Many of the remaining scholarships were from civic organizations of the communities in which the students resided.

Table 3.1
Curriculum: Summary of Instruction (First Year — First Term)

| Subject | Lect. & Discussion | Lab (L) Dem (D) Clinical (CL) Conference (CF) | Total Hours | Weeks of Clinical Experience |
|---|---|---|---|---|
| Anatomy & Physiology | 58 | 46 (L) | 104 | |
| Chemistry | 42 | 30 (L) | 72 | |
| Microbiology (Cont. 2nd term) | 20 | 20 (L) | 40 | |
| Fundamentals of Nursing | 64 | 56 (L) (D) 72 (Cl. Exp.) | 192 | |
| Sociology | 32 | | 32 | |
| Professional Adjustments I | 18 | | 18 | |
| Pharmacology I | 12 | 12 (L) | 24 | |
| Nutrition | 32 | 12 (L) | 44 | |
| Introduction to Medical Science | 20 | 4 (L) | 24 | |
| Christianity I | 16 | | 16 | |
| Total | 314 | 252 | 566 | 26 weeks 2 wks. Vac. |

On Monday, October 19, 1959 the faculty of the Augustana Hospital School of Nursing gave a "Uniform Tea" in honor of the day when the new students wore their uniforms for the first time. Fruit punch and coffee were served from the attractive table; the centerpiece was a doll in a nurse's uniform.

Table 3.2
Curriculum: Summary of Instruction (First Year — Second Term)

| Subject | Lect. & Discussion | Lab (L) Dem (D) Clinical (CL) Conference (CF) | Total Hours | Weeks of Clinical Experience |
|---|---|---|---|---|
| Microbiology (con't.) | 12 | 12 (L) | 24 | |
| History of Nursing | 32 | | 32 | |
| Psychology | 32 | | 32 | |
| Pharmacology II | 32 | | 32 | |
| Diet Therapy | 16 | 8 (L) | 24 | 4 |
| Medical-Surgical Nursing I 158 hours. *Units 1–5* Nursing Rm.) in conditions of the Respiratory. Circulatory, Gastrointestinal, Endocrine, and Nervous Systems | 84 | | 84 | 6 2 (R. |
| *Unit 6* Surgical Technique - 16 hrs. Laboratory Instruction during Clinical experience; includes a Unit on Anesthesiology | 8 | 16 (D) | 24 | 8 |
| *Unit 7* Nursing in conditions of the Musculoskeletal System (Orthopedics) | 16 | 2 (D) | 18 | 2 |
| Medical-Surgical Ward Classes *(Units 1-7)* | | 32 | 32 | |
| Christianity II | 16 | | 16 | |
| Total | 248 | 70 | 318 | 22 weeks 2 wks. Vac. |

Table 3.3
Curriculum: Summary of Instruction (Second Year — First Term)

| Subject | Lect. & Discussion | Lab (L) Dem (D) Clinical (CL) Conference (CF) | Total Hours | Weeks of Clinical Experience |
|---|---|---|---|---|
| Medical-Surgical Nursing II 106 hrs. *Unit 1* Nursing in conditions of the Urinary System (Urology) | 16 | | 16 | 10 2 |
| *Unit 2* Nursing in conditions of the Eye, Ear, Nose and Throat | 16 | | 16 | |
| *Unit 3* Communicable Disease Nursing Acute Communicable (16) Tuberculosis (8) Venereal Diseases (8) | 32 | | 32 | |
| Medical-Surgical Ward Classes *(Units 1–3)* | | 42 (CL) | 42 | |
| Maternity Nursing | 44 | 36 (CL) | 80 | 12 |
| Christianity III | 16 | | 16 | |
| Total | 124 | 78 | 202 | 24 wks. 2 wks. C.S. 26 weeks |

Table 3.4
Curriculum: Summary of Instruction (Second Year — Second Term)

| Subject | Lect. & Discussion | Lab (L) Dem (D) Clinical (CL) Conference (CF) | Total Hours | Weeks of Clinical Experience |
|---|---|---|---|---|
| Medical-Surgical Nursing II (Con't). 61 hours. *Unit 4* Nursing in Conditions of the Reproductive System: Gynecology | 16 | | 16 | 7 2 |
| *Unit 5* Nursing in conditions of the Skin (Dermatology); Integumentary System | 18 | | 18 | |
| Medical-Surgical Ward Classes *(Units 4–5)* | | 27 (CL) | 27 | |
| Pediatrics (Affiliation) | 60 | 60 (CL) | 120 | 13 |
| Total | 94 | 87 | 181 | 22 wks. 4 wks. Vac. |

Table 3.5
Curriculum: Summary of Instruction (Third Year — First and Second Terms)

| Subject | Lect. & Discussion | Lab (L) Dem (D) Clinical (CL) Conference (CF) | Total Hours | Weeks of Clinical Experience |
|---|---|---|---|---|
| Medical-Surgical Nursing III *Unit 1* Emergency and Disaster Nursing | 14 | 10 | 24 | 30 |
| Medical-Surgical Ward Classes | | 48 (CL) | 48 | |
| *Unit 2* Principles of Administration in a Medical-Surgical Unit | 8 | | 8 | |
| Tuberculosis Nursing (if Public Health Nursing is taken, the hours vary) | 42 | 10 (L) 24 (CF) | 76 | 6 |
| Psychiatry | 90 | 48 (CL D) 4 (CF) | 142 | 12 |
| Professional Adjustments II (Trends in Nursing) | 32 | | 32 | |
| Total | 186 | 144 | 330 | 48 4 wks. |
| Vac. | | | | |
| GRAND TOTAL | 966 | 631 | 1597 | 156 wks. for the 3 yrs. |

Table 3.6
Summary of Assignments in the Curriculum (Practice and Vacation)

| | Weeks | Days |
|---|---|---|
| First Year (First Term) — 28 wks. | | |
| Class and Laboratory Practice | 26 | 182 |
| Vacation | 2 | 14 |
| | | |
| First Year (Second Term) — 24 wks. | | |
| Medical-Surgical Nursing I — (18 wks.) | | |
| Medical Nursing | 3 | 21 |
| Surgical Nursing | 3 + 1 d. | 22 |
| Orthopedic Nursing | 2 | 14 |
| Operating Room | 8 | 56 |
| Recovery Room | 2 | 14 |
| Diet Therapy | 4 | 28 |
| Vacation | 2 | 14 |
| | | |
| Second Year — 52 wks. | | |
| Medical-Surgical Nursing II — (19 wks.) | | |
| Medical Nursing | 9 + 1 d. | 64 |
| Surgical Nursing | 10 | 70 |
| Urological Nursing | 2 | 14 |
| Gynecological Nursing | 2 | 14 |
| Central Service | 2 | 14 |
| Maternity Nursing | 12 | 84 |
| Pediatric Nursing | 13 | 91 |
| Vacation | 4 | 28 |
| | | |
| Third Year — 52 wks. | | |
| Medical-Surgical Nursing III — (28 wks.) | | |
| Medical Nursing | 14 | 98 |
| Surgical Nursing | 14 + 1 d. | 99 |
| Tuberculosis Nursing | 6 | 42 |
| Psychiatric Nursing | 12 | 84 |
| Vacation | 4 | 28 |
| | | |
| TOTAL | 156 + 3 d. | 1,095 |

# CHAPTER IV

# THE SIXTIES

A committee was formed to revise the by-laws of the Alumnae Association. The following changes were approved by the membership.

Article X, Sect. 5—"only members are allowed to attend any business meetings."

Sect. 6 be added: "The Director of Nurses shall be an Ex Officio member unless she is an Alumnus."

"In lieu of addition to by-law, Article 3, Section 4,—'consecutive'should be added after "'30 and 40'—years," the Board of Directors has voted to allow everyone the opportunity of paying back any years' dues not paid previously at the current rate ($4.00). This MUST be paid by June 1, 1960. No back dues may be paid after this date, in order to have consecutive membership."

Statistics as compiled in the Annual Report of the Nursing Department was of interest to Alumnae Nurses:

a) The School of Nursing Library had 1698 bound volumes. The library showed continued use evidenced by increased circulations. Our greatest need in relation to the Library was more space and larger seating capacity.

b) Of the 121 graduate/registered nurses on the staff as of December 31, 1959, 68% were Augustana graduates, an increase of 9% over the previous year.

c) Volunteers from the Women's Auxiliary gave a total of 3228 hours in care to patients and in working in Central Service.

The following appeal was again made through the "Augie Nurse".

"We need your help at Augustana Hospital. We need general staff nurses, full and part time. WE WILL GIVE PREFERENCE TO OUR OWN GRADUATES. Write or call: Miss Bertha E. Klauser, Acting Director, 411 W. Dickens Avenue, Chicago 14, Ill. Tel. Div. 8–1000, Ext. 245."

[In late 1961, a letter was received from Madeline Roessler, R.N., President of the First District of the Illinois Nurses Association, stressing the need for general duty nurses in the Army Nurse Corps. Information could be obtained from Lt. Colonel Thelma Munn, Fifth Army Headquarters, Chicago. She or a member of her staff, would be willing to present the facts surrounding the Army's need for nurses.]

The American Nurse Association Convention, held at Miami Beach in May 1960, with a registration of 6460, was a momentous affair. The convention focus was on "Improvement of Practice." At the opening session, a telegram from President Eisenhower was read. One of the highlights was the opening address of Dr. John Krout, Vice President of Columbia University, New York, on "Professional Education and the Humanities." Much discussion centered around Federal Health and Old Age Insurance legislation and the Forand Bill. Perhaps the greatest experience for nurses was the realization that, though we think that our problems are unique, others appear to be beset by the same identical difficulties.

Baccalaureate and Graduation services for the thirty-nine graduates of the School of Nursing were held Sunday, September 11, 1960. Baccalaureate service was held in the St. Johns Chapel in the Hospital and Graduation service at the Evangelical Lutheran Saron Church with the reception following in the Parish Hall.

As of September 12, 1960, Miss Bertha Klauser was officially named Director of Nurses at Augustana. We were proud to have one of our own graduates in this high position.

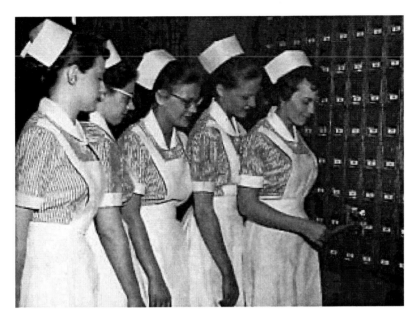

Student Nurses at their Mail Boxes

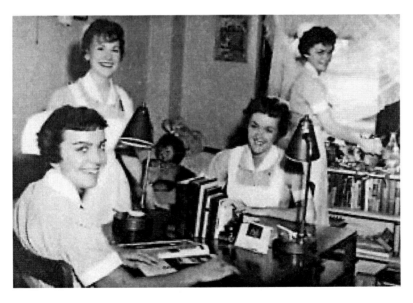

Student Nurses' Room, Circa 1960

The following "Philosophy and Purpose of the School of Nursing" was taken from the 1960 Announcement of the School of Nursing.

The purpose of the School is to select young women with an aptitude for nursing and help them develop their potentials through guidance and direction of the faculty, in a permissive atmosphere, by providing environment and experiences that will accomplish the following:

1. Favor the acquisition of knowledge, skills, attitude and understanding basic to safe, intelligent and comprehensive nursing care.
2. Encourage participation in health teaching and in measures used for the prevention of disease.
3. Broaden one's understanding of the physical, spiritual, mental and social aspects of illness and of the community's resources available for assistance where such problems arise.
4. Provide direction for making satisfactory adjustments in personal and professional matters such as will give emphasis to social and cultural standards, thus promoting high ideals of American womanhood.
5. Provide such instruction in the Christian faith as shall parallel maturing professional knowledge with understanding and practice of the Christian life and worship.
6. Encourage critical and constructive thinking and provide channels for its testing and communication.

It was expected that nurses graduating from this type of program would be enabled to render efficient service in caring for the acutely and chronically ill in general hospitals or allied institutions. Emphasis was given to community nursing.

Sixty-eight students enrolled in the School of Nursing on September 13, 1960. They came from four states: Illinois 48 (20 of these from Chicago); Michigan 14; Indiana 5; Wisconsin 1.

Two Augie seniors, Marilyn Nasberg and Karilyn Sterrenberg, were elected to state offices at the 10th Annual Student Nurses Association of Illinois convention, held in the Pick Congress hotel on October 8, 9 and 10. Another Augustana student, junior, Nancy Johanson, also held a district office. The 1960 convention theme was "Watch Us Grow: Today We Follow, Tomorrow We Lead."

Another Christmas season was launched on December 7, 1960, when approximately 165 alumnae members heralded the festive season in the St. Johns Chapel of Augustana Hospital. Pastor Daniel Sandstedt led the prayers and Viola Anderson, '34, President, welcomed all the members.

Following the Chapel service, a tasty Smorgasbord was served by the Lakeview Catering Service. The roast beef, chicken and the delicious complements to the Smorgasbord were delightfully enjoyed by everyone. The food was eaten in the hospital cafeteria, which was set up with red candles on the tables and lighted Santa Clauses, reindeer and carolers in the windows. Eating by candlelight supplied the mood for friends to chat about many memories. The Social Arrangements Committee excelled themselves for the 1960 Christmas festivities. Each member was given a lapel pin of two lighted candles, which was made by the Committee. It will be long remembered throughout the years.

In 1961, Public Health affiliation was mandatory for Bachelor of Science Nursing students. The pressure from collegiate schools necessitated the Visiting Nurse Association to discontinue affiliation with diploma programs. In 1962 the State of Illinois' financial status caused the discontinuation of the tuberculosis affiliation.

In 1963–1964, students were given one week at the Chicago Maternity Center to observe home deliveries and to obtain clinical experience.

A student loan fund had been established by Mr. and Mrs. Clarence E. Balliett in memory of their daughter Clarice Mae, a former student in the School of Nursing who was fatally injured in an auto accident. Loans were issued in amounts of $50.00 to $200.00. Requests concerning the loan were made to the Director of Nursing.

Scholarships were sometimes available through the generosity of various civic groups and the Women's Auxiliary of the Hospital. Applicants who had attained a good scholastic record

Table 4.1
Expenses: An Approximation of Expenses for the Three-Year Program
\* Total of $500 Is Distributed As Follows:

| Items | First Year | | Second Year | | Third Year | |
|---|---|---|---|---|---|---|
| | *Amount* | *Payable* | *Amount* | *Payable* | *Amount* | *Payable* |
| Pre-Nursing and Guidance Exam. | $10.00 | To N.L.N. when apply-ing for Exam | | | | |
| Registration Fee | 5.00 | When notified of Adm. to School of Nursing | | | | |
| Tuition | 125.00 | Date of Enrollment | $75.00 | Sept. '60 | $75.00 | Sept., '61 |
| Textbooks | 70.00 | Date of Enrollment | $17.00 | Sept. '60 | $10.00 | Sept., '61 |
| Uniforms (Incl. Cape, Caps Bandage Scissors) | 96.00 | Date of Enrollment | | | | |
| Student Act. Fee | 15.00 | | | | | |
| Key Deposit | 2.00 | | | | | |
| TOTAL | $323.00 | | $92.00 | | $85.00 | |

\* Effective with Class enrolling in 1959.

and were in need of assistance to finance their nursing program were at liberty to request a scholarship in their preliminary correspondence with the Director of Nursing.

The Nursing Students' Association had established a scholarship fund and issued a scholarship each year.

The Bess Lang Memorial Award of $25.00 was presented at the annual Commencement program to the nurse in the graduating class whose record indicated highest achievement in Nursing, which included not only academic standing, but sympa-

thetic understanding of the patient, practical ability, professional attitude and conduct.

The Alumnae Association of the Augustana Hospital School
of Nursing offered an annual Scholarship to a graduate nurse
who wished to further her education. [In 1962, this was named
the Ellis J. Walker Scholarship Fund.]

According to the by-laws of the Alumnae Association:

> The committee on the Educational Scholarship Fund shall consist of the Presi-
> dent of the Association, Administrator of the Hospital, Director of the School of
> Nursing, Assistant Director of Nursing Education and three members of the
> Alumnae Association, one elected at each annual election to serve for a period of
> three years.

The Alumnae Association of the Augustana Hospital School
of Nursing offered two $400.00 scholarships in 1961. Appli-
cants had to meet the following requirements: must have been
a member of the Alumnae Association in good standing; was
applying for a scholarship in order to further her nursing education; must have been employed for a period of at least one
year.

The Alumnae received the following correspondence from
Mr. M.H.Hough, Hospital Administrator:

> I have your letter of March 1,1961, in which you tell of the Alumnae
> Association's presentation of $2500.00 to the hospital for use in the Pulmonary
> Function and Heart Catheterization Laboratory.
> This venture of the hospital is one of pioneering in a new field which nor-
> mally would be done by a much larger institution than ours, and it will, there-
> fore, be a considerable financial burden to the hospital and its patients. We are,
> accordingly, more than usually grateful for the interest of the Alumnae Associa-
> tion and for this financial assistance.

Miss Bertha E. Klauser, Director, School of Nursing and
Nursing Services, told the Alumnae of the changes and improvements at Augustana Hospital during the past year. She
pointed out how large the hospital family had grown, the payroll figures showed 267 nursing personnel and an average of
700 employees at the hospital.

For the 11th consecutive year, the Augustana graduates living on the west coast gathered at a luncheon and style show held at Bullock's Wilshire Tea Room.

Captain Betty J. Rothenberg Lynch, '44 Army Nurse Career counselor with the Army Nurse Procurement Program in Los Angeles, was selected "Army Nurse of the Year" for the Greater Los Angeles area by the William Sullivan American Legion Post 617, of Long Beach, California.

The William Sullivan Gold Medallion was instituted to honor the Nursing Profession, was given each year to an outstanding local nurse, alternating between military and civilian.

Captain Lynch entered the Army in January 1945, and after Officer Training at Camp McCoy, Wisconsin she was assigned to the 31st Field Hospital in Okinawa.

The hospital was 150 yards back of the front line. Casualties were carried by litter bearers directly to the hospital that was subject to small arms and artillery fire during daylight and bombing during darkness. Captain Lynch disregarded her own safety and exposed herself to three major typhoons by leaving the protected area to secure medical supplies and water for the patients. Following the Armistice, Captain Lynch worked incessantly nursing the American Prisoners of war, who had been held in PW camps in Japan, preparing them for repatriation.

She returned to the United States in January 1946, and was separated from the Army in March 1946. She was awarded the Asiatic Pacific Ribbon with a Bronze Battle Star. During her eight years of civilian nursing, she distinguished herself by her voluntary and unselfish work among the sick and needy of the county, while continuing her studies at Baylor University in Waco, Texas.

Later she attended the University of California at Berkeley. While there she worked with Dr. Sterling Bunnell, Chief Consultant in Plastic Surgery, and world renowned for his work in plastic surgery of the hand. Captain Lynch designed and applied many new types of splints employed by Dr. Bunnell that were adopted by hospitals. Captain Lynch re-entered the Army in 1954. She served with the 2nd General Hospital in Landstuhl, Germany, for two years.

Upon her return to the States she attended a post-graduate course in obstetrics at Walter Reed Army Medical Center, Washington, D.C. She requested duty at Fort Benjamin Harrison, so that she could take advantage of a scholarship at Indiana University. She obtained a Bachelor's Degree in nursing, and was graduated in June, 1960.

In her capacity with the Army Nurse Procurement program she lectured in Southern California, Nevada and Arizona, presenting the history of nursing and the opportunities for qualified nurses.

In January of 1962, it was announced that Augustana Hospital School of Nursing had lost its National League for Nursing accreditation. We had been put on trial in 1956 and it would be at least two years before we could apply again. The NLN goals were extremely high, and we were commended in some areas. Some of the areas we needed to improve on were: ratio of instructors to students; faculty organization; and students only able to work on shifts where there was a clinical instructor. The loss of the accreditation did not affect the status of state accreditation, transferring to other schools for degrees, or state boards. The question arose regarding Augustana Hospital School of Nursing in relation to State Approval and Approval by the National League for Nursing. For clarification the following explanation was given:

State Approval is essential and Schools in Illinois are visited every two years. Approval by the National League for Nursing is not compulsory and schools desiring this rating apply voluntarily for a visitation. A survey is then made by one or more representatives of this organization. In August 1961, our school was visited and approved by the State of Illinois Department of Registration and Education.

Nurses graduating from a State Approved Diploma Program in Nursing such as that given at Augustana Hospital School of Nursing take the same State Board examination, may obtain licensure by endorsement in any state of the United States, are qualified for the same type of positions, and may enroll in the same college courses as the graduates from schools approved by the National League for Nursing. Our school, although not accredited by the organization, is a member of the National League for Nursing and receives its benefits, including counseling.

Augustana Hospital is fully approved by The Chicago Hospital Council, State of Illinois, American Medical Association, and Joint Commission for Accreditation of Hospitals. The purposes of this institution are: to give excellent care to the patient, to educate nurses, and to provide clinical training for medical interns, residents, theological students, chaplains and other hospital personnel.

The Board of Reviews of the Accreditation Survey mentioned that one of the areas for improvement was that of "initiating a plan for a follow-up study of the graduates of the School to assist in the evaluation of the adequacy of the program to meet the job demands of the graduate nurse."

The Alumnae members had previously asked what they could do to help the School and aid was being sought from the Alumnae Association as follows:

1. To assume the cost of the study, estimated at $100.00.
2. To appoint a committee to assist in formulating the questionnaire.
3. To help address envelopes.
4. To aid in tabulating results.

The Alumnae Association suggested the possibility of a nursery for employees' children, better lighting in the parking lot and someone to escort nurses to the bus as means to attract more nurses.

About 220 alumnae attended the Homecoming Tea in the Lila Pickhardt Lounge. The 61st Alumnae Banquet was held at 7:30 p.m. at the Furniture Club of America after a social hour with 212 alumnae attending the dinner. Rev. Dr. A.R.Kretzmann, the Chairman of the Nursing Advisory Committee of the Hospital Board, gave a short resume of the past standing of the School. Dr. Kretzmann explained the findings of the National League for Nursing Survey in September, 1961, and stressed education of student nurses rather than the ideal of service during the training days. To be able to achieve this standing Dr. Kretzmann called for loyalty of the Alumnae to the School and the Hospital. He appealed to them to either give time to the Hospital so that the patients can go on enjoying the best of nursing care and/or, if unable to do so, help to underwrite the added expense of student nurse education by donations to the Scholarship Fund. To comply with the National League for Nursing guidelines, incoming students were restricted from working p.m.'s and nights, therefore the following ad appeared in the Augie Nurse.

Augustana Nurses Want to Give Good Patient Care, but we need help. Won't you join us?

Openings for P.M. and Night Nurses in Intensive Care, Pediatrics, Orthopedics and Private Divisions.

Starting Salary $2.42 per hour.

Other positions also available.

Salary range for Staff Nurses, $4680-$5220 per year. Free Blue Cross. Paid vacation. Legal Holidays. Sick Leave. Retirement Plan.

At our Alumnae Meetings, we began using the following prayer written by Chaplain Daniel Sandstedt to open our meetings.

O God, our Gracious Heavenly Father, for Thy guidance and care we thank Thee. Thou has called us from many places and different tasks. We have been privileged to serve in many situations.

Bless us now as we meet together. Bless this organization as through it we maintain and renew our friendships. Bless also our efforts as we support and encourage the institution which has shared in all of our lives. Keep us willing to share and serve even as we have received and been served. Use us as Thy hands of healing in this world of suffering and pain.

Hear this our prayer in Jesus Name.

Amen.

Our Augustana nurses were encouraged to talk or write to their State Senator or Representative about the nursing revision bill in committee in Springfield. This was House Bill 143 with companion Bill 144.

Fact Sheet on HB143
Amendments to the Illinois Nursing Act

1.  Modernizes definitions of professional and practical nursing in line with current-day practice.
2.  Makes licensure mandatory for practical nurses.

    After July 1, 1965, all persons wishing to practice practical nursing must graduate from a school approved under the Illinois Nursing Act and pass a state licensing examination. Permits those now in practice to become licensed if they apply before July 1, 1965, and submit evidence of competence to practice.

    Permits those now in practice who do not meet the educational requirements of the law to become liscensed if they apply before July 1, 1965, and submit evidence of competence to practice.
3.  Changes requirements for licensure as a professional nurse:

    Removes minimum age and citizenship requirements. Removes requirement that professional nurse course be minimum of 3 calendar years in length. Length of course to be determined by the Committee of Nurse Examiners, within the Department of Registration and Education, which administers the law. Change is expected to help expand nurse supply by stimulating development of accelerated, 2-year junior college programs now operating in other states. Also provides for flexibility in 3-year hospital diploma schools of nursing.
4.  Changes requirements for licensure as a practical nurse: Candidates must have 2 years of high school, instead of minimum of 8 years of grammar school, removes age and citizenship requirement; deletes requirement that approved practical nurse course be minimum of one year in length.
5.  Adds provision that all schools of practical nursing are governed by the Act. Would make illegal, operation of the commercial schools of practical nursing, which offer

correspondence courses and sometimes classroom instruction.

6. Adds provision that all persons wishing to practice practical or professional nursing apply for a license and receive acknowledgement of application before accepting employment. Designed to aid licensing law enforcement.
7. Excuses nurses registered but not practicing in Illinois from renewal fee payment.
8. Requires Master's degree as minimum academic requirement for members of Committee of Nurse Examiners. Shortens terms from 5 to 3 years. Spells out duties. Upgrades educational requirements of professional nurse staff of Department, Registration and Education. [Now known as Department of Professional Regulation.]
9. Increases from 7 to 8 membership of advisory council representing public, general education and groups associated with nursing education. Shortens terms from 5 to 3 years.
10. Adds to causes for revocation or suspension of a license, unprofessional conduct and willful violation of the nursing act. Raises maximum fine from $500 to $1000.

Supporting Organizations:
Illinois Nurses' Association
Committee of Nurse Examiners
Illinois Hospital Association
Illinois League for Nursing
Illinois State Medical Society
Licensed Practical Nurse Association
Illinois Conference of Catholic Schools of Nursing

This bill was highly controversial. There was considerable opposition to this bill from nurses and also from citizens interested in nursing. The greatest opposition was to the removal of the requirement that the professional nurse course be a minimum of 3 calendar years in length. The argument of some was that it would downgrade nursing education in that a person who has average intelligence can read enough and cram enough to make the necessary passing grade on an examination; but this does not mean that they can perform on the same level as another student who has had both direct teaching and practice and theory. In order to practice excellence in nursing, the nurse must have an opportunity to develop skills, good judgment, tact, diplomacy and ethics as well as theory. It was common knowledge that there was a vast amount of new scientific information being discovered in all fields including the nursing profession. Due to this fact, teachers, pharmacists, doctors and all professions were increasing the length of time which they required to obtain degrees in their profession.

Another prime objection to the bill was the removal of the citizenship clause. A nurse who was not a U.S. citizen would not have the privilege of voting, holding office or being an active nurse in her nursing organizations. Another H.B. 165 was also written to remove the citizenship clause from the Illinois Nursing Act.

Mrs. Esther Nelson '28 reported that those who were working against HB 143 were primarily owners of some nursing homes, and representatives of commercial schools of practical nursing.

In recent years our hospital had grown in size, in service, and in numbers of people involved in its work. In 1961, several church groups with members and local congregations located from coast to coast in varying degrees of density, merged to form the nationwide church known as LCA, the Lutheran Church in America. The greater church was composed of 31 synods, in some cases having geographic boundaries the same as the larger states. In others, two or more states were included in one. Augustana Hospital was owned and operated by the Illinois Synod, which included all of the state of Illinois, as well as part of the state of Missouri. All of the congregations, in all of the merged churches in this geographic area numbered 350, instead of the former 160 congregations, which previously owned and operated Augustana Hospital. This increased number of congregations with 220,000 members was one way in which more people were involved in the work of Augustana. There were now more doctors, more patients, more nurses, and more helping hands throughout the hospital.

In September 1962, excavation began as the first step in a series of ten steps, which were to be completed in September, 1964. The hospital was to have a new heating plant, laundry, kitchen, cafeteria, out-patient and emergency room, and elevator. Alterations to improve the Coffee and Gift Shop, radiology, the Chaplain's Department, the pharmacy, and the business office were also planned. The heating plant and the laundry were completed and put into operation in November.

On December 8, 1962, our students, in costume, danced for the Swedish Day program at the Museum of Science and Industry.

A directive was sent to all students from Bertha Klauser, Director of Nursing, in April of 1963, regarding regulations about standards of dress.

In the Augustana Hospital School of Nursing Manual of Policies—Rules—Standards, page 4, item c, No. 3, it is stated: "The wearing of slacks or similar attire is not permitted anywhere in the hospital. The wearing of slacks will be permitted in the residence lounge only while waiting for escorts." All students were expected to adhere to the above regulations.

In May 1963, in an effort to avoid a Communist Government in Vietnam, the stalemate between the Allies broke and after religious flags were flown in the imperial city of Hue which the Buddhists protected, security troops moved in.

On July 4, the C.I.A. and State Department made plans and committed troops to provide leadership against the Communist Regime. The United States tried to impose our ideas and ideals on a country which was not only divided but not ready for change. President Kennedy stated that unless a greater effort was made to win popular support, we could not win the war.

The U.S. had been warned not to become involved in a war with Southeast Asia. There was no discipline or commitment in that war and we pulled out in April of 1975. It was an unpopular war. Americans had grown suspicious and resentful of events and of its own government. It was believed that due to chemical warfare of Agent Orange, many birth defects had resulted in the offspring of service personnel.[29]

[In the December 1966, issue of "Chart," the official publication of the Illinois Nurses' Association, there was the following appeal from the Agency for International Development, U.S. Department of State. Civilian Registered Nurses are needed in Vietnam. Difficult, possibly hazardous, working conditions; long hours, great responsibility, in remote locations. To work with international medical teams in provincial hospitals of South Vietnam, treating civilian war casualties and villagers needing medical attention, as part of U.S. A.I.D. program.

Applicants must be U.S. citizens for at least 5 years, without dependents, physically fit, and willing to serve abroad for at least 18 months.

Requires Registered Nurse Certificate and at least 2 years ward nursing experience.

Salary range: $6,500-$10,000, plus 25% hardship bonus, housing allowance, and other benefits.

Interviews will be held January 16 through 21 from 11:00 a.m. to 7:00 p.m. at 623 South Wabash Avenue, Chicago, Illinois. After January 21, information may be obtained by writing the Far East Recruitment Division, Agency for International Development, Washington, D.C.]

A Safety Committee at the hospital working in conjunction with the fire department, had a yearly teaching-learning-doing session with the first year students. Heat detectors and alarm

---

29. U.S. News & World Report, Oct. 1983.

giving devices were strategically located both in the hospital and the residence which gave a greater feeling of security.

On October 23, 1963, the Safety Committee sponsored a fire demonstration presented by the Chicago Fire Department. Use of various fire extinguishers and methods of moving patients were demonstrated by student nurses. The fire department also demonstrated the use of its equipment, including evacuation by the use of a snorkel.

Augustana Hospital began a Bowling League in September of 1963. The eight teams met each Monday at 5:30 p.m. The names of the teams were: Cherry Pickers, Unmentionables, V.I.P.'s, Dafs, Clean Sweepers, Jets, Alley Kats and Pillpushers.

The following item was in a December issue of Time Magazine. "A team of surgeons at Chicago's Augustana Hospital has been using autotransfusion for more than two years, with excellent results and no ill effects." The possibility was discussed as long ago as 1883. "Autotransfusion remains a relative rarity," said a leading transfusion authority, "because many doctors still don't know about it." The Augustana team consists of Drs. William Dalessandro, Hiram T. Langston and George Milles."

Esther Schreib '31, wrote the following article for the Augustana Nurse entitled, "Something Old and Something New": [After many years of working in the Recovery Room at Augustana Hospital, Esther J. Schreib retired from nursing in 1971. She died in 1996.]

Wednesday afternoon, March 4, 1964, while returning a patient to her room from recovery, Sven (he probably would not answer if we addressed him as Mr. Lindquist) our orderly and I passed the 8th floor desk. The graduate said, "I'll be right with you." In reply, "You needn't hurry, we'll manage nicely getting her into bed." As we continued on we saw what looked like a strange bed in 822. When we got into 833B there was another of the new type beds I had never seen before. If her husband had not been there to show me how to bring it to cart level, I would have had to call floor personnel. That started a thorough looking over of the three [types of] beds they have on 8th. I began to reminisce about the long way we had come. Take the backrests alone—the portable kind we used in the

Old West Building; (those we would lift in place); to the kind a patient could lean forward, hold onto the loop at the side of the bed and the spring let it join your back. The only trouble with that was the knees also came up, which was not too good for orthopedic patients. Next came the crank model for altering positions and bed levels. Now it is electric and the patient has access to the dial as desired, again an improvement over the push-pull buttons alongside the bed. Central location of the electrical mechanism provides storage area for the side rails which are permanently stored underneath and just swing into position. Remember the boards with metal permanent fixtures that took off the bed's finish each time they were put on or taken off? Then came the all metal swing type with the spring controlled holders—stretch and pull. We got our exercise as well as many a blood blister. Those of us who have worked with all kinds are probably most appreciative of the latest model as well as the patient. So this is the new number AMP MultiMatic all Electric Hospital Bed. The patient control switch is readily accessible to either patients or nurses. A lock feature prevents operation of the bed by the patient if so desired by hospital personnel. Whenever oxygen is being used, the patient's control switch MUST be locked in its storage bracket on the bed frame. There are eight motorizing actions. Every desired position of the bed is operated smoothly, quietly, electrically. The vertical height of the bed can be adjusted from 5" to 30". The adjustment to a low chair height assists patients in entering or leaving the bed. Hospital personnel can conveniently attend to the patient's needs or make the bed without stooping or bending. Three piece posture, firm mattress panel, eliminates the need for boards and is also easily cleaned. Non-skid rubber strips are provided to aid in maintaining the mattress and bed clothes in position. There is a choice of head and foot panels in wood which has the versatility of being either "left or right handed" by being placed on either side of the bed.

Have you heard that the former surgical dressings rooms are no more? They had made way for an elevator shaft. Each floor gave up Room 20 for that purpose. Ah, that old surgical dressing room, how many received burned arms attempting to reach the gauges in the sterilizers. P.M. service had the privilege of making sterile water. Filling was slow for it passed through filters. It was always our aim to get them to the right level and never allow them to blow off as we sterilized.

There have been strange noises, plaster dust, odd looking makeshift enclosures, etc., as the men have worked, breaking through the floors and putting in the new elevator next to the old freight elevator. The old chimney has also been torn down. Some day we will have trouble remembering how it used to be before they started renovating.

I think we take all our disposable equipment for granted. Only to mention a few; syringes come complete with needle (two, six and twelve cc), tuberculin, insulin and needles of all sizes come by the 100 per box. Remember the time-consuming Bunsen burner? We had to boil up needles after having checked them for burrs, sharpened up and wired when not in use. Disposable also are rectal and levine tubes and catheters, both urinary and nasal, douche, bladder irrigation and spinal puncture trays. Many medications come put up in syringes. There are still plenty of places that do not have all of our conveniences.

In the basement just off the boiler room at the end of the hall stands a disposable can and a glass machine. It is a bit of a din when this is in operation. It reduces that type of waste to compact bulk. [A garbage compactor.]

In September 1962, a small pressure chamber was installed on the 9th floor. The Mist $O_2$ Gen Aquasteam Aerosol $O_2$ tent was purchased and it was felt that these fine mist $O_2$ tents were a great boon to the patient who was forced to be confined within one, especially children.

The Hyperbaric Chamber on the 4th floor was put into use in the spring of 1964, with some patients coming to the new location for their 10th and 11th treatment. The Hyperbaric Chamber was a steel vessel in which atmospheric pressure could be raised or lowered by air compressors. This was used to treat patients with circulatory or respiratory problems and to provide hi-oxygen environments for certain medical treatments and operations. [At the May 1965, Alumnae Association meeting, Dr. VanEck of Lutheran General Hospital spoke about the Hyperbaric $O_2$ Chamber. He was chief investigator for the high pressure oxygen research and therapy program.]

The following departments were now on the 4th floor. Electro encephalogram, inhalation office and storage, surgery clinical supervisor's office, Hyperbaric Room, Recovery Room, surgical dressing room, and Intensive Care Area. The remainder of the floor, rooms 430 through 434 were patient rooms which had piped in oxygen and wall suction.

The old surgery wing on the north side through the 1st amphitheater was now physiotherapy. Beyond that was linen sorting and pack making, a waiting room, emergency room and cast room. This brings us to the automatic door of surgery which covers the west side. Coming east along the south side— Pathology laboratory, Drs. locker and shower room, coffee, dictating lounge, nurses lounge, pharmacy and locker area.

The year of 1963, was one of continued growth for Augustana Hospital, with an all-time high in admissions and total patient days. During 1963 we admitted 10,891 patients from 26 different states for 105,101 patient days, took 70,000 X-rays, served 500,000 meals, used 30,000 bars of soap, washed 1,650,000 pounds of laundry, delivered 971 babies, conducted 118,014 laboratory tests, performed 5,602 operations, gave 7,590 physiotherapy treatments and were blessed with 19,674 hours of volunteer time. During its 80-year history, Augustana had admitted 391,944 patients and given 4,245,704 days of care.

Not all of our nurses worked in this type of hospital as demonstrated by the following. Maryann Welton Sharifi '60 wrote an interesting letter from Iran, where she and her husband were working at the Oil Company Hospital, Marjed-i-Sulaiman, Iran.

1964 has brought us some unusually cold weather for the Southern part of Iran. We have had freezing temperatures destroying most of our local crops. (The summer months have temperatures of 110° F. to 120° F.) We have also just had our first snow fall for a record-breaking 40 years!! We also had a small earthquake the day after Christmas. Dr. Sharifi is the first Pediatrician that has ever been to this area. The mortality rate amongst the Pediatric cases dropped 33% about 2 mo. after he started work here and has progressively improved, but it has been a job for him. He has had to make up his own spinal tap trays, sub-dural tap trays, mix all his own IV solutions, has just received his first incubator and is still working without any electrolyte equipment. Our first child was born here a year ago last December, a girl named Mithra. It was an experience to raise her here since baby food and clothing were not available but we had a good time compensating and making our own. My first 6 mo. here were very crowded with learning the language and customs. I can happily say that everyone has been kind to me and accepted my differences. Nowadays, we're looking forward to the arrival of another baby in June and hoping to be able to spend Christmas in the States this 1964.

Another interesting letter was received from Marge Ness Scheel, '50, and her husband, Dr. Richard Scheel from Soddu, Wolamo, Ethiopia, where they were missionaries.

Christmas was a very happy occasion here. The children were all home and enjoyed celebrating Dan's 12th birthday on Dec. 24. We took all the boys on an overnight camping trip, saw gazelle, pig and even hippo. We shot a 150 lb. wart hog with huge tusks. It gave plenty of meat for the whole station. Miriam enjoyed baking in the kitchen. On a wood stove this can be quite a feat. Becky got a nurse's kit for Christmas, so I had a new assistant for 4 weeks. Stephen gave us our biggest scare, he was real sick with pneumonia for five days. He's back to health now, for which we praise God. Bible conference for national Christians has just finished, with as many as 6000 at some of the meetings. What seemed most significant to us was the giving. Some folk took off their coats, others their shoes, in order to make an offering for the work of their national evangelists. And it was done in such a spirit of gladness!

46 more beds were added to our hospital, increasing patient capacity to 101. Ethiopia and Somalia are much in the news. It is a border problem and does not affect us here at Soddu. Our former station of Kallafo is affected and most of the missionary staff have been evacuated from there. Pray that peace will soon come and this border dispute settled. Recently 18 of our student dressers (male nurses) completed their training program and successfully passed their government exam. We feel this is one of our greatest ministries, training Ethiopian young men to give medical and spiritual help to their own people and thus multiply our services.

On January 8 and 9, 1964, a survey was conducted at Augustana Hospital by the Joint Commission on Accreditation of Hospitals. The hospital was accredited for a period of 3 years or until a subsequent survey could be conducted.

The Student Chorus sang at the World Flower and Garden Show at McCormick Place, Sunday, March 8, 1964. Karen Bischoff, senior student, was elected Second Vice-President of the Illinois Student Nurses' Association and Barbara Burkett, Instructor, had an article on "The Relationships of Thought Processes to Methods of Teaching" published in the Journal of Nursing Education.

One of our graduates, Clarice Olsen Rech, '54, wrote the following poem:

AUGUSTANA HERITAGE

Augustana has a heritage, this we all well know—
Ever since our hospital was founded 80 years ago.
In 1884, thru the church it was begun.
The first hospital was the home of Reverend Carlsson.

At that time the beds numbered only 15.
The first patient was a lady, who broke her leg, poor thing!
Then a 3 story building with 26 beds
In 1885 was finally completed.
In the reception room surgery was done

With the rug rolled up, for the table, planks were put on,
The nurses were hardy, and had to be strong,
For the work was hard and the hours were long.

Miss Frejd was the matron in the early days—
The first anesthetist, Dr. Ochsner said in her praise.
The uniforms had white aprons, and were white and blue,
The caps were round organdy with black bands, then, too.

The patients received one bath per week.
The privates got two, which then was a treat.
Each patient had a bell and the nurses had to run
Up and down stairs to find the right one!

Once a week the linen was changed,
And a special drink came into fame.
The Augustana cocktail became very well known,
It was castor oil, served in beer foam!

A new building was erected in 1892.
Reverend Thelander was superintendent, and the chaplain, too.
The first Chief of Staff was Dr. Charles Parkes—
Who was a famous surgeon, it has been remarked.

In 1894 was the beginning of our school.
Miss Pickhardt was the guiding light, she set up the rules.
She was an idealist, with endearing ways.
She was highly thought of, even to this day.

In 1895 came Miss Julia Anderson.
A good nurse and teacher, besides a lovely person.
Graduation, 1896, was the very first one—
The graduates wore the pin with the Good Samaritan.

The first "Augie Nurse" was published in 1903,
One of the finest things ever done by our alumnae.
It was originated by the class of '01—
And in longhand writing the paper was done.

A new addition was added in 1904
With a capacity for 225, more than ever before.
The Red Cross was reorganized that same year,
Many of our nurses joined as part of their career.
Dr. A. J. Ochsner was termed the beloved professor

And Dr. Nelson M. Percy became his successor.
Both men had talent and brought the hospital fame.
And we're proud to remember these two by name.
(Dr. Ochsner organized unit 11 with Julia Flikke in 1915)

There were many who served in World War I—
Our first gold star was for Miss Hokanson.
The base hospital director was Major Nelson M. Percy,
Who served with so many of our "angels of mercy."
Julia Flikke was very active all thru the war—
She was a captain in the Army Nurse Corp.
She was highly thought of and one of our own,
And with the rank of major, became very well known.

There were tornadoes, floods, hurricanes, disasters,
And our Augustana nurses couldn't respond faster.
Our nurses have served as missionaries, too.
They also aided in those epidemics of flu.
(Hurricane in '26—Mabel Josephson '23—assistant chief nurse Amy
Chamberlain—change of flood unit)

The new nurses' residence was done in '22,
Before the nurses lived in homes on Garfield Avenue.
In 1926 the new hospital held its dedication,
And this is where most of us had our education.

Matilda Anderson designed the cap we wear.
The Jenny Lind Chorus provided music rare.
The big sister movement was Margaret Sanger's thought.
Thru the Thalian Drama Club, many plays were wrought.

Dr. Edward Ochsner was admired in the early era.
Drs. Rudolph Oden, Beilin and Nadeau also were there.
Dr. Abrahamson served the board such a long time.
Mr. E. I. Erickson as Superintendent was the finest of his kind.

Of the internes, there were many we all know.
The Drs. Nuzum, Garside and also Crow.
Drs. Hedberg, Grosz, Milles and Duess.
Drs. Crean, Swenson, William Browne and Boice.

The Sick Benefit Fund was started in 1926.
In 1938 came the fund to give scholarships.
Miss Haggman became the director in 1927.
Homecoming Day was her idea even.
During the depression each nurse took her turn.

At working when they could so money they could earn.
In 1934 came our present uniform—
This is the familiar one so many of us have worn.

Vera Leaf was in the class of '24.
She was the first doctor, we hadn't had one before.
Alva Johnson was Augustana's first
To go into a new field and be a sky nurse.
There are so many others I should mention, too—
But due to lack of time and all, I could name but just a few.
Most of the information came from our history book,
And for a time, it's rather fun to take a backward look.

Now let us all do our very best
To insure Augustana's continued success.
There are so many things we all could do
So that those following us will have a heritage, too.

Many years ago a friend of Augustana Hospital and long-time patient of Dr. Carl Hedberg donated the Grass Model III Electroencephalograph to the hospital as a memorial to his parents, Morris and Pearl Dry. In the fall, Mr. Dry joined with the hospital in replacing this machine with the $6,000 up-dated Grass Model 6. This new machine is accurate, dependable and stable for long-term recording.

After forty-two years of service the elevator in the Nurses Residence had to be replaced. The new one went directly east of "Old Unfaithful" and eventually gave way for another new one.

From January to September, Dr. Thomas Baffes had performed 50 open heart operations—36 of these utilized the heart pump—we were quite proud!

On August 26, 1964, an impressive dedication service was held in Room 824 of Augustana Hospital. This attractive, newly decorated and furnished room was donated by Mrs. Gordon Thorne, who had already completed two rooms on the same floor in memory of her husband, Mr. Gordon Thorne, and her son, Montgomery Ward Thorne.

The following report was written by Connie Bezanis about the refresher nursing course.

The morning of September 28, 1964 was the beginning of a renewal of an old love [nursing] and the making of new acquaintances, for Ruth Ellison Swasko '39 and Connie DeMet Bezanis '52, for we began the 16th Refresher Course at MacNeal Memorial Hospital, Berwyn, Illinois. There were 17 "students" who had not worked at their profession from 10 to 34 years. Everyone was amazed at how quickly we fell into routine again, trembling and hesitant but generally knowing what we were doing. The many disposable items, the patient from O.R. via the recovery room awake and responding, the aides and orderlies doing the many not critical patients, and housekeeping making the beds after discharge, surprised and pleased us. The weakest point and most frightening were the many new drugs. We all needed to have a P.D.R. close at hand—might be a good idea to have it like we do our scissors and pens.

Five days a week, for six weeks we attended classes often given by the staff doctors, and we worked on the floors. Each had one day observing in the emergency room (they have 2000 cases a month), delivery room, nursery, and recovery room. Mrs. Sparmaker from the Chicago Council on Community Nursing spoke and told about the new Nursing programs with the Junior Colleges and reminded us that "the Future Not the Past" should be our motto to help improve our profession.

At the end of six weeks the hospital held a tea at which time we received certificates—it was almost like graduating again. A little sadness crept into us for we had gotten to know each other and now we would go our separate ways to Michigan, Southwest Chicago, Dixon, and the western suburbs. Most of us will return to work immediately if only for part time. We urge any of you who contemplate a return, even if you've been away a long time to make the leap, it will be rewarding and you'll soon see how easy it is to get back into the groove.

On April 28, 1965, at the Tri-State Convention at the Palmer House in Chicago, Sister Elizabeth Marie, Chairman of the Presentation Committee and past president for the National Association of Hospital Central Service Personnel, gave an award to Edith Pauline Johnson '29, with the following speech.

The award is presented to the outstanding central service person of the year and the recipient is just exactly that—The outstanding central service person of the year—both nationally and locally.

This person has given of her time and energy since the inception of the National Association without asking anything in return. She has worked hard to promote local chapter activities and to gain recognition for the local chapter as well as the National Association.

She has missed very few meetings of her organization and has taken vacation time and disbursed personal funds to support the organization "closest to her heart."

Our recipient is not one to move in the spotlight but rather she has supported those in the limelight from behind the scenes. She does not seek personal publicity but rather the knowledge that she has promoted central service just one step higher in its aims.

She is one of the early pioneers of this Association and through her almost stubborn belief in central service it has advanced to the role it has today.

This award is but a small token of the high esteem we feel for her.

In 1964, Edith Pauline Johnson '29 assisted in compiling a Manual for the National Association of Hospital Central Service Personnel, for which the Association received a grant from the government. The Manual was published under the auspices of the U.S. Public Health Service.

In December of 1965, the new cafeteria opened. Being in the heart of the main floor we thought we'd miss windows, but we were compensated with mirrors, planters, and air conditioning. Just west of the original front elevator was a room with vending machines and a microwave. The Coffee and Gift Shop had added space for their storeroom and the Business Office, X-Ray and Pharmacy were enlarged and refurbished in a modern pleasing manner. The Outpatient, OB, Medical and Surgical Clinic, and the Emergency Room on the main floor were still in the staffing and setting up process. This meant the majority of emergencies were still handled by surgery personnel on the 4th floor.

The Augustana Surgical Department had an interesting exhibit at the Association of Operating Room Nurses' Congress held early in 1965 in Chicago. The exhibit, entitled "Cardiovascular Surgery in the Community Hospital" was well received and given close attention. This was a credit to Augustana Hospital as no other hospital had anything comparable. Our surgical nurses took turns at the booth and answered questions about the exhibit. The new disposable isolation gown now being used at the hospital was modeled.

Augustana Hospital School of Nursing was one of 18 Schools

of Nursing participating in a televised teaching program. The program resulted from a meeting in January 1964, to explore the use of television in nursing education. Hoping to upgrade curricula and cut costs, the 18 schools each contributed $1,000.00 as a beginning. The project was successful to the point that the U.S. Government saw fit to provide a grant for it.

The U.S. Public Health Service gave a grant for $419,539 to underwrite the costs of the Chicago Area Video Nursing Education project. The grant, made under the Nurse Training Act of 1964, extended over a three year period, ending in 1968. The courses were telecast over Channel 20 and reached 2,500 student nurses. Video tapes and kinescopes of the courses were produced. They were available, along with study guides and other teaching materials, to nursing schools throughout the country.

The project afforded many advantages. Schools with a critical shortage of qualified instructors had the assistance of "master" teachers from other schools in curriculum planning. Bi-weekly conferences for instructors were held to help solve problems which arose; to brief instructors in advance about telecasts so they could prepare students to benefit from them; and to make the "follow-up" a meaningful learning experience. Costs for participating schools were reduced by centralized services for printed materials, machine scoring and data processing of examinations and for TV repairs. (The Alumnae gave a donation of $1,000.00 to this project in September, 1965.)

English 101 was given at the Chicago City College— Amundsen, Mayfair Branch. Pediatric affiliation at Children's Memorial Hospital changed to eight 35-hour weeks with assignments Monday through Friday. Tuition charge for the program was $300 for tuition, fees, and room, meals were obtained on a cash basis. Augustana students remained in the home residence and fees were assessed at $235 plus meals.

Pastor Sandstedt was named a "Fellow" of the American Protestant Hospital Association. He and two hospital administrators were so cited, at their 1966 Convention, during the week of February 4, in Dallas, Texas. He received a certificate designating the honor and including in its wording for "recognition of his outstanding contribution to the field of hospital chaplaincy." (Mrs. Sandstedt is Arlene Johnson Sandstedt '41.)

March 6 was Nurse Recognition Day at Augustana. Tea was served to 200 guests. Students received stripes for their caps at this occasion. Freshmen had a small blue stripe on the corner of the cap, Juniors had two stripes, and Seniors had a long blue stripe across the entire top of the cap. However, when the student was graduated she would turn in her stripe and join the ranks of Augustana graduates and wear our traditional and honored white cap.

The following were guidelines for student employment as set forth by the Director of Nursing Service.

1. Students may work for pay one 8-hour day per week.
   a. Senior students—days, p.m.'s or nights
   b. Junior students—days or p.m.'s
   c. Freshmen students—only as directed by the School of Nursing
   EXCEPTION:   On a holiday week—16 hours of employment permitted.
2. Students employed must sign up in person in the Nursing Service Office. Notes are not accepted.
3. Students off due to illness after signing up for employment, must notify the Nursing Service Office to remove their names from the employment book. Not eligible for employment for one week if off ill on a class day or clinical day.
4. A cancellation of employment date will not be accepted within two hours or less of assigned time.
   EXCEPTION:   Only if the student who is canceling provides a replacement.

5. When a replacement is not provided, the student will have her employment privileges taken away for one week.
   a. Second cancellation—employment not allowed for two weeks.
   b. Third cancellation—employment not allowed for four weeks.
6. Students employed assume the role of nurse's aides.
7. Lunches will not be provided for students employed on p.m.'s or nights as of January 19, 1966.

On April 19, 1966, the Annual Meeting of the Chicago District of the Illinois Nurses' Association was held at the Continental Plaza Hotel. Mrs. Zercher, President of the Chicago District, told of the change of the name from 1st District to the Chicago District, of the renovation of the headquarters and of the activities of the various committees.

Dean Emily Holmquist of the School of Nursing at the University of Indiana spoke on the "American Nurses' Association's Position on Education for Nursing." She stated "that all practitioners of nursing will within the next thirty years, be prepared at the B.S. level and that technicians possibly will be doing each procedure as a specialist. But who will be caring for the patients? Nurses must come together and agree where they are going and what their purpose in nursing is to be. The Diploma School is the backbone of this country but more education is stressed, especially for those who are qualified to move ahead into the graduate level of college." Dean Holmquist said that nursing would never return to the way it was before World War II. She stressed there must be an interdependence between the medical and nursing teams and that Nursing must find its central purpose in its relationship to patient care. She urged all to contribute to professional groups by taking part in the organizations.

Open House and Dedication was May 15, 1966, for Augustana Hospital. The new Emergency Room and Outpatient Dept., Payroll and Personnel Office, Chaplain's Office and

Conference Room were only a few changes. Also seen were additions to the Pharmacy, X-Ray Department, and Business Offices.

A description of "A Hospital" was written in the Extension Magazine in 1966.

> A hospital is a mercy mission. It always has its doors open and unlocked. It offers hope and refuge to the ill, injured, infirm and mothers-to-be. A hospital is a highly technical workshop. Its personnel are specialists. Each is expert in some phase of patient care. A hospital is a storehouse of scientific vision, medical know-how, expensive equipment and surgical instruments. A hospital is a City. Regardless of political views or party lines, its inhabitants team together for the same merciful purpose. Its communal spirit is the closest thing on earth to brotherhood and charity. A hospital is a hot-bed of revolution. Research within its walls is unending. Progress in patient care, relief of pain, surgical and post-operative techniques are continuous. A hospital is a daring adventure. It takes courageous, strong and dedicated souls to engage in its activities. It cannot accept on its staff, a physician or surgeon who isn't willing to question the unknown. A hospital is a court of final appeal. Its doctors and nurses never give up. No patient is forsaken as hopeless. As a business, a hospital is a financial failure. It makes no profits and distributes no dividends. Sometimes it operates at a loss. It is owned by no one, which means everyone. A hospital is founded on faith and sustained by hope and charity. It's a haven to the worlds' hurt. A hospital is a chapel. Its works are a constant prayer watched over by a merciful and indulgent God.

Meryl Redpath Linquist '61 wrote from the mission field in June of 1966.

> She and her family arrived in Africa in July of 1965. They had been in Obo for the past nine months. The climate was pleasant, never sultry, even though the wet season usually lasts for nine months. The terrain is gently rolling hills dotted with neat African villages. The coastal towns were not clean but in the inland everything is. The mission (Africa Inland Missions) had 4 stations in the Central Africa Republic manned by 25 missionaries (this includes children). Meryl ran a small dispensary—saw about 50 patients a day and her husband, Don, did everything from preaching, teaching, building and repairing equipment. "It is day to day living and working in every sphere among the people." The nearest store was three days away so their storeroom looked like a grocery store. They lived off the land as much as possible. Meat had to be hunted and this included elephant, buffalo, antelope and wild hogs. The children, Bruce 4 and Carolyn 3 seemed to thrive on living in the mission field and except for an occasional bout of malaria had been very healthy. In closing, Meryl wrote "If any of you are passing this way, please come and visit us."

The annual Christmas program was held in the Chapel at 7:30 p.m., on Wednesday, December 7, 1966. Rev. Sandstedt conducted the service and read the Christmas Story. Several students from the School of Nursing joined in the festivities. Wearing colorful Swedish dress they sang selections as each Advent candle was lit. The service was followed by refreshments in the Lila Pickhardt Lounge. Everyone now had an opportunity to see the many new pieces of furniture and lamps which had arrived only a week before. The lounge was grouped in a series of conversation corners and each group was in use with members catching up on news from their classmates and friends. During the conversation we busied ourselves eating delicious sandwich loaves and butter cookies, washed down by what every Augie nurse loves, good hot coffee! After all was quiet and the lounge empty we could hear in the distance that familiar call of departing members, "Merry Christmas!" Another Christmas season was under way—and it started for many members with the Alumnae Christmas Program.

In January 1967, the newspaper headlines read: "Record Snow Grips City;" "Schools Close;" "Motorists Stranded;" "Transportation at a Standstill;" but there was no moratorium on sickness. Hospital patients required care and we were proud to say, they received care.

Out of the "Big Snow" grew an operation—good will. The nurses residence became a haven for the many R.N.'s, L.P.N.'s and aides who remained to devote additional time to hospital work. Mr. Hough, several doctors, and a number of other hospital personnel took up sleeping quarters on 4-East.

Shortages developed in areas other than personnel. From the deep freeze came English muffins, apple turnovers and waffles to substitute for bread. Milk and coffee supplies were at an all time low. Delivery of formulas for babies was made by fire truck. Some surgery was canceled but there could, of course, be no delay in the maternity division. One expectant mother walked two blocks to the ambulance which transported her to Augustana Hospital.

There were many, many unsung heroines and heroes; the members of the nursing personnel who worked sixteen hours and then returned in eight hours to work another long stretch; those who arrived for work in spite of stalled transportation (many walked for miles, some rode part of the way on snow plows, garbage trucks and in squad cars); the students who assisted; the sister and wife of a doctor who helped serve patients food; the firemen and Boy Scouts who helped dig us out; the policemen who aided in innumerable ways; the non-nursing personnel who, too, gave so much of themselves; the patients who were very understanding; and the neighbors who called to volunteer services. The events of these days will long be remembered.

Our members inquired from time to time about purchasing Augustana nurses caps. The only Augustana caps available at that time were permanently starched and prefolded, and were priced at $1.75, plus $.35 postage for one cap, or $.65 postage for two.

A fashion show was held on April 7, 1967, at 7:30 p.m. by the student nurses. It was held in the recreation room of the nurses residence, with tickets sold at the door—price $1.00.

"On Wednesday, March 15, 1967, the Illinois State Medical Society held a Public Symposium, "Medical Implications of the Current Abortions Law in Illinois." Eight doctors presented their views about abortion. They represented both sides of the issue of making it legal to perform abortions if medically advisable under H.B. 715 in the Illinois Legislature.

In the January 1968 issue of the Augustana Nurse, an appeal was made for nurses to come back to nursing. The hospital wanted to open up their new Coronary Intensive Care Unit but could not because of the shortage of nurses. Base pay on days was $3.17 per hour and on P.M.'s and nights $3.57. The Hospital now paid for Blue Cross and a group life and accidental death policy at no cost to employees. Twelve sick days were allowed and six paid legal holidays per year.

More than one hundred of our Chicago area Lutheran Church in America churches had been visited since the beginning of 1967, according to Fred Shearer, Director of Development at Augustana. They in turn had provided names of potential student nurses, patient and doctor referrals, active men interested in helping the hospital by serving in a group of "Associates," and those who could be approached for contributions to the Development Fund.

According to Mr. Shearer, this had resulted in some fine financial support for the long-range program of Augustana Hospital. The first phase of modernization was completed early in 1966, when the improved service utilities such as the laundry, heating and power plant, kitchen, cafeteria and other facilities were dedicated. Phase II was in progress, involving architect's plans for a proposed new wing, and additional parking area. Lincoln Park No. 1 Urban Renewal Project permitted Augustana to keep pace with the progress of the city and of other hospitals in the general community. Forward looking steps were under way to maintain the fine image of our hospital created at the time of founding eighty-five years earlier, all in keeping with the outstanding reputation of surgical and medical patient care over the entire period.

For those of you who remember the President Hotel—where the early Augustana Hospital was located—it was now completely down to the ground—the first step in development by Urban Renewal.

Shirlee Anderson Nemec '53, wrote thoughts and notes on Private Duty Nursing.

Working in New York and doing Private Duty for the first time, I must speak about this and nursing in general. Hospitals are short of help and nurses are overworked and underpaid, especially in city hospitals. We may be called baby sitters, but more often than not, it may mean the difference between life and death; comfort or misery. Many times blood pressures, temperatures and treatments are fotgotten because nurses are not attentive to patients' needs. Nurses sometimes lower the standard of our profession instead of raising it. Respect and common courtesies between the nurse and doctor no longer exist. Doctors often spend precious time looking for a nurse to assist him with a procedure. How about thinking of why we became nurses?

The Augustana Hospital School of Nursing developed an accelerated program in nursing education. The first class was admitted in September 1968, and for the first time one male student and two African American students were included. This 24 month diploma program offered many challenges and advantages for the student who was interested in a professional career in nursing.

The aim of the program was to help the community meet the increasing need for nursing services by offering the student the opportunity to participate in a curriculum designed to prepare the student to become an R.N. and function as beginning staff nurse in the hospital or other comparable agencies.

This two year career program offered clinical experience in three Chicago area hospitals. Psychiatric courses in nursing were taught at Augustana Hospital School of Nursing, and students affiliated at Veterans Administration Hospital at Downey, Illinois and Children's Memorial Hospital. In addition, students attended a branch of the Chicago City College for courses in the social and biological sciences as well as the humanities. Approximately 23 transferable college credit hours were earned during these two years. The school also participated in the Video Nursing Program for courses given via television. The program was open to all qualified men and women, seventeen years of age and over, who were interested in nursing as a career. Tuition was $750.00 per year. Clinical and housing facilities of Augustana Hospital were used by 15 Lutheran General Hospital students from July to November.

The long-awaited Coronary Care Unit opening took place with a ribbon-cutting ceremony on Monday, September 16, 1968. Mr. John Sward cut the ribbon with bandage scissors borrowed from Miss Gloria Trebets, Head Nurse of the unit.

Miss B. Klauser, Director of Nursing, and Miss I. Magnuson, Supervisor of the Intensive and Recovery areas witnessed the ceremony. The unit had a ten-bed capacity, nine of these beds were filled by the end of the first day. Twelve nurses had been allocated to staff this unit; this included the head nurse. Dr. William Delessandro served as the medical director of the new unit.

The following directive was sent to Nursing Personnel from Bertha E. Klauser, Director of Nursing on February 17, 1969:

"Nursing Personnel returning patients from Recovery Room, Intensive Care, Coronary Care, or Emergency Room, must be met by an R.N. who is to accept the patient, receive a report, and assist in placing him/her in bed. This is a legal and moral responsibility.

"Should a nurse not be at the desk, a ward clerk is to locate one."

During 1968, the Unit Management program at Augustana came into full maturity with the hiring of six unit managers. The work of these men, all college graduates, was coordinated by Mr. William Wiesmann, the Coordinator.

During the day, each manager was responsible for the administration of two floors of the hospital, an area of approximately 102 beds. In the evening each of the two managers was responsible for one-half of the hospital, and the man on nights was responsible for the entire house. Each unit manager was the personal representative of administration in his assigned area and was responsible for everything that occurred except actual nursing care. The young men supervised and followed through on a myriad of activities for administration in their assigned areas. This was not only done for the purpose of better administration of the business of the hospital but for the immediate goal of better nursing care. The registered and licensed practical nurses were relieved for important patient nursing functions instead of investing their time in administrative and clerical duties.

An important person in the unit management program was the Ward Clerk. The women who were ward clerks were easily recognized in their crisp blue smocks as they handled the complete clerical function in the floor station. From transcribing doctors' orders to handling phone messages, the clerks put in a full and busy day supporting the nursing teams on their floors.

Elda R. Peters '54, a graduate of Augustana, was a member of the Lyric Opera of Chicago Chorus and was participating in the production of "Norma" at Chicago's Civic Opera House. She also sang in seven other operas during the 1968 season and sang at our Alumnae Banquet in June. Miss Peters, an alto with the supplementary chorus, had been with Lyric for five years and was also a church soloist. During the day she was an office nurse.

The following article is a reprint from the Daily Times of Ottawa, Illinois, Thursday, September 26, 1968.

Astrid Carter '30 wrote of her experiences with the State Department and her tour of duty to serve in the American Embassy in Afghanistan. She spent a month in Washington which included 2 weeks in the Foreign Service Institute and 2 weeks in the Department of State Medical Division.

In 1968 there were no railroads in Afghanistan. Transportation was by plane or car. The terrain of that part of the country compared to that of Santa Fe, New Mexico. The Afghan people are characterized by their pride, toughness, religious devotion, hospitality, conservatism and frugality. The afghan owes primary allegiance to his family. Most are Muslims and religion pervades all aspects of life. It was necessary to boil all water and fresh produce had to be soaked in detergent and then washed with boiled water. Amoebic and Bacillary Dysentery were very prevalent.

Besides the embassy, the United States Information Service, The Agency for International Development and the Peace Corp were represented there. The medical personnel at the State Department kept immunizations up to date for the approximate 660 people in the Department; and the nurses dispensed prescription medications. There was a tiny hospital in the building. The local Afghans hired by the various agencies were given first aid in the dispensary. At times the medical personnel witnessed interesting superstitions. The Afghan people believed that Allah would take care of their needs.

Some improvements made at Augustana were not related to construction. Computer programming was being initiated at Augustana in the business office and three west became the Stroke Rehabilitation Unit.

Twenty-three foreign languages, spoken by 61 individuals, were featured on the interpreters' list at Augustana Hospital. This list was used whenever a patient who did not speak English was brought to Augustana.

German, Spanish, Filipino, Swedish and Italian were the most common languages. Also listed were some less known languages such as Assyrian, Estonian, Russian, Serbian, Sioux, Thai, Tagalog and Yugoslavian. Twelve of the interpreters were on Augustana's nursing staff.

Each fall, freshman students at Augustana studied cultural and sociological aspects of the ethnic and racial groups which comprise Chicago's northside community. Through this study, the students acquired a better understanding of black and Appalachian cultures. Classroom sessions were followed by walking tours of the community of which Augustana was an integral part.

Augustana Hospital received a shipment of 20 new units of furniture, featuring the newest in electric beds, dressers, over-the-bed tables and side tables. These beds allowed the patient to adjust his own positioning without calling a nurse to crank him up. The beds had rods for intravenous medication and attached side rails.

The following article was printed in the June, 1969 edition of the University of Illinois Medical Center News:

"DR. HEDBERG RECEIVES MEDICAL ALUMNI AWARD.
"A former president of the Medical Alumni Association, Dr. Carl A. Hedberg, was named the group's 'Alumnus of the Year' May 20, 1969, during Medical Alumni Day. Dr. Hedberg received a B.S. degree in 1924, and an M.D. degree in 1926, both from the University of Illinois. During 1958-1959, he was the Association's president. He has served on the Association's Board of Councilors for 18 years.

After graduation from the College of Medicine, Dr. Hedberg joined Augustana Hospital in Chicago as an intern and remained there for his residency. As an internist, he has been a member of the hospital's attending staff since 1932 and presently is chairman of the Department of Medicine there. He is past president of the hospital's attending staff.

He also is treasurer of the Institute of Medicine of Chicago and a member of its Board of Directors, former president and member of the Board of Directors of the Diabetes Association of Greater Chicago and member of the Nu Sigma Nu and Alpha Omega Alpha. When his schedule permits, Dr. Hedberg's hobbies are golf and travel."

Miss Stella Dytko '41 was named Augustana Hospital's Employee-of-the-year for 1968. Along with employees of other Chicago hospitals she was honored at a Chicago Hospital Council luncheon in the International Ballroom of the Conrad Hilton Hotel. Miss Dytko worked in the x-ray department as a technician. Popular with all her co-workers, she was nominated not only for her kindnesses to patients and fellow workers, but also for her gentleness with patients. Often she stayed after work to do whatever was necessary for the welfare of her patients. A graduate of our School of Nursing, Miss Dytko had been employed by Augustana since 1943. Her twenty-five years of fine service to Augustana undoubtedly was an important factor in her selection.

Betty Thomson '63 wrote the following description of her work with researcher Dr. Frances E. Knock.

The majority of her work dealt with the chemotherapy treatments of Dr. Knock. The day began with the preparation of the various medications in their specified amounts. The main medications were results of Dr. Knock's research. All of these treatments were given intravenously five to six times a week. Besides the in-patients there were many out-patients, many of whom were back to work full-time, who came two or three times a week for chemotherapy injections. Giving treatments in the hyperbaric chamber was also a part of the day. Daily records for the government had to be accurately kept as to medications given and laboratory results since some of the research was supported by special grants.

Dr. Knock, author of "Anticancer Agents" and founder of the Knock Research Foundation saw her theories accepted in many other countries but not by the American Medical Association. Dr. Knock stressed that individualized cancer therapy, adjusted to each patient's own chemistry can now be offered. She believed that a surgically removed cancer should be immediately submitted to sensitivity tests with various chemicals to learn which one it best responds to.

Dr. Knock graduated Phi Beta Kappa from the University of Chicago at the age of 18 with a bachelor's degree in chemistry. She received her medical degree from the University of Illinois. She served on the staff of Augustana, Rush Presbyterian-St. Lukes and Hines Veteran Administration Hospitals. Dr. Knock was a pioneer in chemical and radioactive traces studies and published over 100 papers on cancer research. She conducted spectrometer experiments with Dr. P.R.C. Gascoyne of the National Foundation for Cancer Research in Woods Hole, Massachusetts. She was a licensed physician in three states, was a certified medical examiner, was trained in acupuncture and had a degree in hypnosis.

An interesting article was sent to us from the August 31st Sun Telegram newspaper published in Richmond, Indiana. At this time much research was being done with dialysis and artificial kidneys.

Phyllis Richie Dudas '61, had given much of the information about her husband's condition to the paper. He had a rare kidney condition diagnosed as oxalosis which necessitated the removal of his kidneys. In this condition, crystals and stones would again form in transplanted kidneys. Researchers were working on drugs that would inhibit the continual formation of crystals which are caused by an enzyme imbalance.

There was a two month training period before they could bring the unit home. Dialysis treatments were taken from 9 p.m. to 7 a.m., 4 days a week. A plastic tube was connected to an artery and one to a vein. The blood was pumped into the machine where it removed impurities and out again making the complete cycle with the machine doing the work of the kidneys. The machine was equipped with an alarm mechanism which would sound if the machine was malfunctioning.

# CHAPTER V

# THE SEVENTIES

The By-Laws of the Alumnae Association state: "The objectives of this Association are to stimulate mutual help, improvement in professional work, and good fellowship among the graduates of this school, to advance the interest of the Augustana Hospital School of Nursing, to assist needy sick members, to promote the professional and educational development of nursing in cooperation with First District of the Illinois Nurses' Association, and the American Nurse's Association."

As of 1970, the Alumnae Association had nearly 1000 members. At our winter meetings the following news was received. Miss Klauser reported that the last of the three year students will graduate in June. The first of the two year classes will graduate later in the summer. It was reported that Augustana Hospital is now recognized as a corporate entity under the leadership of Mr. Bennett and Dr. Hall. Mrs. Stevens is now Director of Nursing Education. A colored television was donated by a relative of one of the student nurses and was placed in the lounge.

A letter was received from Doris Bruce '46, who was working as a missionary at the Makunda Leprosy Colony, Assam, India. Excerpts from her letter were as follows:

"The Word of God is being held forth and slowly we can see evidence of the Lord visiting some of the young people with heart-searching and self-examination and we believe we will see more changes. This fall we plan to start a special work among the young people where they will plan and carry out their own meetings with our sponsorship. They will also have practical teaching assignments

283

to better prepare them as useful servants in spiritual matters. We thoroughly enjoy teaching nursing but it is far more rewarding to be allowed to help mold lives for spiritual gain."

Members and friends of the Augustana Hospital staff were cordially invited to attend a spring dinner dance at the Belden Stratford Hotel on May 9, 1970. Sponsored by the Employee Public Relations Committee in cooperation with the medical staff, the "Enchanted Evening" proved to be just that for all who attended. Guest star James Wesley Jackson was on hand with his special brand of "here and now" humor. An excellent orchestra provided musical entertainment for all and tickets were $6 per person.

Representatives of Augustana Hospital met with community residents for the purpose of determining the unmet needs of the Lincoln Park area and the best possible ways of responding to them. These dialogues proved helpful to our institution in that we recognized that community controlled health centers were both desired and needed in the area. Augustana responded to this need by cooperating with the Citizens' Health Organization in establishing a free neighborhood health center located at 2747 N. Wilton and called the Fritzi Englestein Free People's Health Care Center. This receiving and clearing center provided general screening, inoculations, and routine treatment in the areas of prenatal, pediatric, and general adult care. Emphasis was placed upon preventative rather than crisis oriented care. Those patients needing more extensive treatment were referred to area hospitals. This center was community controlled in that a Citizens Advisory Board was responsible for determining operational procedure. Augustana recognized and encouraged this participation. The doctors that staffed the center were responsible for decisions relating to the quality of care administered.

Dr. C. Anderson Hedberg of the Augustana Hospital medical staff, was formally inducted into the American College of Physicians at its annual meeting in Philadelphia. A 1961 graduate of the Cornell University Medical School, he specialized in internal medicine at Augustana for one and a half years.

Letters and newspaper clippings were received from Verna Cavallo Thompson '58 and Florence Hedman Belden '32 telling us of some nursing history that was made forty years ago. The article from Verna Thompson from the Chicago Tribune in part read:

"When passenger service was inaugurated by Boeing the original plan was to have men stewards. My understanding of the reason for the change from stewards to stewardesses (graduate nurses) was the decision of Mr. Boeing himself and Mrs. Boeing, who had been greatly impressed by the qualifications and character of Miss Church, who had nursed the Boeing children when they were hospitalized in Seattle, then the home base for Boeing Air Transport. The original nurses we employed at Chicago were graduates of Augustana Hospital School of Nursing, all highly rated in their profession."

The article from Florence Belden was printed in a California newspaper. Florence was a stewardess for American Airlines from 1937 to 1944. The article in part said:

"In the chilled dawn of May 15, 1930, eight pretty girls in identical green capes swept onto an air-strip ready to make aviation history. 'And then the motors went haywire', recalls Harriet Iden, one of the eight. 'It took them three hours to fix the plane while we sat in the greasy spoon across the street drinking coffee. When they took off, the ladies launched a new career for women. They called themselves Stewardesses. Now on the 40th anniversary of that flight, some 50,000 young women work at the occupation.

"'Being a stewardess now couldn't be as exciting.' says the Glendale housewife, now in her 60s. 'Don't forget we were landing in cow pastures when the weather was bad.' They were also doing chores foreign to today's miniskirted stewardesses-such as cleaning the plane's chemical toilets, hauling baggage and, when the plane broke down, baby-sitting with it until mechanics arrived."

Realizing that as an outstanding hospital with a proud heritage, the Board of Directors of Augustana Hospital appointed in March 1970, Walker G. Bennett, President. He had a background of research, development and management for over 20 years. Prior to this appointment, he was Project Manager for Northrop Space Laboratories. Also announced by the Board was the election of Martin Hough, longtime administrator of

Augustana Hospital, to a newly created position as vice president for administration. In this role, Mr. Hough would concentrate his attention in a crucial, widespread area of administrative responsibility.

In planning for the future of Augustana Hospital, Mr. Bennett constructed a Master Plan which set goals in the following areas to be accomplished in four years.

1.  Intern-Residency Program and Teaching Hospital in Internal Medicine and Surgery, affiliated with the Medical School of Northwestern University. Also to have an extensive out-patient preventive medicine program.

2.  Support of Community Health Clinics to whatever ex tent necessary to ensure their success. This would include support of the Augustana Nursery for Retarded Children as well as establishing an active counseling program for young people interested in pursuing medical-nursing careers in cooperation with the Chicago Public School Sytem.

3.   Affiliation with a university to provide AAN (Associate Arts in Nursing) and BSN degree programs, plus establishment of a separately managed Master Degree Program for physician's assistants, dovetailing with the nursing pro-gram.

4.  Establishment of a training/intern program for clinical chaplains of all faiths, specializing in treatment of stress that underlies many cases of illness and accidents.

5.  Development of an MBA degree program and a semi nar program in Health Care Management.

6.  Reduce patient costs significantly below national levels by
    a) charging patients only for services rendered and their administration and facilities.
    b) development of subsidiary corporations.
    c) system management/cost centers.

7.  Enhance the Percy Research Foundation for part-time

pre-liminary research on selected medical programs, by practicing physicians, engineers and scientists nationwide in an informal atmosphere.

8.  Construction of a small auditorium, cafeteria, multistory parking garage, professional office building, apartment building and a new hospital building. Refurbishing that section of the old hospital which is less than forty-five years old as an education and research facility.

Mabel Haggman, a retired registered nurse, died on November 13, 1970, after a long illness. She was a graduate of General Hospital, Kansas City, Missouri. During her career she was Superintendent of Nurses at Grace Hospital, Detroit, Michigan and Augustana Hospital, Chicago, Illinois.

Mabel was a very capable woman, pleasing conversationalist and always ready to give her help to anyone. She recognized the worth of each individual. Through her direction and counseling, students in nursing were inspired to give of themselves to the patient and to the hospital. She will remain in loving memory of all those who received her guidance.

Bertha Klauser retired in December, 1970. For 38 years, she had given of her time and talents to the service of Augustana Hospital and to the School of Nursing.

Miss Klauser graduated from Augustana Hospital School of Nursing in 1933 and received a B.S. in Nursing Education from the University of Chicago and a Master's degree from Columbia University Teachers College. She served as an Instructor of Nursing Arts and Medical-Surgical Nursing and as Clinical Instructor for the School of Nursing. In 1953, she was appointed Assistant Director of Nursing Education and since 1960 had held her current position of Director of Nursing of Augustana Hospital.

Her gracious manner, devotion to nursing, and true Christian concern for her fellow man stood as a shining example of what it truly meant to be an Augustana Nurse.

The appointment of Mrs. Barbara Stevens to the position

of Director of Nursing Service was announced on December 17, 1970 by Mr. W. Bennett. Mrs. Stevens received her M.A. Degree in Education from DePaul University in 1970 and had Bachelor of Philosophy and Associate Arts in Nursing Degrees from Northwestern University and St. Petersburg respectively. During her more than seven years at Augustana she held positions of responsibility which included Faculty Instructor, Co-ordinator of Nursing Education, Assistant Director—Nursing Education, and Director—School of Nursing.

Mrs. Genevieve Carb, R.N., M.A., A.B., was appointed Director of the Augustana Hospital School of Nursing. Mrs. Carb had been with the American Hospital Association as Assistant Director of Nursing. Prior to this, she held the position of Executive Director of the Chicago Council Community Nursing; Director of the Tutorial and Cultural Project, Cook County School of Nursing; and staff consultant on many assignments in the health care field. In addition, Mrs. Carb served as Instructor of Mental Health and Psychiatric Nursing at Logansport State Hospital in Logansport, Indiana. She received her M.A. in Nursing Education from Columbia University, and A.B. in Sociology and Psychology from Hanover College. Mrs. Carb received her nurses training at Cook County School of Nursing. The Augustana Hospital staff and students of the School of Nursing extended a warm welcome.

A letter from Mrs. Carb stated in a letter to the Alumnae Association that it was her intention to continue to achieve excellence in the school in the 1970's.

The V.A. Hospital in Downey, Illinois was unable to furnish housing for affiliating students anymore, so the Psychiatric affiliation was now given at Chicago State Hospital—Reed Zone Center. Grant Hospital facilities were used for some of the maternity teaching and Cook County Hospital for some of the orthopedic teaching.

A letter was received from Sadie Holm '31 telling of Marit Moe Droivoldsino's exciting and interesting life since she graduated from Augustana. The letter read:

"Marit has had a varied and most interesting career in her nursing. She was born in Norway and taught country school after high school. She came on a year's visit to her uncle's in Muskegon, Michigan and decided on nursing as a career. She had been accepted by several Chicago schools but decided that Augustana had the most to offer and Miss Haggman was so nice to her. For the time being, she worked for a family who took her under their wing to help her with her English and grammar. As a student nurse, she 'scrubbed' for Dr. Percy which in those days was a singular honor.

"Since graduation she has been in Public Health, polio nursing, Norwegian Red Cross and Army Nursing, a ship's nurse on the Norwegian America Line, nurse for Norwegian Public Health in Brooklyn, staff nurse in the American Hospital in Paris, x-ray technician and private duty nurse in New York.

"She was in Norway during the Nazi occupation and she and another nurse escaped to Sweden on skis where they were interrogated for weeks and finally 'the underground' transported these two, plus 60–70 Norwegian soldiers practically around the world. Russia, Africa, etc. and finally to a base in Scotland. She worked there and then in Finland and Iceland.

"In 1947 Marit came back to the U.S. during which time (1947-1968) she did private duty nursing, Norwegian Public Health Nursing in Brooklyn, V.N.A. in Brooklyn and Minnesota. She had gotten her B.S. degree from the University of Minnesota. The last ten years she was employed by the U.S. Government, Department of State and was an embassy nurse in Korea, Rome, Sudan and Somalia. Now she is retired and lives in Norway with her mother. She, of course, is an American citizen and hopes to come to visit the U.S.A. again some day."

Doris V. Ummel '55 (Mrs. Richard Ferguson) wrote a work book for Anatomy and Physiology for use with Basic Human Anatomy and Physiology by Charlotte M. Dienhart, Ph.D.

A newspaper article was received telling us that Beth Bystrom Ford '46 was appointed director of nursing services for Morningside Hospital in Northern California.

Highlighting her professional experiences have been a head nurse's role at the Henry Phipps Psychiatric Clinic of Johns Hopkins, a medical-surgical supervisor in the Guggenheim and semi-private pavilions of Mt. Sinai Hospital in New York City, and directorship responsibilities at three northern California hospitals.

An accomplished singer, Mrs. Ford was a soprano soloist in the Augustana Hospital Nurses Chorus, besides singing operatic roles with the Baltimore Symphony Orchestra, the Bethlehem Bach Festival Chorus and at the Peabody Conservatory of Music. Sharing her interest in singing is her husband, formerly a well-known professional opera and light opera singer with major companies in the East, Midwest and Southwest.

In March of 1971, in a section on fifth floor of the hospital, a new program and facility was set up. This was called the Hematology Oncology Center (HOC) and according to its director, Dr. John Louis, it was the only such operation in the United States at that time. The philosophy of the program was "The Total Welfare of the Patient."

The HOC program was a coordinated and team approach to every aspect of the patient's life. The inpatients were persons with malignancies requiring Chemotherapy, reversible complications from malignant disease, complications from Chemotherapy and hematologic disorders which required close monitoring. Physicians on Augustana's Medical Staff could admit qualified patients to the 12-bed unit, as long as they continued to remain the primary physician and complied with HOC procedures.

The center's staff hoped to be able to return the patient to his own environment in as normal a state as possible—usually within 10 days. Socializing was gently encouraged and various amenities were introduced such as games, buffet dinners, movies, etc. Psychiatric and social service professionals as well as other resources were asked for their services in keeping with the philosophy of the program.

The hospital also had a School of Medical Technology and was affiliated with:

American Hospital Association
Illinois Hospital Association
Chicago Hospital Council
Lutheran Hospital Association
American Protestant Hospital Association
National League for Nursing
Mid-North Association
Welfare Council of Metropolitan Chicago
American Management Association.

Augustana was approved by:
    American Medical Association (for training interns and pathology residents)
Augustana was accredited by:
    The Joint Commission on Accreditation of Hospitals
Augustana was endorsed by:
    Chicago Association of Commerce and Industry
    Blue Cross and Blue Shield
The School of Nursing was approved by:
    Department of Registration and Education, State of Illinois
The School of Nursing was accredited by:
    National League for Nursing
The School of Nursing was a member of:
    Council of Member Agencies of the Department of Diploma Programs, National League for Nursing
The School of Medical Technology was approved by:
    The Board of Registry
    American Society of Clinical Pathologists

Since the primary business of a hospital is patient care, both for in-patients and out-patients, the steps taken during 1971 at Augustana to improve the quality of care were significant. Development and continuing education of the Medical Staff stood out. A "medical officer of the day" program was instituted with well-trained physicians available in the hospital around-the-clock every day. Meetings of the Joint Conference Committee (Hospital Board and Medical Staff) were especially helpful in establishing better communications and understanding of mutual problems. This communication was further strengthened by the addition of four staff doctors plus the President of the Medical Staff to the hospital's board itself.

An active Stroke Team, composed of various elements of hospital personnel, was functioning so well that other hospitals sent representatives to Augustana to observe this model performance. Occupational therapy was added to Augustana's already existing programs of physical and speech therapy and the three were coordinated to provide a full range of care seven days a week.

In August of '71, Augustana made available facilities and equipment to the Easter Seal Society for treatment of their patients by their therapists, thus becoming the first hospital in the Chicago area to provide such service.

Our surgical department re-established the Surgical and Tumor Clinic and completed a major study, setting standards for surgical privileges at Augustana. With the aid of Systems Management, the Cardiopulmonary Resuscitation Team re-evaluated its procedures, with doctors and nurses spending many hours educating all personnel involved in methods of responding to cardiac arrest.

Chart Audit, Quality Control and Forms Committees were functioning in Nursing Service by late summer. Additionally, skills-training classes for Nursing Assistants, orientation programs, for newly hired R.N.'s and L.P.N.'s, eight-week internships for beginning nurse practitioners, along with weekly classes on the nursing units to keep staff up to date on techniques and equipment were held.

These advances enabled Augustana nurses to give better care than ever to 106 patients in the stroke rehabilitation program; 261 in coronary care, 798 in intensive care, 2241 in the clinics, 6872 in the emergency room, 2747 major and 2964 minor in surgery. Also better care was given to 907 mothers in the labor, delivery, and postpartum phases.

In 1970, our School of Nursing began observance of the 75th Anniversary of its first graduating class. A time of expansion and stabilization, 1971 saw the school make available two neurological units for student experience—one at Hines V.A. Hospital, the other at Whitehall Convalescent and Nursing Home. Students also received obstetrical experience and clinical instruction in urology and general surgery at Cook County Hospital. Thus was Augustana Hospital and Health Care Center (the name was changed in 1971 too, from Augustana Hospital) at the close of the year. Augustana's motto was "To Strive in Faith, To Innovate with Reason, To Achieve by Sharing."

The Magazine section of the Chicago Tribune had a feature article on May 9, 1971 entitled "Healthy hearts: getting there by way of the bypass." It featured Dr. W. Dudley Johnson who had been an intern at Augustana in the '50's. Following are some excerpts.

The new operation, which was perfected by Dr. W. Dudley Johnson at St. Luke's [Milwaukee, Wisconsin], has eliminated the need for most heart transplants. The surgeons operate on an average of one patient each week who would have been considered a good candidate for a heart transplant in the days when transplants were being done wildly.

Dr. Christiaan Barnard, the Cape Town, South Africa, surgeon who performed the world's first heart transplant in 1967, visited St. Luke's last year to learn the bypass technique. He remarked then that two of his early patients would not have received transplanted hearts if the Milwaukee procedure had been available.

Well over 200 heart surgeons from the United States and other countries have traveled to St. Luke's to study the technique, which some estimate may benefit 9 out of 10 patients with severe coronary artery disease, more commonly known as hardening of the arteries.

Various attempts have been made to bring new blood supplies into the heart to overcome the blocks but they have met with limited success. The pioneer in the field is Dr. Arthur Vineberg, a Montreal surgeon, who 35 years ago [1936] first detached the internal mammary artery, which feeds the chest muscle, and hooked it up to the heart muscle. But this procedure took up to six months for the implant to grow into the unplugged sections of the coronary vessels, too long for seriously sick patients.

Several years ago a number of surgeons, including Dr. Johnson, hit upon the idea of using the spare leg vein, called the saphenous vein, to bypass a single block at the top of the right coronary artery. But Dr. Johnson's pioneering operation to bypass blockages in the top of the right coronary was useful in only 5 to 10 percent of the cases because most patients had blocks in their left coronary artery or farther down in the right one. Heart surgeons dreaded to operate on the left coronary or go beyond the top section of the right one because earlier attempts using other techniques ended in disaster. Most of the coronary arteries were considered off limits for surgeons.

One July morning in 1968, Dr. Johnson made a momentous decision. While performing a routine heart surgery [removing a weakened section of the left ventricle that was interfering with normal function], he discovered that his patient suffered a major block in the lower part of his right coronary behind the heart. It probably would have been a fatal heart attack if he had not been on the heart-lung machine at the time. With the heart already weakened and no blood flowing to the back side of the left ventricle, the ventricle would not pump and the patient would not live. Dr. Johnson had been experimenting with the saphenous vein bypass on animals, and he decided to try it on his dying patient. There was no other chance. Swiftly he cut into the patient's leg and removed a long section of the vein. With fingers that refused to tremble, he sewed one end of the vein into a tiny slit in the aorta, turned the heart around and made another slit in the coronary artery below the block where he attached the other end of the new "pipe." The vein turned reddish as the life-saving blood surged thru. It worked. The chamber began pumping.

Dr. Johnson decided on the daring operation because he knew something that probably no other surgeon knew. During his animal experiments, the coronaries had to be shut off in order to stop the flow of blood so the vein could be sewn on. Dr. Johnson had discovered that the coronary arteries could be clamped shut for up to 20 minutes at a time without damaging the heart. But the patient had to be on the heart-lung machine and his heart not doing any work.

He and his associates tried more operations. The first year the death rate was 17 percent, but this was considered acceptable since without the operation, most of the patients would certainly have died. Last year [1970] the team performed 483 bypasses, and the mortality rate dropped to only 10 percent. These patients included many who had been turned down at other centers because the risk was considered too great. Now most patients receive two, three and even four bypasses routinely. The reason is that 60 percent of the patients with coronary artery disease have blockages in two or three of their main arteries.

"We know we have been able to prevent heart attacks because the number of attacks among the patients after the surgery has fallen off dramatically compared to the great number of attacks they had just before the bypasses," Dr. Johnson explains. Most victims don't know they have heart disease. Even with a major coronary 95 percent plugged up, a person can "feel" healthy and most routine medical tests will fail to uncover the potentially lethal situation. To overcome this difficulty, Dr. Mason Sones of the Cleveland Clinic in 1959 developed a technique called angiography, which for the first time gave cardiologists a way of looking directly at the coronary arteries to determine if they are healthy or diseased.

The difference in the patients after the operation is stunning. "I do everything now," a patient beams. "I don't get tired, there are no more pains and I don't run out of breath. I feel wonderful. I would gladly go thru the operation again if I had to."

# The following is reprinted in part from an article printed in the Chicago Tribune.

The streets surrounding Augustana are lined with quaint townhouses and chic apartments representing the ultimate urban lifestyle. Just a few blocks away however, live thousands of people who can scarcely afford one visit to the doctor's office. Augustana stands within the Near North drug culture and just a few blocks away a physician performed Chicago's first legal abortion.

In short, Augustana could serve as a 365-bed microcosm for the entire medical crisis facing metropolitan areas. "It is involved in a creative struggle to hammer out new answers," said a brochure which appeared on college campuses all across the country, and the brochure went on to invite students planning a career in medicine to take part in a summer program there.

Augustana served as a kind of classroom for the 15 students who ended up in "Urban Medicine, Super '71," as the program was called. They took fulltime, nonprofessional jobs aiding nurses, balancing the books, filing and typing and plugging in machines. They also attended seminars, asked the staff a lot of questions and generally poked and prodded and confronted Augustana's system. For several of the students, the summer at Augustana was their first brush with the reality of sickness and death, and they could not get used to the professional detachment that seemed to surround it.

In a couple of ways, Augustana had already begun reaching out. It provided laboratory support for a store-front clinic run by a coalition of North Side movement organizations ranging from the "Concerned Citizens Survival Front" to "Rising Up Angry", a radical offspring of "Students for a Democratic Society", Augustana provided the funding for a unique ambulance service organized and managed by the grassroots Citizens' Health Organization. People stricken ill and with no place to turn, no doctor available, could call a special "Communiphone," and the operator then called emergency rooms at Augustana, Henrotin, Grant or Children's Memorial to determine which one could take the case most quickly. A driver was dispatched to pick up the patient.

At our October alumnae meeting we learned that on September 13, 1971, Dr. Rudolph J.E.Oden, internationally renowned surgeon and devoted member of the Board of Directors of Augustana Hospital, passed from this life.

At the same meeting the following recommendations for setting up a student loan program were read: (1) a maximum of two scholarships of $100 each (2) one loan for $500 to be repaid within one year of graduation (3) all monies to be repaid to the Alumnae if the student does not complete the program. The committee established criteria for awarding scholarships according to need. Applications were drawn up and the school was informed of loan availability.

More than half of Augustana's patients underwent surgery during their hospital stay. Ten operating rooms and one large recovery room, all on the hospital's fourth floor, were the scene of bustling, skilled and disciplined teamwork devoted to the care of some 550 surgery patients a month. This vital service normally took place from 7:00 A.M. to 7:30 P.M., Monday through Friday, but in cases of immediate need, an on-call team was ready for action within 15 minutes during after-hours or on weekends.

Over 30 physicians regularly performed operations at Augustana. The back-up force consisted of about 30 nurses who received at least a year's in-service training in operating room procedures, plus numerous paramedical assistants, aides and orderlies. Our Augustana students also played a role, assisting in pre and post-operative duties and learned by observation of the actual operation. Supervisor Anarose Palumbo stated, "Augustana can handle just about any kind of operation. We have excellent equipment. Our annual budget for it is over $500,000. We also have fine relations with the other hospitals in this area, so if we need special instruments we can pick them up at a moment's notice."

A letter was received by the Alumnae Association from the Graduating Class of 1972 concerning their desire for a change in the Augustana Nurse's Cap. As this was a matter of concern to each Augustana graduate, the letter was printed in the Augustana Nurse.

"The graduating class of 1972 would like the approval of the alumni to change the tradition of graduating with the plain white cap, to graduating with the cap with one blue velvet stripe on it. We realize that the cap you now wear signifies your years of hard work and we are by no means asking you to change your own cap. However, as seniors we were given a blue stripe which has come to mean a lot to us. We feel we would as a class value the school cap more if we could graduate with the stripe."

The Alumnae Association requested its members to consider this matter carefully, vote, and respond before June 1, 1972, with comments.

The results of the voting were as follows:

YES (add a blue stripe)—52 votes

NO (do not change the cap)—151 votes

There were three votes to change the cap for the 2-year graduates only and two votes for an entirely new cap.

Because it was an important issue to each of us, the Board of Directors felt that the decision had to be made by the Alumnae members themselves.

Many wondered when and why the student cap was changed. The blue stripe was added in 1966 to differentiate between the various student levels and was a decision made by the student body and the School of Nursing. The Alumnae members could make decisions about the graduate cap only.

The Board felt, as did many of the alumnae, that if we allowed a change for this class, we could be allowing our cap to be changed each year in some different way and soon we'd have dozens of "Augustana caps." We are all graduates of the same school and the caps should all be the same.

> That cap the nurse on duty wears
> Is costlier than the bonnets gay
> Worn by the wives of millionaires
> Regardless of the price they pay.
> Tis something she herself can make,
> A bit of linen, trimmed and turned.
> The right to it (for mercy's sake)
> Was with three years of training earned.
> That uniform of spotless white
> Was costlier than a lady's gown,
> T'was bought with care by day and night
> For those with illness stricken down.
> The royal robes show royal birth

But every nurse's simple pin
Is emblematic of her worth;
A symbol she has toiled to win.

Oh, Gracious Spirit, love indued
That can such tender care accord,
Perhaps it is, the gratitude
Must always be your best reward.
Now out of gratitude appears
This tribute done in simple verse,
Unto the dedicated years
Of all who choose to be a nurse.

—From the writing of Edgar A. Guest

In the early 60's, three Chicago physicians founded FOCUS (Foreign Ophthalmologic Care from the U.S.), an organization providing free or very low cost eye-care service to the people of Haiti, whose living standard was the lowest in the Western Hemisphere. One of those founding physicians was Dr. Arthur Light, President of Augustana's Medical Staff. He was quite active in FOCUS until his death on March 31, 1990.

The annual tour of duty for the approximately 90 participating doctors was 3 or 4 weeks, which managed to cover every month of the year on a continuing basis in Haiti. The program was expanded to serve a clinic in Guatemala, also in dire need, for 2 months of the year.

FOCUS used the facilities of Public Health Hospitals; the doctors donated their services and paid their own transportation costs. Over 3,500 operations (for trachoma, glaucoma, cataracts and pterygia) were performed annually in Les Caya and the two other Haitian locations where the project was in effect. Cost to the patient was twenty cents for a consultation or four dollars for surgery.

Dr. Light said most of the doctors in FOCUS were from the Chicago area, but some were from other parts of the U.S. His enthusiasm for the work was contagious and there were plenty of reasons for Chicagoans and Augustanians to be proud of this manifestation of medical concern and leadership.

A letter from missionary nurse Mary Ellen Bulander Adams '48, read:

"Our flight to Nigeria on May 25th was one of intrigue and suspense. With the talk of 'Hi-jackers' and 'Ski-hikers' buzzing in our ears, a discreetly worded message from a pretty airline hostess increased the buzz! Some 37,000 feet over the Atlantic, she politely informed us that we were flying in the same plane that had been hi'jacked to Tel Aviv just a few weeks earlier! Would history repeat itself? The reason for the meticulous and thorough security measures taken at the Brussels Airport suddenly became apparent, although at the time most embarrassing. Twenty-three hours after leaving O'Hare we landed in Kano, only to learn that for 30 minutes we had been circling the airport because someone had forgotten to switch on the runway landing lights. It was a dark night. The temperature was a hot and steamy 95 degrees and when the perspiration started rolling we knew we were back in Kano. "Brenda [my daughter] and her talking doll, 'Smarty Pants' both looking forlorn and travel weary, were the center of attraction at Immigration. The intelligent pre-recorded answers 'Smarty Pants' gave to Brenda's equally intelligent questions simply fascinated the Officials. The brilliant performance set the stage for a problem-free passage through Immigration."

The Augustana Student Nurses' Association, which conducted a "Christmas-Needy Fund Drive," was delighted to have 22 dolls to distribute, which were made and donated by neighbor, Mrs. Mary Viertel. Student Nurse Association President, Janet Miller, paid a visit to Mr. and Mrs. Viertel to express a special thanks for the dolls. Canned goods were also collected and distributed.

Collecting gifts from Augustana employees for patients was done for the first time in 1971, and it was successful in brightening the occasion for many. Each employee was asked again in 1972 to buy a gift or to donate $2 to brighten our patients' spirits.

David Archer, organist for the Chapel, since 1966 had gained a reputation as a fine chorus-master around Chicago. He was a native Chicagoan and a graduate of Northwestern University.

He organized a glee club for employees, volunteers, student nurses, auxiliary members, and friendly neighbors who wanted to join. [He died September 14, 1995 at the age of 54.]

On November 28, 1972 at 10:00 a.m. a bulldozer severed the power cable of three area hospitals, but Augustana slowed only briefly. Although Augustana was without full power for nearly three hours, vital routines continued. Immediately the Intensive Care Unit, the Stroke Unit, and Surgery switched automatically to auxiliary power. Emergency lighting—enough so that critical areas were well lit and the rest of the hospital was dim but not dark—came on. Two of the nine elevators switched over to emergency power and exit signs went back on. Two persons were caught in transit in elevators and were rescued by the engineering department.

There was a flurry of activity among the engineering and maintenance crews. Although emergency gas came on to continue heating the hospital, the boilers had to be restarted. The OB Department required emergency power lines to be run over to the incubators. Some departments employed battery-powered lanterns. Anarose Palumbo, Surgery Coordinator, explained that five major operations were in progress, and three minor ones. "We were only delayed on our normal surgery schedule for the day by a half-hour, and that was because the sterilizers were off for a while," she said.

Dishwashers were off in Dietary, patients received their lunches on disposable plates. The electric tray line leading from the stoves to the food elevator was not on emergency power, but this proved no major problem. "We just shifted around our personnel and hand-passed the food to the elevator," said Phyllis Andrews, Food Service Manager. "And because of all the extra cooperation on the floors," she added, "the patients were fed all in an hour. Usually it takes at least an hour and fifteen minutes."

On December 20, 1972, the S.S. Hope completed her tenth medical teaching-treatment mission and returned to Baltimore from northeast Brazil. Karen H. Madsen, '43, served as a member of the Hope staff during the ten month say in Natal. Karen served as an operating room nurse during the voyage. Just prior to the Hope's departure for northeast Brazil, she served as a staff nurse with Project Hope's health education and career training program on the Navajo reservation at Ganado, Arizona. During the Hope's mission in Natal, 1,410 inpatients were treated aboard the hospital ship and 7,092 outpatients received care; 1.727 major operations were conducted and 74,375 people were immunized. Over 500 persons from Natal and other nearby communities participated in Hope education programs, with over 24 health facilities in and around Natal. Hope was involved in assisting the community in the development of an intensive care unit, improvement of operating room facilities, expansion of laboratory services, and the institution of a medical record system. Hope personnel remained in Natal to conduct an extensive land-based follow-up program.

The following article was taken from the Chicago Tribune, December 28, 1996:

Dr. William B. Walsh, who founded and led Project HOPE, a non-profit program that provides medical training, health education and humanitarian assistance around the world died Friday, December 27, 1996, at his home in Bethesda, Md. He was 76 and also lived in Tucson.

Since it was founded in 1958, Project HOPE (Health Opportunities for People Everywhere) has worked in more than 70 countries on five continents, including North America. More than 5,000 health professionals have donated their services to the project, and it has trained more than 1.3 million health workers and provided aid to millions of people, project officials said.

Dr. Walsh said he saw the need for the program while serving as a Navy medical officer aboard a destroyer in the South Pacific in World War II. He was particularly affected by the illnesses and deaths of children who could have benefited from simple medical care, he said.

Speaking of the people of the South Pacific, he told an interviewer in 1994: "Some of them had never had any real medical care in their life. I promised myself that if I ever got the chance, I wanted to do something about that sort of thing."

The chance to do something for them came in 1958, when, as a young cardiologist, he was called in as a consultant after President Dwight Eisenhower suffered a heart attack. Eisenhower took a liking to Dr. Walsh and asked him to become co-chairman of the Committee on Medicine and the Health Professions of his People-to-People program, intended to assist developing nations.

Soon Dr. Walsh proposed what became the first peacetime hospital ship. He led a successful effort to raise $750,000 to refit a gray, mothballed, 15,000-ton hospital ship loaned to the project by the Navy. On Sept., 22, 1960, a fully equipped white "HOPE" ship left San Francisco on its first voyage to Indonesia.

Dr. Walsh spent time on the ship but also publicized its efforts, writing several books, and raised money. He was chief executive officer and medical director of Project HOPE's parent organization, the People-to-People Health Foundation, from 1958 to 1992 and president from 1958 to 1991.

At the April, 1973 meeting of the Alumnae Association, the finance committee suggested that we publish 6 copies of the "Augustana Nurse" yearly instead of 9, and that we find a less expensive way of having it printed.

Connie Welch '68 returned from a 6 month trip to Africa where she lived and worked with Meryl Redpath Lindquist '61 and her husband. Her trip took her to OBO in the Central African Republic. It is approximately 60 miles or a 5-1/2-6 hour drive to the Sudan and a 5 day trip to the capital of the CAR.

In telling about her experiences there, she says, "A typical day begins with our rising between 4:30 and 5:00 a.m. We arrive at the Dispensary by 7:00 a.m. and see anywhere from 40 to 100 patients and usually return home by 11:00 a.m. On Tuesday mornings we do circumcisions on infants and older boys. We mixed all our own liquid medicines. I helped mainly with paper work and pharmacy duties. We had two African men who dispensed the meds. The rest of the morning we would be busy around the house. We had a cook and laundry boy, but we helped as much as we could because Meryl and I both loved to cook. During the morning also, Don, Meryl's husband, would do construction, teaching and maintenance work.

"Lunch was always at noon, then a siesta until 1:30 or 2:00 p.m., because the temperatures were so high. Our afternoons were spent making village trips or sewing for the family and the boys in the trade school. Don taught in the school.

"We made village medical trips Thursday morning, Thursday afternoon, Friday afternoon, and Saturday morning. We went out on Mokylette's (like a small Honda) and Meryl carried a 30-40 pound box of meds on the back of her Mokylette. In the villages we would see anywhere from 15 to 100 people and on some Thursdays we'd see over 200. I dispensed the meds and dressed sores and gave shots while Meryl recorded their names, age, complaints, meds and treatments. The people pay for injections—50 francs or about 20 cents.

"Dinner was usually around 5:30 p.m. We had electricity from 5:15 to 8:15 p.m. while the Diesel engine operated the generator. Our evenings were spent reading, writing and listening to the stereo and we usually went to bed early.

"Every Wednesday afternoon we had Maternity clinic—prenatal and well-baby. Two girls worked in Maternity and could handle normal deliveries. We had a 4 bed maternity unit with a delivery room and cribs just like the ones in the Nursery at Augie. There was also a 12 bed sick house and the Dispensary which consisted of Pharmacy, Meds and Treatment Room and an Examining Room.

"We had running water during the rainy season and during the beginning of the dry season, but by the beginning of February, water had to be hauled from the stream. We grew what vegetables we could and we also had 60 orange trees and grapefruit and bananas were plentiful too. Don has 43 head of cattle, beef and milk, so there was fresh beef at intervals and milk, cream and butter. We also raised chickens so we had eggs too.

"During the dry season, Don goes hunting and supplies wild meat—buffalo, elephant, warthog, baboon, guinea fowl and others which supply real variety.

"Being a nurse in a foreign country includes more than just nursing. Some of my other duties were helping teach English, making uniforms for the students in the trade schools, cooking and planning the Senior Banquet, setting broken legs on kids and on cows, and chick sitting with new baby chicks."

Augustana Hospital donated the use of its newly acquired property on the west side of Lincoln Avenue for the fourth annual 43rd Ward Tent Party on Sunday June 3. Thousands of people came from all over the city and paid $2.00 for an afternoon of all they could eat and drink. There was live entertainment and an impressive list of guest speakers and well-wishers.

Ardith Gannon '63 gave us some statistics on the new class that entered Augustana in September. There were 39 members in the class: 4 were men, 30 had some college background, 5 had degrees, 8 women were married, 2 men were married, 28 were between the ages of 20-30, 2 were over 40, 1 was an OR Tech., 2 were LPN's, 2 were Social Workers, many had been Aides, and 21 lived in the Nurses Residence. It was announced that the first male Alumni Association member joined in September of 1973.

In an effort to increase use of community resources for enhancing clinical experience, Augustana students used facilities at Chicago Lying-In, Grant and Hines for training in several specialties.

The Seventy-Sixth graduating class had 31 members. Admitted in September was a new class of 49 students selected from

150 applicants. Over 3,000 inquiries about the school were answered.

On receiving its renewed 7-year accreditation from the National League of Nursing, the school was praised for its outstanding library and its excellent faculty-student relations.

Scholarship funding was received from the U.S. Department of Health, Education and Welfare, State of Illinois, Allstate Insurance Foundation, Dr. John I. Perl Scholarship fund, Augustana Alumnae and the Augustana Auxiliary. [Dr. Perl, a general surgeon, was on Augustana's Medical staff for 33 years. He died July 25, 1972.]

A special committee was engaged, during the most of 1972, in evaluation of the curriculum, with special concern for clinical evaluation, placement of basic sciences, and emergency and disaster nursing.

At the suggestion of the Chicago Heart Association, Augustana began a program of providing a free service of taking blood pressures every Wednesday from 1-3 p.m. in the hospital lobby. The goal of the program was to reduce the complications of high blood pressure by early detection. Anyone with an elevated pressure was advised to see a doctor for treatment.

Ten Augustana R.N.'s volunteered their services, under the direction of Ina Magnuson '36, and made the program a success. On the average, they took between 40 and 50 blood pressures each time.

About this time attention had been brought to the move going on to make continuing education for nurses mandatory. While theoretically, the idea that nurses should constantly update their knowledge in the health-care field is sound; in actuality, it could place an undue burden on many nurses or drive many out of nursing entirely. Furthermore, "continuing education" had not actually been defined, leading to the possibility that each state would come up with a different definition and different laws governing it.

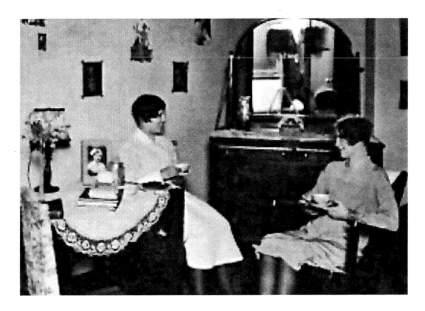

Student Nurses' Quarters, Circa 1930s

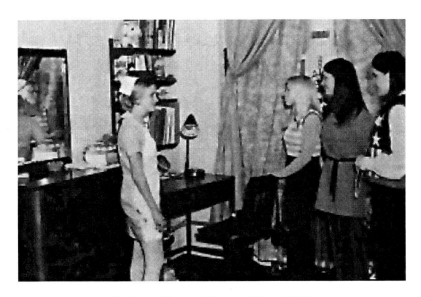

Student Nurses' Room, Circa 1970

The editors of RN Magazine urged leaders in nursing to act to keep laws off the books at this time and to hold a national meeting to discuss vital questions concerning continuing education. They further urged all nurses to make their views known.

The statement of the Illinois Nurse's Association to the Health Care licensure commission on September 13, 1972 read in part:

Regarding the issues of continuing education for continued licensure peer review, it is the position of the Illinois Nurses' Association that participation in planned learning experiences beyond the basic nursing education level is essential to the effective practice of nursing. This will ensure that: 1) the quality of patient care will be enhanced by narrowing the gap that exists between what is known and what is practiced in nursing; 2) those who are the recipients of nursing care will have some guarantee of competency and quality; and 3) nurses themselves will be stimulated, gratified through self-edification and currently knowledgeable—all of which can only serve to increase their professional competency.

As is often the case when a new and sound idea is conceived, faulty planning caused by impatience and/or pressure from the need to see tangible results, leads to the premature demise of the entire venture. In the case of continuing education, the strongest factor leading to this demise would be to make it mandatory for continued relicensure before guaranteeing easy accessibility and rewards.

In September, the Alumni voted to cancel future January and February meetings since the weather was so undependable.

In the early 1970's the female student uniform was changed to a mini A-line dress, with a light blue back and white front and a Peter Pan collar. The male students wore white slacks and tops. The students worked 4 to 8 hours a day, 3 or 4 days a week, depending on their class load, and tuition was $700.00 per semester. The affiliations were Hines Veterans Administration Hospital, Reed Mental Health Center, Childrens Memorial Hospital, Lying-In, Columbus and Grant Hospitals. The specialties of obstetrics and operating room were each 8 weeks. There was no diet kitchen experience but a nutrition class was taken at Loop College. Also taught at Loop College were language arts, biological sciences and social sciences. Basic courses in nursing were taught in Augustana and were so arranged that theory and practice were concurrent. The class of 1973 graduated the first male students.

On Wednesday, January 6, several tables were set up in the first floor hall, West Wing, displaying and selling the products of the Blindskills Association. Augustana is one of 400 organizations in the Chicago area that has these displays each year. We are glad so many employees stopped by and helped support the Association.

In 1974, Augustana joined 3 other hospitals in Chicago in supplying the "Meals on Wheels" program. It supplied two meals per day, one hot and one cold, to persons throughout the city. By mid-March, Augustana supplied meals for about 30 persons per day. Arrangements for this service were handled through the Social Service Department.

This program began at Augustana as a federally funded project of the Community Services of Metropolitan Chicago. In mid-August Federal funds ran out and the Mayor's Committee on Senior Citizens agreed to continue the program. It took a month and a half for this committee to get their project going and during that time, many people in need of this food went without it. Seeing the need, Augustana decided to continue "Meals on Wheels" as a hospital program. It took about a week to set up the procedure, and on August 19, the hospital began supplying the service on its own. Augustana paid for the food, preparation and packaging and the services of a delivery drive. About half the cost of the food was returned through the payments of the people served and the rest was paid totally by the hospital.

The week of March 10–15, 1974, was National Nursing Week. At Augustana Nurse Recognition Day was celebrated on Wednesday the 13th, with a tea honoring the hospital's R.N.'s. Mrs. Genevieve Carb, Acting President, was appreciative of the hospital's nursing staff. She said that Nurses were a vital element in running the hospital and they kept the quality of patient care high. Many of the nurses were Augustana graduates.

The Augustana Hospital West Coast Alumnae met for a luncheon at Bullock's Wilshire Tea Room in Los Angeles, California on April 28, 1974. They have been meeting over twenty years.

The 73rd Annual Tea and Banquet of the Alumni Association was held on June 1, 1974. The Annual Tea with 290 in attendance was held in the Lila Pickhardt Lounge of the Nurse's Residence. We adjourned to the Furniture Club of America for the Social Hour and Banquet, where we dined lavishly on Deviled Seafood Encoquille, Athenian Salad with Anchovy Dressing, Sirloin of Beef Cubes, Mushrooms En Brochette, Rice Pilaf, Green Asparagus Polonaise. Our lovely meal came to an end with French Cream Cheese Cake with Strawberry Sauce.

After dining, we were welcomed by Joyce Herter '48, President. Greeting to the Alumnae was given by Genevieve Carb, Director of Nursing, and various members of the special classes. Entertainment for the evening was presented by Elda Peters '54 who sang several lovely vocal selections accompanied on the piano by Betty Thompson '63. [Elda performed at LaScala Opera in Milan, Italy with the Chicago Lyric Opera in January 1978.]

Eleven hospitals of the Lincoln Park-Lakeview community participated in an areawide disaster exercise on Thursday, Sept. 19 at 10:00 a.m. The disaster was the simulated collision of two chartered buses at Dearborn and North Avenue, resulting in injuries to 67 persons.

Cooperating for the disaster program were Augustana, Childrens, Columbus, Grant, Henrotin, Northwestern Memorial, Norwegian American, St. Elizabeth, St. Joseph, St. Mary and Walther Memorial Hospital. Each hospital had a specific role in the exercise and all area hospitals were placed on a disaster alert. Five hospitals received casualties in the exercise: Childrens, Columbus, Henrotin, St. Elizabeth and St. Mary.

The purpose of the drill was to coordinate emergency medical services in the Lincoln Park-Lakeview hospitals and to review the medical capability for providing on-the-site emergency care to save lives in the event of a real disaster.

Since Augustana did not have a completed Disaster Plan until Sept. 17, our role in this exercise was on a stand-by basis only. As soon as our Disaster Plan was approved, we held our own disaster drill to test its effectiveness. All areas of the hospital were involved and everyone was informed of their function in the drill beforehand.

Dr. Carl A. Hedberg made a different kind of rounds on Sunday, September 29, greeting guests at Augustana's 90th Anniversary Open House on the newly-renovated 8th floor. Over 2000 people showed up to share in refreshments, wished us a "Happy Birthday" and saw the results of Renovation.

People began to arrive at 12:45 p.m., even though the invitation stated the Open House began at 1:00 p.m. The flow throughout the afternoon was steady and people were still viewing the lobby and the 8th floor at 6:30 p.m..

The first greeting, as guests entered the newly-carpeted and furnished lobby, came from several nursing students, on hand to guide our guests to various points of interest. The 12 panel, picture history of the hospital was in the lobby, along with a table loaded with souvenirs and mementos of the hospital, past and present. From there, guests were led to the express elevator in the East Wing, to go directly to the 8th floor. Near the elevator, a 13 minute slide-tape presentation, "The Exercise of Mercy" ran continuously through the afternoon. Just down the hall from there, the new Special Procedures Room in X-ray was open for viewing.

Upstairs, the main attraction was the 8th floor itself. Newly-renovated, about to be opened for patients, the floor showed all the features that would make Augustana a much better care and treatment facility when the entire Renovation was completed. The floor had a new nursing station, new room furniture and patient bed consoles, treatment and exam rooms, better lighting and a completely new "look." "It looks like a different hospital" was a quote heard often throughout the day.

There was a brief program at 3:00 p.m. which attracted several hundred people to the already crowded solarium. Board Chairman, Jerry H. Pearson, presented former Board member, Ralph A. Powers, with a plaque in recognition of his initial work on the Renovation program. Acting President, Genevieve Carb, presented many records and documents from Augustana's past to The Chicago Historical Society. Rev. Harry Victorson, Chairman of the 90th Anniversary, read greetings and congratulations from the King of Sweden, Senators Percy and Stevenson, Mayor Daley and Dr. Gerald K. Johnson, Illinois Synod President. Finally, Chaplain Philip Anderson introduced 12 Chicago area senior citizens who came to celebrate their birthdays with us.

That year at Augustana, the two fall ceremonies for the School of Nursing took place at the same time. Capping for the freshmen and striping for the seniors were held on Monday evening, September 30 at St. Paul's Church, Orchard and Fullerton. 30 seniors and 35 freshmen, along with many relatives and friends, joined in these ceremonies beginning the new school year. Both groups were addressed briefly by Ms. Genevieve Carb on the responsibility of nurses and administration to excellent patient care and the exercise of mercy among the suffering.

The Vietnam War ended in 1975 and had cut across American politics, economy and ideals. We lost more than 57,000 men in this conflict. It left Vietnam in shambles, and the Communists aggravated the devastation following their victory. They suppressed private entrepreneurs and interned 300,000 South Vietnamese officials and army officers in brutal "re-education" camps. Hundreds of thousands of lost people fled the country as a result of persecution as well as proof that the economy was breaking down. (Source—U.S. News and World Report and Smithsonian Magazine, 1996.)

The Graduation Awards of the School of Nursing were presented annually at the Commencement Ceremony. At this time with the changes that were putting the school on a more collegiate level, it was felt by the faculty that more recognition should be given to students who excelled in various areas. Graduation with honors was given to those graduates who consistently maintained a 3.50 or better grade point average in both theory and nursing performance as a student. The faculty award was presented to the individual with the highest scholastic achievement of the graduating class.

The Bess Lang award was given for high achievement in Nursing which included not only academic standing, but sympathetic understanding of the patient, practical ability, professional attitude and conduct. This award was given back in the 1960's.

The Alumnae Association Award was given for intelligent and compassionate care of patients. In the late 1970's two new awards were added, the coordinators' award for personal growth toward professional excellence, [The term coordinator was now being used instead of head nurse or supervisor] and the Chester L. Crean Memorial Award. This was given to the graduating nurse who demonstrated the internalization of values and philosophies that were most reflective of the role of the professional nurse-values appreciated and fostered by Dr. Crean and those physicians who continue to practice the art of medicine.

The Alumnae's pledge to the hospital of $10,000 for the glassed-in nurse's stations was completed in December 1976. This was accomplished in two years. The total amount of donations collected was $11,270.

In the mid-1970's the Internal Revenue Service began checking in depth into the funds of not-for-profit organizations. The amount of money in our Sick Nurses' Benefit Fund was accumulating interest and the Association was told by our auditor that we would have to disperse the excess funds or pay a substantial income tax.

Legal counsel was sought and some money was given to the hospital, which was used for buying casters for the bedside tables, audio-visual equipment for continuing education, a Stryker Frame Bed, several wheel chairs and two Holter Pumps. Some money was put in the general fund and legal fees were paid. We continued to accept donations for sick nurses and distributed it at Christmas time and as the need arose.

Augustana had installed a brand new system in the delivery area on 2 West. It was the Imed Fetal Monitoring System. When a mother began labor, a microphone-like disc was secured to her abdomen. It remained there through labor and delivery. The disc monitored the baby's heart rate, making it visible on a screen and audible in the labor room. In the hall there was a monitoring unit exactly like the one next to the mother's bed. With this duplicate monitor, nurses could keep track of labor progress while attending to other duties. An alarm, which would sound or flash if any trouble developed, was included in the system.

About this time the Federal Drug Administration believed that a study of the long term effects of the cementing substance used to fix an implanted joint should be available prior to its release for general use. During that time, Dr. Thomas Hall became familiar with the procedure through his work on the faculty of Northwestern University and at the Veteran's Administration Hospital. A 10-year F.D.A. study showed the apparent effects of the cement to be innocuous during that period. Restrictions were removed and the procedure was made available in this country. At considerable expense, Augustana obtained the specialized equipment required for this procedure.

Augustana was one of the only six medical centers in the United States to study the use of a total hip replacement without using cement. This procedure, called the Sivash Hip was developed and implemented in the Soviet Union. The Sivash Hip was used at Augustana in those cases determined unsatisfactory for the use of the cement procedures.

The 1976 Class of the Augustana Hospital School of Nursing joined the ranks of the nursing profession at graduation exercises held Friday evening, July 9, at St. Paul's United Church of Christ. In her remarks, Mrs. Carb addressed the seniors about the preparation to be professional nurses: "May I remind you that nursing is not a job; it is not a position. It is a commitment that will enrich your life. Our good wishes go with you."

Dr. Alton Ochsner, nephew of world-renowned Augustana surgeon Dr. Albert J. Ochsner (1858–1927), was honored in New Orleans by former students on the occasion of his 80th birthday. Dr. Alton Ochsner served his internship and residency at Augustana under Drs. A.J. Ochsner and Nelson Percy. Nearly 3,600 men and women trained in surgery under Dr. Alton Ochsner, including heart surgeon Dr. Michael DeBakey. Dr. Ochsner no longer performed surgery, but was active in teaching, which he once described as his central aim: "To teach students how to think under stress, to think quickly and correctly, and to back up every decision they make."

Current legislation in Springfield was brought to the attention of those present, so the Senators could be contacted regarding one bill in particular, namely House Bill #564, which would authorize Physicians Assistants to be employed by the House of Corrections. It was pointed out that Legislators were not all aware of the wide variety of preparation of the P.A.'s. There were legal implications since nurses could not legally follow orders written by P.A. nurses. It was felt that the State Senators should be advised to vote "Nay" to that Bill.

The annual Tea and Banquet was held on Saturday, June 3, 1978 at the Furniture Mart. Ms. Margaret Biemolt, Interim

Director of the School of Nursing, was introduced and spoke about our changed and changing school. The changes began in the 1950's, with the educational-type program. Science classes were taught in the Jr. College system, and 27 transferable credits were given. Students no longer worked P.M.'s and nights, and were no longer in charge on any shift, Instructors had 6-7 students to supervise and went to all 15 affiliating institutions with the students. On state boards the graduates had consistently ranked in the upper third of all 3 types of graduates. All faculty either had a master's degree or were enrolled in a Master's Program.

Ms. Biemolt then introduced a senior student who would graduate on June 30, 1978; Ms. Chris Aubert, who, had maintained a 4.0 average. Ms. Aubert stated her reasons for coming to Augustana at age 28 after previous education and work as a social worker. She noted her age was close to the average, since most students had already had previous "work and living experience in other areas" rather than being right out of high school. The large percentage of students were self-supporting.

The 2 members present from the 60 year class of 1918 were warmly welcomed. Once again we were privileged to have Hilda Dickenson, 1914, with us; she had attended over 20 banquets. She read a poem for happiness in which a garden is planted, and left us with the message that to love and be loved is one of the biggest joys of life.

# CHAPTER VI

## THE EIGHTIES

The seriousness of the low attendance at Alumnae Meetings was discussed at the Board meeting in April 1980, and presented to those present. The suggestion was made to hold only four meetings a year—a spring meeting, the tea and banquet, a fall meeting, and a Christmas meeting; or possibly only have the June banquet and Christmas meeting.

At the June 1980, Alumnae Banquet at the Swedish Club, President Bea Ruble '51 first introduced the officers and board, then the guest speaker, John Jezierski, coordinator for the School of Nursing. He had been on the faculty for 5 years and had served in the present position for 1 year. He noted that the 1980's would be dynamic for nursing and nursing education. The goal of the school was to be sure that the nurses trained were as concerned and competent as they were in the past. The school was faced with increased costs, decreased enrollment, and the challenges of nursing itself. On June 27, 1980, 26 seniors would graduate and 30 would advance to their senior year. Forty were expected in the new class. Only 16 lived in the residence, all on one floor. Mr. Jezierski served on the Nursing Executive Board and the school was again part of the hospital nursing service. He extended an invitation to all Alumnae to come and see what was going on in the hospital and school. Ms. Ruble noted it was good to see the school and hospital being reunited.

Mary Ellen Adams '48 wrote from Jos, Nigeria that she was acting as a dormitory parent at Kent Academy, which was a

boarding school for missionary children. She cared for first and
second grade children.

From the Joliet Herald News, November 1980—Hilda
Dickinson '14 celebrated her 93rd birthday and 86 people of
all ages were there. Hilda's secret for longevity was love. She
said, "It doesn't matter how old you are, you can develop skills
you never knew you had." She made Raggedy Ann and Andy
dolls for gifts and for sale. She said about nursing, "Once your
heart is in nursing, it never lets go."

> Her niece Betty Sundin wrote this song for her:
>> "How many people have known the touch of your hand?
>> Nursing their suffering, meeting their every demand.
>> And your compassion is like a ray from above.
>> May the Lord bless and keep you
>> For the way you show His love."

In the fall of 1980, Augustana successfully placed the largest debt issue in its history to underwrite the $11 million cost
of its current building program. The total project included not
only direct patient care areas, but the 20 doctors' offices and
the 400-car parking structure. (Alumnae and auxiliary members were allowed to park free.) To help pay for the emergency
room, outpatient area, lobby and other facilities that did not
normally produce any revenue or enough revenue to pay for
their construction, the Board of Directors had authorized a
public appeal for $2 million to help the hospital repay the loans
it had made.

This appeal, called "Partners in Caring," was conducted under the co-chairmanship of Dr. and Mrs. Carl A. Hedberg, who
both had long and distinguished records of concern for the welfare of Augustana Hospital. Leaders of the Board of Directors,
the Medical Staff, Administration, the Auxiliary, Nursing
School Alumnae, the Lutheran community and other key men
and women associated with the hospital were working with Dr.
and Mrs. Hedberg to secure gifts for this capital fundraising
venture. Individuals, corporations, charitable foundations, com-

munity residents and other groups were invited to consider becoming "Partners in Caring." In doing so, they would be making an investment in the future of patient care in one of Chicago's best known community hospitals.

Augustana Hospital established one of the earliest schools of nursing in the Midwest in 1894. Since the first class graduated in 1896, some 3,000 Augustana R.N.'s entered nursing careers in the hospital itself or in other hospitals, industry, the military, overseas missions and public health service. Through the years, the school had gained a wide and enviable reputation for the high quality of nurses it produced.

As was true of most educational institutions, tuition paid for only a part of the annual cost of over $300,000 to maintain the school. The costs included faculty salaries, equipment and other elements necessary to educate future nurses. With other expenses essential to a modern hospital and with decreasing federal assistance, Augustana had to include some of its school of nursing's operating costs in its appeal for assistance.

Another famous Augustana program, now in its seventh year, was the Seniors' Health Program. This community activity provided health education and demonstration of 20 specific topics to thousands of Chicago's elderly each year. It also offered hundreds of health care workers specific training seminars in geriatric care. Begun as a program to educate seniors on the proper use of medication, it provided them with information on topics such as sleep, high blood pressure, nutrition, arthritis and exercise. Two R.N.-health educators, physician-specialists and geriatric social workers met with groups of seniors in churches, schools, libraries, senior centers and other sites all over the Chicago area. Because the government did not reimburse the hospital for this community program, gifts from private sources had to be secured annually to supplement its budget. It was our hope that substantial philanthropic funding would be obtained to insure the continuation of the Seniors' Health Program.

LaVerne Oerke '49, our own Asst. Editor, represented Augustana at the annual Chicago Hospital Council Luncheon, on May 13, 1981, at the Conrad Hilton Hotel, honoring those "candlelighters" (those working night shifts). LaVerne was chosen because of her consistently professional performance, often above and beyond the call of duty. She was a model representative of those nurses, who when the rest of the world was asleep, must be constantly vigilant and alert to the needs of their patients. The nursing administration nominated LaVerne with pride and spoke of her as a very dedicated nurse. LaVerne served as charge nurse on the 11-7 shift for 11 years at Augustana. Her devotion and dedication was rightly recognized, as we in the Alumnae Association were well aware of how much of herself LaVerne put into all of her endeavors.

A memo was sent to the students in June 1981, from the financial aid officer.

"We would like to alert you to the possibility that the Illinois State Scholarship Commission will reduce its 1980-81 second semester grants and scholarships by $100.00 for many students. We have not been notified officially that this will occur or which students will have their awards cut this semester. Since Augustana has already allowed credit on student tuition accounts for Illinois State Awards as they were originally announced, such reductions in State Awards will result in a balance due on the accounts of those students affected by the grant reductions. We are alerting you of this possibility now so that you might plan for this additional expense should it affect your grant award."

As of August 1981, tuition was $2500, room $1000, meals (approx.) $750, activity fee $25, library fee $25, health fee $50 and liability insurance fee $15.

In 1982 the Tax Equity and Fiscal Responsibility Bill was signed into law. This brought about the D.R.G.'s (Diagnostic Related Groups) and all the problems related to it. There was much confusion and to this day we witness much unfairness.

An issue facing Augustana and other Illinois hospitals stemmed from the 1981–1982 limitations by the State of Illinois on all Medicaid procedures and imposed a quota on Medicaid patient cases for which public funds provided reimbursement. Limitations were based on 1979 figures. Because the number of Medicaid patients was increasing, great financial damage was being done to Illinois hospitals that had heavy Medicaid clientele.

In 1981, the Joint Commission on Accreditation of Hospitals gave Augustana a full 2 year approval for its high-level standards of quality for patient care, physical plant, safety requirements and medical records.

Irene Shymaniv, RN, MSN of our Augustana's Dept. of Nursing Education, wrote in a "Nurses Notes" editorial regarding the responsibility of nursing to shoulder the blame for some of the causes of the nursing shortage. She named two problems: patient education and peer orientation as being two areas in which nursing should begin healing itself. She stated that we as nurses must earn our patients' respect by planning their care beyond the mechanics of pill-passing and daily care, to include the health education and discharge planning essential to the understanding and management of their care at home. The other problem was that we neglect our own peers by not accepting and helping new graduates in their orientation, causing them to be discouraged and leave the profession.

On Wednesday, November 4 at 7:00 p.m., the Alumnae met at Northwest Community Hospital Treatment and Health Center located at Lake Cook Road and Rte. 83 in Buffalo Grove, Illinois. It was an ambulatory care facility designed to treat non life-threatening illnesses and injuries when your physician was not available. Our speaker for the evening was Clarice Rech '54, nursing administrator of the free standing unit, located about eleven miles from its "parent" Northwest Community Hospital in Arlington Heights. The first fiscal year ended October 31, 1981, and over 19,000 patients were treated there while 55,000 were seen in the main hospital trauma center. This

concept in providing health care was well received by the surrounding community. Patients needing hospitalization were
transported to NCH by ambulance.

Clarice had a staff of 30 that included registered nurses, laboratory, and x-ray personnel. All were CPR certified. All nursing staff must have had either critical care nursing or emergency
room nursing to qualify for employment. This facility, open
24 hours a day, 365 days a year was also staffed with an experienced emergency room physician. The staff rotated to NCH
trauma center for two weeks every six months to keep their
emergency room skills up to date. With a skeleton staff on at
night, the night nurse carried a beeper for immediate help from
police if needed.

Finance Chairman Marie Ruehrdanz '26, presented some
new business which hopefully would motivate alumnae members as it had in the past. The Hospital was again looking for
money. The goal was $2 million, of which $1,500,000 would
be spent on the new building. The School of Nursing was to
receive $250,000 with the same amount going to the Seniors'
Health Program. The anticipated donation from the Alumnae
Association was $20,000 over a 3 year period. There was
$961.60 left from the last fund drive for the glass-enclosed
nursing stations, and $17,719.00 in the general fund. The
motion was unanimously approved to give $961.60 and
$4,038.40 for a total of $5,000.00 to the Hospital's "Those
Who Care" drive at this time. The remaining $15,000 would
be donated by the membership.

Joint projects with neighboring hospitals included a successful benefit at Adler Planetarium for the Five Hospital
Homebound Elderly Program; Augustana was one of the five.
The continuing publication of FYI (For Your Information), the
Six Hospital Consortium's semiannual newsletter, which was
mailed to Lincoln Park and Lake View residents was part of
the joint project. The consortium also sponsored a health careers day for high school students in the area. Highlight of the

event was exhibits by 20 health-related groups featuring the attractions of their professions. The American Association of Blood Banks after an extensive on-site inspection, gave a two-year accreditation to Augustana's Blood Bank.

Augustana began performing outpatient operations on a limited basis in 1973. By 1982, when Augustana's ambulatory care center opened, the case load had grown to over 900. The Chicago Hospital Council found that 27% of all Chicago area operations were performed in an outpatient setting. On the national level, 7 of the 10 operations performed most frequently were one day surgeries.

The tremendous growth in one day surgeries was traced to the advent of government and private insurance policies that covered outpatient operations. The federal government listed over 95 operations which Medicaid and Medicare would cover if performed as one day surgeries. This policy trend was the direct result of technological advances in surgical equipment and anesthetic methods. New equipment allowed surgeons to operate while making smaller incisions, and often in a non-invasive manner. This led to the increased use of local, rather than general anesthetics. Commonly performed procedures ranged from simple removal of ingrown nails to more complex reconstructive plastic surgery, skin lesion excisions, and sterilization. The CHC predicted continued growth in the number and type of operations performed as one day surgeries.

The Alumnae Association decided to accept the Birthing Room as a project and through pledges from Alumnae members, donated $5,000.00 to the hospital.

Augustana Hospital was looking for nurses, retired or active, who would be interested in donating time on a regular basis. Volunteers were needed in all areas of the hospital.

Augustana Hospital's new ambulatory care center opened and accepted patients in mid-1982. These facilities increased Augustana's available services to its community and were expected to heighten the hospital's attractiveness to physicians.

Ambulatory care was gaining importance in the United States as a more suitable setting and less expensive means of treating many health problems than admission to inpatient care. Most people entered the health care system, received preventive and primary care, early detection, and routine treatment in doctors' offices, clinics, hospital outpatient areas and neighborhood health centers.

Augustana had been providing quality medical care and health education to Chicago area people since 1884. In adding to its capacity, without increasing its number of beds, the hospital was continuing this proud tradition of service to humanity.

Sharing the ground floor of the three-story structure with the new ambulatory care services was a lobby and gift shop/coffee shop. The Lincoln Avenue frontage of the building became the main entrance to the hospital, replacing the Dickens Avenue entrance. Offices of the chaplaincy and social services were also remodeled.

In the emergency department there were five treatment cubicles, a cast room, an observation area, separate ambulance and walk-in entrances, reception and triage areas, nursing stations, supply and equipment storage space, on-call rooms and a lounge.

The outpatient department had centralized registration and a separate waiting area, both located next to the front entrance and main lobby. There were six examination rooms, an ophthalmology room, a proctoscopy room, a major treatment-minor surgery room, and associated support areas that included a physician charting area, nursing work stations and storage space. It was expected that increased emphasis would be placed on the use of the surgicenter, so its patients would have dressing rooms and locker facilities. A laboratory specimen collection station, EKG facilities for inpatients prior to admission and for outpatients were located adjacent to the patient registration area, just off the main lobby.

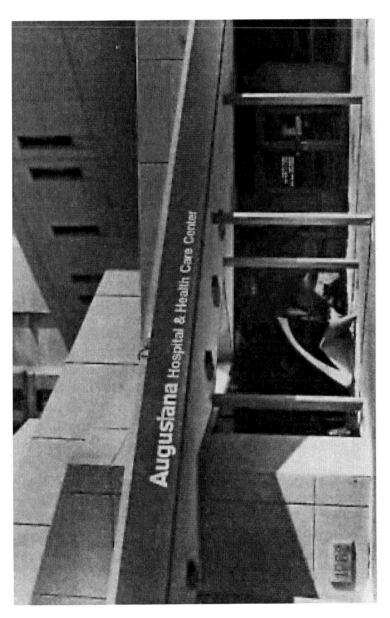

Lincoln Avenue Entrance to Augustana

Close to the emergency and outpatient departments and connected by a corridor restricted to patient traffic were both the radiology and radiation oncology departments. Other areas under construction were an elevator tower, corridors, laundry plant, freight receiving area, standby boiler and incinerator. Especially interesting to many friends of this religious hospital was a lift that enabled patients in their wheelchairs to attend religious services in the Chapel, which was below ground level.

"Ask the President," a live interview program featuring Augustana President John Rice made its debut on the patient television channel in September. During this once-a-month program, patients could phone their questions from their rooms and watch the chief executive officer answer them live.

The hospital, through the volunteers department, brought to the patients 'BINGO" via their television sets. The hospital's closed circuit system aired the game every Wednesday afternoon and was only one of a handful of hospitals across the country using closed circuit TV for patient information. It was hoped that this system could also be used for patient education.

The following news items were announced at Alumnae meetings during 1981.

The plaque for the Lila Pickhardt lounge noting it was furnished by the Alumni Association was put in place in June of 1981.

There was now only one housemother on duty from 9 a.m. to 4 p.m.

Roland and Tanya Frazier both of the class of '79, welcomed to their family their first born son Roland Davis Jr., born March 13, 1981.

Librarian Betsy Clausen of the Carl Hedberg Memorial Library requested us to bring her any nursing journals that we were through with, so that the students could have more than one copy for their studies.

Joy Smith Catterson '61 and co-author Karon White Gibson of the '67 graduating class of Mt. Sinai Hospital proudly an nounced the release of their non-fiction novel "ON OUR OWN" published by St. Martin's Press in New York.

Three hundred fifty employees and community residents attended a 2-day Safety Fair at the hospital. Sponsored by the hospital safety committee, it stressed fire and on-the-job safety and careful use of prescription medicine. In the interest of public health education, the hospital conducted three "stop smoking" clinics, free blood pressure monitoring, diabetics testing, stress seminar for women and classes in cardiopulmonary resuscitation. A six-week LaMaze class began July 30 at Augustana. Held Thursday evenings 7:30-9:30 p.m., in the Hickey Room, the class demonstrated breathing techniques and relaxation exercises, and discussed the birth process from conception to fetal development.

Augustana's school of nursing Audio/Visual Resource Center was available to all Augustana employees. Typical patrons of the resource center were medical technology and nursing students, nurses, dieticians, surgical assistants, medical technologists and respiratory therapists. Subjects ranged in diversity from cancer, nurse-patient interaction, an introduction to radiation and holistic health to nursing fundamentals, CPR and stress. Started in 1976, the resource center had continually expanded itself to be able to offer several hundred educational programs in its location on the third floor of the school of nursing building.

The 29th Annual benefit of the Augustana Hospital Auxiliary, which sponsored a performance of the 1982 Ice Capades, netted $30,000 for the "Partners in Caring" building project.

Some of the honors bestowed upon Augustana medical staff members during the past year included: Dr. Anderson Hedberg who had been elected president of the Chicago Society of Internal Medicine, vice-president of the Chicago Society of Gastroenterology and vice president of the Institute of Medicine of Chicago. Dr. Peter Werner was serving as clinical professor of Pulmonary Diseases at Loyola University and Dr. Joshua

Oden, had been elected Fellow of the American College of Utilization Review Physicians.

An invitation was received from the School for the striping and capping ceremony on December 17 at 7:00 p.m.

A funeral was held on January 20, 1983 for Eleanor Olsen Schallmoser '50 who passed away at Augustana Hospital on January 17. Her entire nursing career was devoted to Augustana, holding positions of staff nurse, head nurse, supervisor, Assistant Director of Nurses and for 1 year (1977–78) was Acting Director of Nursing. She retired in the summer of 1982. Her professional life was dedicated to Augustana and its well-being, and to upholding the Augustana Nurse tradition of giving excellent patient care.

Augustana Hospital continued to adapt to the times by upgrading its facility and equipment. In 1983, Augustana installed an argon laser for treatment of eye disorders and improved laboratory testing with the purchase of the latest state-of-the-art equipment. Also in 1983, Augustana added to its radiology department digital vascular imaging, a Computed Axial Tomography scanner and a mobile nuclear medicine unit.

The Oncology Nursing Society announced the election of Judi Johnson, R.N., PhD '58 to its Presidency for a two year term. The election results were announced at the organization's Eighth Annual Congress in San Diego, CA, May 18–21, 1983. At this time, Dr. Johnson was the Oncology Coordinator at North Memorial Medical Center in Minneapolis, MN. Dr. Johnson received international acclaim for the development of the I CAN COPE program for cancer patients and their families. The Oncology Nursing Society was incorporated in 1975 and had a membership of over 5000 nurses. It was dedicated to promoting the highest standards of oncology nursing as well as encouraging nurses to specialize in this field.

Augustana's spirit of caring sometimes took surprise turns. In 1983, an anonymous donor gave $130,000 to promote quality nursing care and education in honor of Dr. C.L.Crean, who died in 1980. Dr. Crean served with distinction on Augustana'a medical staff for over 50 years. During his career, Dr. Crean showed a reverence for life and the patient, and he was dedicated to improving the care provided by student and professional nurses. The Dr. C.L.Crean Memorial Award was used for student scholarships and for awards to outstanding student and professional nurses.

A strategic plan had been devised to guide Augustana. The 1983 affiliation with the Lutheran Institute for Human Ecology, the parent organization for Lutheran General Hospital, Lutheran Center for Substance Abuse and now, Augustana, strengthened the institution and added to its resources. Augustana saw its greatest strength in its people and in its relationship as a church hospital that was committed to primary care and to the community.

An informative videotape on Diagnostic Related Groups was available to key hospital personnel, including physicians in charge of clinical management. Produced by the Center for Educational Development at the University of Illinois at Chicago, the videotape was entitled "Implementing DRG's: Developing Effective Strategies." It was based upon the final Federal regulations published January 1, 1984.

By 1984, in keeping with quality assurance and ambulatory care, a questionnaire was sent out to patients who had been served. Some questions were asked about why they chose Augustana and were they satisfied with the care. The questionnaire also asked the recipient of care to rate the courtesy of the staff.

Banners bearing Augustana Hospital and Health Care Center's name and logo flew on Michigan Avenue as the hospital kicked off its centennial Feb. 25 of 100 years of caring with a formal ball in the Ritz-Carlton Hotel.

Over three hundred eighty staff, auxiliary, alumnae, and

friends of the hospital attended the magnificent affair. A delicious meal of soup, salad, prime rib and baked Alaska was followed by music and dancing in the Grand Ballroom.

During the program, Dr. Andy Hedberg served as Master of Ceremonies. A welcome was given by Mrs. Marion Victorson, Co-Chairman of the Centennial Committee and the invocation was given by her husband, Rev. Harry Victorson, also Co-Chairman. The following people spoke during the program: Rev. Paul E. Erickson, Bishop of Illinois Synod LCA; J. Arthur Gustafson, Chairman of the Board of Trustees, Augustana Hospital; Dr. Luis Mella, President of the Medical Staff; the Honorable Lars Arno, Consul General, Sweden; Jimmy Sorenson, Lutheran Institute of Human Ecology; and Rev. Robert Shaner, President, Chief Executive Officer, Augustana Hospital.

A number of Alumnae members were in attendance and were asked to stand in recognition. Mrs. Joyce Herter '48, President of the Alumnae Association was thanked for her help in organizing the Ball, and Mrs. Hilda Sundeen Dickinson '14, received a hand of applause as the oldest living Alumnae member. Her many years of interest and service to the Alumnae Association were well known.

A Centennial Book printed in honor of the celebration gave a very thorough, condensed history of the hospital and nursing school from its inception, through the war years (I and II), the post-war expansion and remodeling, to the hospital of today with its continued commitment and ministry to the health of the whole person.

For Nurses Week, there was a display of models of past uniforms and memorabilia in the hospital lobby. Five Alumnae members modeled Augustana Hospital student nurse uniforms of the last century at the Nurses' Tea held in honor of Illinois Nurses' Week on Thursday March 8, in the Lila Pickhardt Lounge. All personnel, Auxiliary and Alumnae members were invited to attend. Those modeling uniforms were Ina Magnuson

'36, with a 1956 uniform and cape; Ingrid Olson Stalle '64, a 1948 uniform; Doreen Gromik Pelnar '63 with a 1900's uniform made by Caroll Anderson Fagerman '63; Janice Carlson Young '62 with a 1948 scrub gown and cap; and Carol Stegall '63 modeled a 1947 cadet uniform.

The hospital also planned a Eucharist Service in the hospital chapel May 7 and a September Health Fair. A seminar on social, ethical and economic issues was held Oct. 10 in the hospital, featuring speakers of national and local prominence. Panel discussions were held on such subjects as the status of community hospitals, care of the aged and the ethical issues of life support systems. The seminar was open to all interested health care personnel.The Women's Auxiliary held a centennial luncheon Nov. 3 at the Westin Hotel. The year culminated with a centennial concert by the Swedish Glee Club Dec. 2 in the hospital chapel.

On Saturday, June 2, 1984, the Augustana Alumnae held its Annual Tea and Banquet. A Chapel Service was held at 1:30 p.m. in the Hospital Chapel with The Rev. Phillip Anderson officiating. The Tea followed in the Lila Pickhardt Lounge where over 200 alumnae visited and reminisced about "old times." Tours of the hospital were given by Mr. John Jezierski, Coordinator of the School of Nursing. There was an interesting collection of memorabilia from the 100 Years of Caring. Centennial Booklets, published in honor of the 100 year celebration were available to all. There was a presentation on Col. Julia Flicke '15, the first military nurse to be commissioned Colonel in the Army Nurse Corp.

A dream of long standing came true on Saturday, September 8, 1984, when the first reunion of Augie grads currently living in the Upper Peninsula of Michigan was held in the King George Room of the House of Ludington in Escanaba, Michigan. After such coordinating of plans, 35 of 49 grads who were contacted were able to attend the reunion. They represented classes from 1925-1979. The program was a do-it-yourself with self-introductions, Augie anecdotes and reminiscence of years gone by. Many Lutheran women from the central and western parts of the Upper Peninsula trained at Augustana because it was easier to come home from Chicago than from other parts of Michigan. Many Lutheran pastors hearing their young parishioners planning a nursing career automatically said, "You will attend Augustana." Augustana benefited and so did each graduate as could be seen by this wonderful reunion.

In honor of Augustana Hospital's 1984 Centennial, the Auxiliary hosted a Luncheon and Centennial Fashion Show, "Vintage Views" on Saturday, November 3 at the Cotillion Ballroom of the Westin Hotel on Michigan Avenue. The event began with a social hour at 11:30 a.m. followed by lunch at 12:30 p.m. and the fashion show at 1:30 p.m. Renee Chaden, Fashion coordinator for the show and owner of "Sincerely Yours, Renee" directed the show presenting fashions from her collections, including lacy Victorian dresses, white Edwardian tea gowns, fringed flapper dresses, war uniforms and wedding gowns from the 20's and 40's. Auxiliary members, nursing alumnae and doctors' wives modeled styles from 1884, when Augustana was founded, to the present.

The Centennial Sculpture Exhibition was one Centennial Event. There were unusual goings on in the hospital lobby since December 9. Augustana Hospital and Health Care Center and the Chicago Sculpture Society presented the Centennial Sculpture Exhibition through February 28. Many unusual and intriguing works were there; steel, bronze, aluminum, acrylic, wood and other materials. There was a wide range of interest, something for everyone.

We had many difficulties with trying to plan a place for our Banquet. With the Swedish Club of Chicago gone and The Furniture Club gone we were not getting the same considerations that we did because of having had our Banquets there so often. We found a very elegant place in 1985 at the Saddle & Cycle Club. It was a private club and we were able to have our banquet there through the courtesy of Dr. Anderson Hedberg. It was a new place for us and we were anticipating the enjoyment of new and elegant surroundings. The real enjoyment was seeing classmates and renewing acquaintances with our friends from our student and early years.

A farewell reception was held in the Lila Pickhardt Lounge on Wednesday afternoon, February 27, for Dr. Anderson Hedberg. "Andy" accepted a position at Presbyterian-St. Luke's Hospital. Our good wishes went with him.

The following news items were in the summer issue of The Augustana Nurse.

In a previous Augustana Nurse an appeal was issued for Board members and Committee members to serve in 1986. Our Alumnae Association was organized July 12, 1901. 1986 will be our 85th year. It will be a good beginning for this anniversary year if those of you in the area will come to our first meeting this fall.

A majority voted to have a luncheon instead of an evening banquet. The Lila Pickhardt Lounge would be open for visiting, and tours of the hospital would be offered in the afternoon.

The school of Nursing held its 90th Commencement on July 12, 1985. There were 26 graduates, 23 women and 3 men.

You could now have surgery in the morning at Augustana and be home in the afternoon—all done on an outpatient basis. Following surgery and time in the Recovery Room for wake up you went to the Surgicare unit and were with family and friends until you were able to be discharged. Should it develop you needed further care you would be admitted to the hospital for overnight care.

Health and Harmony was a new paper published by the Seniors' Health Program of Augustana. The first issues appeared the summer of '85 and the paper was published quarterly.

Augustana was now associated with three Health Maintenance Organizations (HMO)—Maxicare Illinois, Compass Health Care Plans and HMO Illinois. Augustana was part of the Lutheran General Health Care System (LGHCS). LGHCS and Evangelical Health System (EHS) formed a new joint venture company to operate the seven hospitals owned by the two health care systems. Beside Lutheran General and Augustana, the other hospitals were: Bethany, Christ Hospital and Medical Center, Good Samaritan, Good Shepherd and Woodlawn. These two large organizations had a good deal in common. Both were church affiliated, both were committed to the understanding care of human beings as whole persons. This joint venture made LGHCS/EHS more attractive to HMO's and employers because of the geographical coverage and the range of services available. Also, cost savings were realized by sharing and combining services.

Charlotte Benson Campbell '46 wrote:
Back in 1946 when we were the bright-eyed, sparkling graduates of the year, a 40th anniversary of our graduation from Augustana seemed not only remote but totally removed from reality. We had just completed 3 years of training that progressed from the overwhelming procedure of giving a total bed bath to the competent performance of the duties of "charge nurse" of a 51 bed floor—including 3rd floor on those frantic times of the non-stop Percy operating days.

Where would we be 40 years from that magical moment—besides alive and able to sit up and take nourishment?

Many of us were newly engaged and anxiously awaiting our wedding day, most were leaving the glories of life in Chicago to once again bask in the sweet, clean air of places like upper Michigan; each of us was bursting with excitement to put into practice in a job all we had learned and to emerge from our rooms clad in glowing white from head to toe, the famed blue and white striped uniform having been ripped off our backs a short time before.

We had daughters of nurses in our class and from those present 5 offspring chose nursing as a profession. We had a wide variety of nursing experience for those ancient days and members of our class have distinguished themselves in functioning professionally in a broad spectrum of ways.

Those of us who chose to lead a lower profile professionally found that there are unsung moments of glory in filling the role of neighborhood nurse, keeper of the family health, as well as that of every friend and neighbor who discovered the existence of a real live nurse in their midst. Owning our own personal sphygmomanometer became our badge of honor—helping out in Red Cross Blood drives our contribution to the health and welfare of mankind. Yes, we owe all this to our 3 year high level, gripe-infested, fun-filled, super learning experience from 1943 to 1946 in the hallowed halls of Augustana Hospital School of Nursing. But we owe so much more...

Our memories of associations with appealing, clean-cut, young women from small towns and cities all over the Midwest who became our dearest friends and in many cases remain so to this day are precious to us. The halls of the 7th floor of the former Nurse's Residence must still ring with laughter, screams and an occasional groan from the days when we were growing in love and friendship and in the fine art of becoming a nurse.

A distinguishing mark of our class was that in 1943 we were the first group of nursing students to be enrolled in the Nurses Cadet program and many of our members happily donned the snappy gray uniform and enjoyed an evening with Service people at the local U.S.O.

We had fine examples of dedication in our teachers, supervisors and doctors but, perhaps, it was the essence of what we absorbed from Augustana that was not always directly taught to us that became the priceless gem of our years of nurse's training. We were exposed to a consistent high degree of personal Christian dedication and concern for the total welfare of the patient, every ounce of our energy being directed to that end. Because of the World War II timing, we were never over-staffed and, thus, were given and accepted responsibilities far beyond the context of the term "student." As a result, we developed rapidly in skill and reliability and carried these traits into future jobs.

We thank you, Augustana, for all that you gave us that fills us with pride. We are happy to leave with you at this time of our 40th anniversary a gift symbolizing our interest and union with you. Always we give you our loyalty and love and the hope that you can share this pride in the nurses of the class of 1946.

Dolores Fischer Aleksandras, '51 brought us up to date on the status of The Nurse Practice Act. LPN's would be "grandfathered" in if they had taken or passed an accredited Pharmacology course.

In 1986, we had three official groups of Augustana nurses in addition to our Alumnae. They were the Florida, California and Upper Peninsula.

There were a few additions to the hospital since the luncheon in June. The Pharmacy opened an Outpatient Department just off the lobby. In addition to routine pharmaceuticals many medical supplies could be purchased. The new Coffee Shop was also ready to serve you with a tasty breakfast in addition to sandwiches and snacks. The new Gift Shop solved many a problem as you looked for that distinctive gift. Now open and in operation was the new Orthopedic Wing located on 3 West. The new and expanded Physiotherapy Unit served all of our patients' needs. Soon after, our Extended Care Unit was opened, as was our Substance Abuse Unit. Bea Ruble '51 was in charge of the new Observation Unit. Here patients were observed for up to 23 hours without being officially admitted to the hospital. These patients were post-surgical, possible coronary, injuries, asthmatics, or any other medical or surgical cases requiring attention.

The following notice appeared in The Augustana Nurse.

Sadly, we must report that the Augustana Hospital School of Nursing did not accept a new class this year and the last class will graduate in 1987. As past graduates of our beloved School this is a very sad time for us. The years of nursing tradition are coming to an end but our loyalty to Augustana and our devotion to each other will never end. What we have in memories will last forever. What we learned is a part of us forever.

Augustana Hospital School of Nursing is just one of so many diploma schools to close. Another sister school graduated its last class in December 1986, The Evangelical Deaconess Hospital Training School for nurses awarded its 1,746th diploma and after 67 years closed forever. Deaconess is in Milwaukee but might well be in Chicago or any other city in the nation. There is only one hospital nursing school left in Wisconsin.

It might be interesting to assess why. This material is taken from an article in the Milwaukee Journal sent by one of our members: "Hospital nursing schools have been dying out gradually during the last decade, victims of women's advances in business, a more technical medical profession and changing national economy. Women's advances in other professions have left a void in nursing. Today, many schools are unable to fill nursing classes. Also, nurses need to know so much more today. Nurses entering the field today are encouraged to have a bachelor's degree. Perhaps the biggest blow to hospital nursing schools was the change in how they were financed. After 1987 the government will no longer give financial aid. The cost of operating a school is just too expensive for the hospital."

The Annual Christmas Party was held on December 3, 1986 in the Lila Pickhardt Lounge. It was a gala night—the weather was fine—the Lounge beautifully decorated.

Elda Peters '54 and her friend, pianist Lois Ladage, presented a program of Christmas readings and song. The lovely presentation was a wonderful beginning of our Christmas season. Refreshments, including salads and cookies, provided by each member attending, plus other assorted goodies were served by our Social Arrangements Committee. A free will offering was added to our Sick Nurses Fund.

The following letter was received from Carol Hucko '55.

With the changes in nursing and the health care field, many new opportunities have developed and are available for nurses today. I would be interested in learning of or hearing from any Augustana Alumnae who have done some entrepreneuring or are involved in special interest areas. With Augustana nurses spread across the country, I feel it would be of value to the alumnae to share these experiences which could open new doors for others.

Some of my special interests included reaching out into the community. Examples: blood pressure screening; CPR programs for various ages, other health screening or wellness programs; assisting the elderly or anyone with special needs to remain independent in their home; enrichment of the home environment and check for safety; community or out-patient education; liaison between the hospital, doctor, community, and agencies such as the Heart Association or Cancer Society; health education and support for women; teenage pregnancies, new mothers, divorced or widowed, also for the middle-aged woman (but not limited to) who is the primary caregiver; and health education and support for "males only" of all ages.

We were very sorry to hear of the death of Rev. Daniel H. Sandstedt on February 24, 1987. Many of us remember our former Chaplain who served Augustana and her student nurses for 18 years. We expressed our sadness to his wife, Arlene Johnson Sandstedt '41, and his family.

If you were a Chicago area resident, age 65 or over enrolled in Medicare Parts A and B with an acceptable supplemental insurance policy, you would never have to pay an inpatient Augustana Hospital bill again. It was all part of Senior Passport coverage.

For those caring for a relative who needed supervision, often the most difficult aspect was being tied to home, unable to take a vacation or just have a weekend without responsibility. To address this problem Augustana offered Respite Care to provide temporary 24-hour-a-day care for the elderly and disabled in a safe, secure environment. While Respite Care was designed to provide family caregivers a chance for rest or vacation, it could also be used by older adults who lived alone and may have needed extra care before or after surgery. Guests had the assurance that if an emergency arose, all the services of the hospital were available. Respite Care service was provided within the skilled nursing unit under the supervision of a registered nurse. It could even be arranged for the family doctor to visit on the unit.

A note from Bertha Klauser '33 was read at the Luncheon. "Dear Alumnae Members: As you gather today I am confident all of you are experiencing mixed emotions—sadness at the closing of the school that has influenced our lives, happiness in being with cherished friends, and pride in your many achievements. We have much for which to be grateful. It is most appropriate at this time to pay special tribute to the members of our Board. Their arduous work and sincere dedication have been the lifeline of the Alumnae Association. To all in attendance and to the many graduates unable to be present I wish for you God's richest blessings.

All graduates of our beloved School of Nursing were invited to attend the last graduation ceremony. It was held Saturday, July 11, 1987, at 1:00 p.m. in the Chapel.

Ardith Gannon '63 wrote of the Graduation—

July 11, 1987 dawned sunny, hot and humid with an air of anticipation and excitement. Today was graduation for five young women who had survived the rigors of their nursing program. They had passed their theory and clinical practice and had earned the diploma and pin of the Augustana Hospital School of Nursing. They are joining a long list of past graduates. In fact 3,245 students have graduated from the School since it began in 1896. Augie grads are proud of their school and the education/training they have received.

Graduation was held in the Augustana chapel and attended

by family and friends of the graduates as well as honored guests; member of the Board of Directors, medical staff, faculty, hospital administration and friends and many past graduates and alumnae. Rev. Arnold O. Pierson gave greetings from the Board of Directors with an emphasis on farewell, not goodbye, but to go forth doing well and to remember God is with you. Anna Waino Henningsen, '60, brought to the graduates the Commencement Address and encouraged them to continue to learn as their education is not ending but beginning. They will be a vital part in the nursing profession and to take an active role in its future. Joyce Herter, President of the Alumnae Association, was on hand to welcome the graduates into the Augustana family and to encourage them to become active members of the association. David Jensen, President of the Augustana Hospital and John Ruckauf, Acting Director of the School of Nursing, brought greetings and presented the graduates with their diplomas and pins.

The graduates' response was given by Romaine Rothstein, a member of the graduation class. Her speech was very emotional as she related the struggles of the past two years, but believes they have gained the skills and knowledge to face the nursing challenge so "Look out world. Here we come!" She also related the friendship and camaraderie the class had experienced, but this has been a vital part of the Augustana Nurses throughout the School's history.

Following the ceremony, everyone enjoyed a champagne buffet in the courtyard under a yellow and white canopy. It was a time for congratulations and picture taking for the graduates and for the Alumnae members to "remember when." Thus the graduation day came to a close and the Augustana Hospital School of Nursing would graduate no more students, but not before Augustana nurses have made their presence felt in every state and many foreign countries. The Augustana tradition lives on. So, as Rev. Pierson stated, "It's not Good-bye but Fare-Well."

# EPILOGUE

Augustana Hospital was taken over by Lutheran General December 31, 1987 and closed December 8, 1989.

Lutheran General Health Care System still served the community by keeping the Doctor's offices open until the building was demolished in 1993.

Some of the Augustana Hospital Chapel windows were moved to and dedicated at the A.D. Johnson Memorial Chapel of Lutheran General Hospital on December 5, 1991.

The following article is taken from "North Loop News," December 7, 1989:

## DEATH OF A HOSPITAL

(Editor's note: The following is a tribute to the employees of service provided by Lutheran General-Lincoln Park Hospital, which will close on Dec. 8. It was written by Dr. James C. Arrington, recipient of the hospital's 1989 "Spirit" award.)

Some years ago, while still a medical student, I experienced the loss of a patient. He was a young man with sickle cell anemia. The fine line between life and death became all too real for me. The tears I shed for that young man are vivid in my mind; his spirit still lives in my memory.

Several nights ago, as I sat in my car in the parking lot of a small North Side hospital, my eyes once again began to moisten. The same feeling of loss I felt at the death of my patient came upon me.

For more than 100 years, this hospital has gone quietly about the business of administering health care. This hospital, like so many before it and those that are surely to follow it, is yet another casualty of a changing medical environment.

Even at its demise, this long-standing institution, which impacted the lives of so many in Chicago, received just a few paragraphs of type in Chicago's major newspapers.

Since my patient was not a man of great importance, no doubt, his death was not mentioned in any paper. Yet, he, like this hospital had worth; they both deserved more.

The people of this hospital went about the daily routine of providing care to patients, without fanfare and without many, if any, accolades.

Like to many of us who go about our daily routines, doing our jobs as best as we can; at death, our total existence is often comprised of just a few lines in the obituary.

I think sadly of the time my patient confided in me that he felt a burden to his family, and questioned the worth of his existence. He, like this hospital, should never question the worth of his-or its-existence. We, in Chicago, speak of a surplus of hospital beds, but fail to address the deficiency of personal health care.

Following the death of my patient, he underwent an autopsy, to learn the cause of his death so that others might benefit. There will be no autopsy for this hospital. Perhaps its death was caused by the fact that no patient in need of care, regardless of ability to pay, was turned away. Maybe too much attention was paid to the care, comfort and concern of the sick, and not enough to the bottom line.

As doctors are sworn to do in the face of death, the doctors at this hospital attempted to save it. Purchasing the hospital would have allowed the doctors, and the more than 600 employees, to continue their commitment to caring for the sick. The doctors, more than 40, reached into their own pockets; willing to risk financial loss for the chance of new life into the hospital. Ultimately, the decision was not ours to make. Our proposal for saving the hospital was rejected. Still I'm proud of my fellow colleagues for trying; there is no shame in failure, if the effort has been valiant and true.

In the final analysis, just like the human body, I would like to believe that this hospital, a temporary physical structure, housed a more important spirit, some might call it a soul.

The soul of this hospital will live on, like the patient whose spirit touched me and lives forever in my memory. For more than 100 years at this site, babies were born, the sick were comforted, cared for and cared about. This hospital was a wonderful place to work and I worked with wonderful people. Whether the walls of this hospital are replaced by high-priced condominiums, an exclusive geriatric center, or the most modern of surgicenters, the spirit of this hospital will live on.

Since care is a team approach, from my fellow colleagues, to the maintenance men, to the nurses, to the ward clerks, to the phone operators, to all in the hospital who endeavored to involve themselves in care to mankind, your spirit will forever live.

In its last days, this hospital's name was changed from Augustana to Lutheran General-Lincoln Park. To those who worked here for years and grew to love it, however, its name will always be Augustana. Tomorrow the doors to Augustana will close forever. If a hospital can have an epitaph, let it be said of Augustana: "Seldom have so few, served so many, for so long, so well."

# PART III

POEMS BY OUR ALUMNI

# HOME COMING

Tis love that brings you home today,
To fill all hearts with joy
A loving memory points your way
To Augustana's door.

The memories of former years
And friendships hallowed ties
Both bind us to our school so dear
It's high ideals we prize.

We love the memories made by you
And ever pray that we
A worthy group of comrades true
To you will always be.

We honor our departed ones,
Their memories we revere
Their influence will with us remain
And ever pray that we always hold them dear.

—GRETTA NESHEIM, '13

345

## MY OLD GRAY DRESS

I lay it down. I lay it down, my uniform of gray
Which I put on unwillingly one far-off summer's day.
I have talked of it and rated it and freely spoken my mind
Of the people who invented it, and called them most unkind.

But when at last I go to put that uniform away
I find my heart grown tender toward that old dress of gray.
All intertwined with thoughts of it are thoughts of other things;
Of joy, of sad and glad days, that memory forward brings.

Sad days when all around me were suffering with pain,
And wounded men who never would be well and whole again;
All glad days when the cheery boys, forgetting every ill,
Would laugh and talk with many jokes, and could never
    be kept still.

And those who worked around me, clad in gray dresses too,
Numbers of splendid women so unselfish, kind and true,
That memory of their splendid work and comradeship so fine
Seems to glorify that old gray dress of mine.

And now at last I put away that simple old gray dress
Which I have worn through many a day of work, and strain,
    and stress;
And my little cap with cross of red, beside it too, I lay
But the memories intertwined with them will last for many a day.

—CLARA LAWSON, '14

# MY HATES

Oh, how I hate the crowds of city ways
With never ending noise; the subway maze
And roar; the elevated's din and crush,
The smell as dirty bodies homeward push.

All noises devastating peace of life;
As rap of rivet hammers, shriek-like fife
Of steam, the clank of clams that dig the earth
Where flowers grew, and children ran in mirth.

The sight and smell of garbage cans, a lair
For rats and flies, polluting morning air.
The beat of jazz, the mawkish sentiment
Of ragtime songs, with vacant laughter spent.

And cats—their shrilling screech unearthly weird,
Like souls in torment, vaguely known and feared.
The dirty snow; the piercing cold; numb feet;
And winter winds which whistle sharp with sleet.

The crowded tenements, discouraged trees
In parks and squares, brown grass, a vagrant breeze
Which fails to cool the throngs; a wailing child.
I hate it! Give me country undefiled!

—HELEN E. OLSON, '16

## WAR TIME

We pause on the time-worn threshold
Where so many before us have paused,
With a feeling so strange, unexpressed.
Sometimes we almost feel lost.
Silent we stand at the gateway,
Knowing not where the path will lead.
The past we will leave behind us.
The future we cannot perceive.

The years that are coming before us.
Demand energy, self-sacrifice, strength.
We stand ready and willing to give it
On the field of unlimited length.
We'll be called to fight life's battle,
Be it here or on foreign shore.
It will call forth our very best efforts.
We'll give it-how can we give more?

The days we have spent in our training
Are days we will never regret,
They have fitted us better for the trials,
Which the future will not let us forget.
It has made us far better women,
And shown us humanity's need.
We can answer the call of the nation,
And of that we are proud indeed.

—MABELL HOLM, '18

## LOVE WELL THIS WORLD

Love well this World—
A birthright given me when I was placed here.
So should I, with it, a strong friendship rear
Which, 'spite dire rage, foul horror, and deep fear,
Holds power to love this World.

Love well this World—
Its coffers mountain high and valley deep,
Treasure rare beauty which is mine to keep,
And bring as homage through the years that creep,
To show I love this World.

Love well this World—
Whose each great swirl through time, keen fraught with
    pain,
Gives need for hateless touch, that it may gain
A growing reach toward strength, so peace will reign
To help us love this World.

Love well this World—
For it holds quiet places which welcome me;
Sanctums where it, and God, and I: We Three,
Pledge deep, anew, in one close Trinity,
To ever love this World.

—ELLIS J. WALKER, '19

## A PRAYER

God give me sympathy and sense
And help me keep my spirits high.
Give me calm and confidence,
And please, a twinkle in my eye.

—RUTH (ECKWALL) OLANDER, '23

## GOD'S GIFT

We travel through life at such a pace
And we wonder why it's such a race.
We push our limits with all it takes
Then all of a sudden we step on the brakes.
If we slowed down to see what we missed
We would wonder how we could really exist.
There are so many things along life's way,
Moments of pleasures that we threw away.
God gave us love that we might forgive,
He gave us health that we might live,
He gave us patience to understand,
He gave us faith and a helping hand.
He gave us courage, for He has said
"I'll always be with you, there's nothing to dread."
He gave us wisdom that we might know,
He illumined our way so we know where to go.
He gave us prayer for strength that we need.
He died on the cross that we might be freed.
We do not deserve all these gifts from above,
But we're healed and set free because of God's love.
So please slow down and look around
For the precious gifts that you have found
When you stepped on the brakes along life's way
And found God's gifts that we threw away.

—SOPHIE LUND ROBERTSON, '25

## FOREWORD TO THE YEARBOOK OF '26

During the school year of 1926 just gone by,
We've kept a record, very sly
Of the things we've said and done
The interesting work as well as fun.

As we now present to you
Some of our thoughts and doings too,
The "Our Book" staff hopes you will hold dear,
All of these memories of the school year.

If we can link your future with the past
And form a bond with our Alma Mater that will last
Then we shall surely be content
And not begrudge our time and labor spent.

—CARRIE TWITCHELL, '26
Editor of Year Book 1926

## REMINISCING

We came in classes large and small
Some were short and some were tall
Some were fat and some were lean
Others just came in between
But we all learned together.
We worked so hard for little pay
But after work we had our play
We came for knowledge, not for gold
'Twas not for them whose heart was cold
When we all got together.
Some worked day and some worked night
So we managed quite all right
Some worked slow and some worked fast
But we all got thru at last
For we all work together.
Our training days have long been o'er
Gone the stripes that we once wore
But tho we're Mrs. or we're Miss
How we like to reminisce
When we all get together.

—EDA RINGSTROM, '26

## FOREWORD TO THE YEARBOOK OF '27

This volume now goes out,
That it may bring to mind
The memories of a happy past.
The things we've left behind.

Our gratitude goes with it,
To those who lent a hand,
That we might tell in passing
The things for which we stand.

Loyalty to Alma Mater,
Service where'er we go,
Ideals of life and conduct,
Just things worth while and so—

If, when it's finished you have found
That joy and beauty lurked,
Then surely we've accomplished
The things for which we've worked.

—MARY WEGNER, '27
Editor of Year Book 1927

# AUGUSTANA

A is our Aim, the highest in life.
U seful to be, some good in the strife
G race to do what we are told
U niformity always is our goal
S is Sincerity, we work with a will
T rustworthy and loyal our tasks to fulfill
A bility, too, in our profession,
N eatness in work, a worthy possession
AUGUSTANA "The Great Confession."

—AUTHOR UNKNOWN
From the 1928 Year Book

## REUNION OF THE CLASS OF '29

Charles Lindburg crossed the ocean
So did Amelia Earhart
A friend bought a Stutz-Bearcat
But it wouldn't start.

"When Day Is Done" was a well known song
A new fad was a game called Mah Jong.
William Tilden and Helen Wills—
Tennis was their game.
Notre Dame and Knute Rockne—it will never be the same.

Finally uncovered was the tomb of King Tut
The gold shined out, the door never shut.
Aimee' Semple McPherson poured out her charms
Ernest Hemingway wrote "A farewell To Arms."

A massacre happened on St. Valentine's Day.
The stock market crashed—what could we say.

The 1920's had many headlines
But at Augustana and its confines
The greatest news in 1929
Was the graduation of students—they had done fine.

And as nurses they went out the door
To do all jobs—including war.
And now in '79 again we meet
What a handsome group—ain't that a feat?

We wonder what the future will hold.
Whatever it is, we'll all be bold.
God will watch over us in what we do
So good luck, good health to all of you.

—Author Unknown
Found on a slip of paper in
a 1928 Year Book

## THE NURSES' PRAYER

Lord, help me to live from day to day
In such a self-forgetful way
That even when I kneel to pray
My prayer shall be for "Others."
Help me in the work I do
To ever be sincere and true
And know that all I do for you
Must needs be done for "Others."
Let self be crucified and slain
And buried deep; and all in vain
My efforts be to rise again
Unless to live for "Others."
And when my work on earth is done
And my new work in Heaven begun,
May I forget the crown I've won
While thinking still of "Others."
"Others," Lord, yes, "Others!"
Let this my motto be.
Help me to live for "Others"
That I may live for Thee.

—AUTHOR UNKNOWN
From the 1928 Year Book

# INTERMEDIATES

October the first in the year twenty-six,
How well we remember the day;
To 427 in taxis and trains,
We were all making our way.

We were sixty in number and with baggage and pack,
We sure were a regular storm
When all of us came from the east and the west
To make our new home in the "dorm."

There were real tiny girls such as Lois and Ruth;
Others were larger like Gay.
"They have the variety—let's hope as much brains"—
That's what we heard all the girls say.

When we first came in training we rose with the sun,
Which of course we don't do any more.
We studied and studied both evening and morn,
Learning words we'd not heard of before.

At first we were homesick and felt rather blue,
Some were packing their trunks to go back.
But when "Big Sisters" gave the big party for all,
We decided we'd rather not pack.

At the Hallowe'en party we all sure had fun
Among faces so ghastly and weird;
The "Blind Orchestra" fiddled with life and with pep
The old pieces that everyone cheered.

But of all the events that had passed on before,
The one that impressed us the most

Was the day we were changed to a uniform nurse,
As the symbols of standard we boast.

Altho many have left, we are still forty strong,
Struggling to reach the great height,
We are willing and ready to do our small part,
And to boast our dear school with our might.

—AUTHOR UNKNOWN
From the 1928 Year Book

## SPONGING IN C

Five-thirty already? How can it be!
Well, I gotta get up—I'm sponging in C.

Then into the kitchen some toast you grab
And with it some coffee—that's all to be had.

Up in "C" they're scrubbing like mad
And you dash for supplies that you never have.

You pile up your sponges and towels galore
And you know all the time they'll be yelling for more.

"My instruments are ready, please hurry do,"
The internes are scrubbing—Dr. Percy too.

"Tie my gown" in imperative tones
And your teeth all but grind like broken bones.

"Call that order. Is that patient asleep?"
You're rescuing a sponge under Dwyer's feet.

"Your brush can is empty, the soap dish too,
And gloves in the sink, that's no way to do."

The sponges on the bench—that worry is past,
"More instruments hurry, I've given my last."

"No needles? There must be, I just sent some out"
And you hunt and you hunt, 'till you're ready to shout.

"I'm low on sponges and sheets and towels"
And your shelf is empty—won't pay to howl.

"Miss Erickson"—Whoopie!" Everyone stops
Now what is it our young hopeful wants.

It's sutures or sponges or maybe a light
Most likely the suction—There I'm right.

Then in the midst of the din and hum
Dr. Percy opens an empty drum.

And you feel like a worm and wish you could crawl
Right off to the first little crack in the wall.

There's never a word just one mild stare
While others we know would rave and glare.

"Now watch your sponges," the scrub nurse warns
"The count is open," she sharply informs.

"More catgut," she whispers, "and buttons I need"
You reach for the jars, "Sponge count" indeed!

You glance at your board with one wild stare
And try to count your sponges there.

But you've got to touch 'em one by one
In order to get the correct sum.

Then into the midst of all this confusion
Somebody whispers—"A blood transfusion."

Then tables and benches are pushed aside
And doctors and internes from far and wide

Gather around to work or to be
Right in my way it seems to me.

Your brush can is full and (germicidal you'll get)
Scrub nurse contented—everything set.

You dodge back and forth while trying, too,
Not to contaminate and still get through.

Some get excited for they hate to wait
Their gowns aren't tied but it's not too late.

And while you are trying to tie them all
You hear the familiar—"Toot, toot—Alcohol!"

"Sponge count O.K."—you reach for the chart
The orders to write and place on the cart.

Transfusion's over, the donor is out
The room's in a mess—things thrown about.

You try to clean up and wait on 'em too—
(But run like a fool is all you do.)

—And you wish in your heart that those who rave
Would learn to do it "The Percy Way."

—AUTHOR UNKNOWN
From the 1928 Year Book

## THE CHARGE NURSE

To be a "Charge Nurse"—it sounds quite good—
But this is one person who's misunderstood.
She must keep her patients all content
And friction among students she must prevent,
And with the supervisor she must know
Just how things on the floor must go
And inform the doctor when he makes his rounds
Of things important, and make them sound
Not too ridiculous, for it's easy for such
At a time like that to say too much.
She must see that the orders are all carried out
And be able to know what they are all about
And not wake up in the mid of night
And worry and wonder if 'twas all right—
You can see that a "Charge Nurse" is hard to be,
And still be friends with you and me.

—AUTHOR UNKNOWN
From the 1928 Year Book

## JUST A PROBIE

Yes I know I'm just a probie,
Just learning how to face
The problems and the sorrows
That confront our race.

I try to help where'er I can,
I am so dumb, oh, dear!
But I can scrub and clean and run
Messages far and near.

I can't do much for aches and pains
With medicines and pills,
For I don't know a single thing
Of curing human ills.

For a headache I fix the pillow
And an ice bag I apply,
And for the other pains
A hot water bag I try.

I try to make them comfortable
By doing little things,
And try to do it cheerfully
—What pleasure it brings.

To know that at the close of day,
After working hard and long,
Your cheery way and helping hand
Has helped the work along.

I don't do much these first four months
And won't for quite a while,
But though I'm just a PROBIE,
I at least can smile.

    —AUTHOR UNKNOWN
    From the 1928 Year Book

## AFTER THREE LONG YEARS OF TRAINING

After three long years of training
There are things we'll ne'er forget.
All our faithful worthy doctors
Which no where else we could have met.
Always we shall remember Dr. Oschner's $H_2O$ and lime
Yes, of course, it must be given right on the dot of time.
Dr. Percy, our surgeon, who rights the wrongs
We're glad to tell you he to Augustana belongs.
His clever assistant, Dr. Hedberg
Is a most brilliant man from a Michigan burg.
Oh! Dr. Frick prefers the hot pack roast
Specializes in diets of milk and toast.
For cystoscopies Dr. Nadeau knows best
He knows all about them just ask the rest.
In a rush comes in our Dr. Nuzum
Set up right away for a blood transfusion.
Dr. Crile the best bone setter
Couldn't find one any better.
Of all diseases of the chest
Dr. Hedblom can do the best.
The famous obstetricians, Drs. Lundgren and Falls

Welcome the newcomer's first earthly calls.
If a gastric hernia you should suspect
Dr. Oden's diagnosis will sure detect.
To keep in best order eye, ear, nose and throat
Everyone for Dr. Murray will vote.
See Dr. Weigan once in a while
Whenever your baby refuses to smile.
Dr. Beilin, he makes the X-Ray business boom
If you fail to find him just call the drug room.
Dr. Kremer the lab technician
That's not all, he too is a musician.
Dr. Christenson must be about
When nurses need their tonsils out.
Although it doesn't take so long
They all must sing a little song.
As a reward on New Years day he treats
All senior nurses to the best of eats,
Even the internes there with us mingle
But alas! none of them seem to be single.

—MATHILDE DENEF, '29

## WEST BUILDING

Ye are but blind—
Who cannot see the beauty in its veiled brown walls,
Ye are but cold—
Who cannot feel the warmth contained therein
Could ye but see—
At dawn, a tiny sunbeam playing down those old, old, stairs
Or stop to hear—
The faint sweet whisper of a morning breeze come whistling'
    round the corner
To catch a glimpse of some new baby's face, or fan an old
    one as it lies there waiting—
Can ye not see that there is life—
That they have dreamed as you and I have done, that they
    have loved as you and I are doing—
Friends, can ye now see—
That some day we'll be waiting too, longing, dreaming, and
    hungering for that last great rendezvous
With God.

                                    —HORTENSE FORTNEY, '30

# A ROSEBUD—A ROSE

My Lord

You gave me a rosebud
    to tend and to touch
As I gazed at this small waif
    I thought, "He's not much
of an infant to care for," and
    then I touched him.

His response was to move
    his small body toward me
delighted, I knew
    I knew—"he'd improve."
Such a small life
    A meaning to my life.

Days into weeks, he robustly grew
    and filled out quite well
with tender love he knew
    and understood, but could not tell me,
for his words were silent
    but his body movements were
electrifying responses to my touch.

The day has arrived to
    announce his gestational age
It is time to depart
    and start a new page.
I now can reflect
    I was the liaison,
the surrogate mother
    of his growing life.

My Lord

To tend and to touch
    these parents you chose
I now give to them
    a beautiful rose
for all of their lives.

I touched a rosebud
    I held a rose
This is my life.

    —Irene A. Peterson, '46


## THE WEARY WAY

Here's to the girl in surgery
May she always be on top
She not only learns to scrub
But also swings a mean mop.

Don't pity your friends in D.K.
Life down there is a dream
Little work and much fun is their schedule
Then fill up on juice and ice cream.

In O.B. life is much different
Twenty-four hour call is quite wearing
To get your 15 with one hour between
Is an experience not worth sharing.

To the service room we long to go.
That's where you rest if you're feeling low.
It's easy to learn their ration system
And Miss Carlson sees that you properly list 'em.

To C.M.H. we proudly trot
We're Juniors now and know a lot.
But over there their ideas differ,
With books and kids, could life be stiffer?

In V.N.A. life isn't all rosy
Many a soul thinks you're just being nosey
And there's the rain and snow and muddy paths
But the glory of doing, detracts from these wraths.

Now we're out at Downey—the long waited last
Our young years of training far in the past—
Our minds are mature and emotions stable
For the task of aiding others we're willing and able.

—AUTHOR UNKNOWN

From the 1947 Year Book

# A SENIOR'S REFLECTION

It is hard to find words with which to say
The way we all felt on our first day
But to be a good nurse was our intent
And to reach that goal three years we've spent
Studying and working and doing our best
To meet every problem and possible test.

The day we were capped no one will forget
For we were so proud and happy, but yet
We knew it was just our first great step
Toward reaching the goal which we had set
Determined we worked, at times when discouraged
With a smile and kind word we soon were encouraged.

As the Augustana family we all lived together
Sharing in things we'll remember forever
Our troubles and joys, the laughter and tears
We'll cling to and cherish throughout coming years
Though leaving our training with feelings of sorrow
We look forward to being the nurse of tomorrow.

—DORIS HOLMGREN, '52

## THIS IS MY PRAYER

Oh dear Lord, hear my prayer,
and harken to my plea,
Help me to recognize the good
I sometimes fail to see.

I want to live for others,
and whatever I may give,
Let my gifts be noble ones,
A Christian life I want to live.

When I am tempted, intervene,
Keep my thoughts from going wrong,
For I want to live for others,
Keep my virtues ever strong.

Be with me always,
in whatever I may do,
So I may live according to
my everlasting faith in You.

—JEANNE BALKE, '54

# LORD, GIVE ME STRENGTH

Lord, give me strength to pull that sheet
As tight as it can be;
For when Thy back rests on that bed,
I'll want it wrinkle free.
Lord, give me love that I might care
Just what is wrong with Thee;
Then with this knowledge I might know
Just what Your treatment will be.
Lord, give me understanding, too
That I might give Thee rest:
I know what peace of mind can mean
Before important tests.
Lord, one thing more I ask of Thee,
And this in humbleness;
To know that when I soothe a brow,
It's Yours I've really caressed.
And with these traits and others, too
That only You disperse;
May I become and, yes, deserve
The name given to a NURSE.

—CATHERINE RODERICK, '56

## NURSE'S PRAYER

Help me to make my beds in the smoothest way
Help me to make more tempting every tray
Help me to sense when pain must have relief
Help me to deal with those borne down with grief.
Help me to take to every patient's room
The light of life to brighten up the gloom
Help me to bring to every soul in fear,
The sure and steadfast thought that Thou art near.
Help me to live throughout this live-long day
As one who loves thee well, Dear Lord I pray,
And when the day is done and evening stars
Shine through the dark above the sunset bars
When weary quite, I turn to seek my rest
Lord, may I truly know I've done my best!

—AUTHOR UNKNOWN
From the 1958 AugieLog

*A History of the Augustana Hospital School of Nursing*

# PART 4

LISTING OF MISSIONARIES AND
AUGUSTANA GRADUATES

*A History of the Augustana Hospital School of Nursing*

# IN MEMORIAM[30]

Their terrestrial training
In the problems of living,
Taught them patience and faith,
And the joy of giving.
May they have their reward
In that haven above,
Where God supervises
With infinite love.

Those who have preceded us into the Great Beyond have been plucked from the road of Life as a child picks her flowers. One moment she picks a young, tender bud, the next, her choice is fully matured, lovely rose, then her little hands eagerly clasp the drooping petals by the wayside.

Each departed one has left behind her a memory—a memory with which she alone can be identified. May the ideals, loyalty, and enthusiasm which characterized those who have been called from our ranks, be our inspiration, and a memory to be cherished.

To those whom God hath called
To grace His throne above,
We bow in meditation,
Reverence and love.
—MABELL E. HOLM '18.

---

30. Written in memory of the Augustana graduates who have answered the last roll call. [Copied from the 1938 History Book.]

# AUGUSTANA MISSIONARIES

Hedvig Wahlberg Lindorff, 1897
  Rajahmundry, India, Honan,
    China
Alice Holmberg Lange, 1897
  China
Andrea Hanson Winter, 1899
  India
Anna Heistad, 1898
  Marcy Center
Ellen Carlson McDaniel, 1899
  Petchaburi, Siam
Amelia Swanson Eckardt, '02
  Rajahmundry, India
Annie Grover, '08
  Wellington, South Africa,
    Syabei, Kenya County,
    East Africa
Minnie Nelson Benson, '13
  Honan, China
Esther Nelson Unis, '19
  Honan, China
Johanna Peterson Olson, '22
  Peking, China, Surichafu,
    North Manchuria
Margaret Samuelson Tessberg, '27
  Iambi, Tanganyika, East
    Africa
Mildred Kratz, '28
  Bananal, Brazil
Esther M. Nowack Hess, '29
  Koelin Liangchow, Kansu
    Province, North China

Sigrid Walback Koven, '33
  New Delhi, India
Dorothea Nicholson, '43
  Nigeria, West Africa
Clara Lima, '45
  West Borneo, Indonesia
Doris Bruce, '46
  Assam, India
Lois Benson Gotass, '46
  Venezuela
Elaine Anderson Holm, '47
  Eket, Nigeria, West Africa
Mary Ellen Bulander Adams, '48
  Kano, Nigeria, West Africa
Marijean Nelson, '48
  Tanganyika, Africa
Kathryn Gruber, '49
  Peru, South America
Marjorie Ness Scheel, '50
  Africa
Frances Poole Markham, '51
  Africa
Shirley Osborn O'Donnell, '55
  Sleetmute, Alaska
Doris Ummel, '55
  Nigeria, West Africa
Margaret Redpath-Lindquist, '61
  Central Africa Republic

# AUGUSTANA GRADUATES

## 1896

Louise Bylander
Hilda Hedin-Rydell
Anna Johnson-Helt
Emily Johnson-Lewis

Ingeborg Johnson-Fowler
Josie Oberg-Lofgren
Louise Wensjö
Mary Younggren

## 1897

Hulda Carlson
Augusta Erickson
Alice Holmberg-Lundblad
Marie Hvidberg
Amanda Johnson-Edwards

Alida Johnson-Quinlan
Christine Johnstone-Swenson
Tillie Rydell-Johnson
Hilma Swenson
Hedwig Wahlberg-Lindorff

## 1898

Lilian Benson
Anna Berg
Hildur Blomstrand
Axelia Engstrom-Westerlund
Anna Forsman-Mussallem
Anna Heistad

Eva Holm-Wikner
Sadie Johnson
Vera Nelson-Carlson
Anna Peterson-Nelson
Hilma Wold
Anna Younggren-Davidson

## 1899

Marie Anderson
Ellen Berg-White
Emma Burk
Ellen Bylander-Voss
Ellen Carlson-McDaniel
Christine Carpenter-Hughes
Josie Hallden

Andrea Hansen-Winter
Emma Isaacson
Ida Isaacson
Mamie Johnson
Almida Peterson
Clara Seaburg

## 1900

Ida Blade-Olson
Ingeborg Egland-Knutson
Jennie Gummeson-Lundquist
Olga Hultman-Anderson
Hilma Johnson-Anderson

Olivia Kempe-Rosenberg
Katherine Knudson
Minnie Lundgren-Emmons
Mathilda Olson-Hanson
Hilda Swenson

### 1901

Augusta Bjork-Nelson
Alma Borg
Nanna Hallbom
Carrie Larson
Augusta Lindahl
Beda Munson-Lundgren

Ida Nelson-Wright
Johanna Nelson-Hanson
Josephine Oberg-Mattson
Amanda Swenson-Schyles
Celia Wiholm-Nelson
Mary Youngren-Elmquist

### 1902

Augusta Anderson-Sachrison
Hanna C. Anderson-Kelly
Alfrida Billings-Getschell
Agnes E. Danell-Erickson
Rosala W. Freeman-Lewis
Mathilde Hjelm
Josie M. Jacobson-Iverson
Alma Johnson-Christenson

Cecile M. Juhl-Thorndahl
Rebecka Johnson Mellin
Selma E. Lincoln
Frida S. Meyer-Lemair
Anna C. Peterson
Julia A. Swanson-Eckhardt
Clara Tederstrom
Emma C. Wahlberg-Westerlund

### 1903

Mary Ahrman-Pihlblad
Sophie Anderson
J. Amelia Dahlgren
M. Marie Frederikson
H. Marie Fritzen-Meyers
A. C. Johnson-Johnson
Carolina Johnson-Johnson
Ingrid C. Johnson-Sebelius
AnnaB.Johnson-Kronberg

Jennie Johnson
Ella G. Jorstad-Strandness
Hulda Kilstrom-McCoom
Blanche A. Lindorf
Thyra Lorentzen-Anderson
Maja Sabelstrom
Amy O. Schjolberg
H. Naomi Skogberg

### 1904

Hilda E. Berglund-Ranseen
Nancy Ekstrom-Amour
Clara Enerson-Gibson
Anna Forsblom-Buchanan
Esther T. Jackson
Anna M. Johnson-Lindstrom
H. Evelyn Johnson
Christine Jorgenson-Reese
HuldaLarson-Hough

Elsie Lund-Leddy
Christina A. Nelson
Hattie S. Nelson
Hulda E. Norrman-Strutz
Hildur Newberg-Anderson
Agnes M. Paulson
Esther S. A. Peterson
Anna B. Pierson-Ellison

### 1905

Hulda Alm-Clauson
Anna C. Andreen-Swanson
Jennie Benson-Nordgren
Jennie L. Christenson-Burke
Emma M. Erickson
Hedvig A. C. Gronbeck-Strandell
Augusta A. Johnson
Hulda E. Johnson-Leviton
Anna Kilstrom-Titus

Erma Larson-Dorist
Cecilia Linden
Anna S. Olson-Sullivan
Emily C. Olson-Lindberg
Esther B. Olson
Clara A. Peterson
Johanna Peterson-Einarson
Sophie M. Rosen

## 1906

Vina Allen
Anna C. Anderson-Anderson
Agnes Bard
Anna M. Carlson
Teckla A. Fosberg
Almida C. Green-Green
Ada Grip-Edgren
Frances W. Heinrich

Inga Hetland-McConville
Emmy C. Hofstrom-Clevensen
Clara Kittelson-Goldsmith
Anna G. Lofgren
Anna C. Nelson-Blamey
Olga Nelson
Jennie F. Nilsson-Graff
Ebba V. Thorsell-Eckholm

## 1907

Anna C. V. Ahlstrand
Sara M. Bengston-Schwamb
Ida Marie Benson
Emma M. Berggren-Johnson
Ada M. Carlson

Theckla Dahlgren
Charlotte Johnson-Carlson
Anna Metha Jorgensen-Hoff
Eva Nord-Lockwood

## 1908

Hannah Dorothea Aalberg-Suhs
Emma Anderson-Grotness
Charlotte R. Anderson-Stranberg
Ira M. Arvidson-Olson
Sophie Bang-Rache
Alice E. Berg
Emma Bockemeier
Flora P. Bowman
Anna E. Boren-Byquist
Anna L. Brevitz
Victoria Carlson
Marie S. Christensen
Anna Ericson
Annie Ranella Grover
Wilhelmina C. Holmberg-
  Treichler

Emma M. Holmquist
Gertie Jacobs
Frieda E. Johnson
Cora Muntinga
Alma C. Nelson-Hawes
Agnes Katherine Norbdy-
  Fynboe
Bertha Outzen-Lamberton
Sena Fredrika Peterson
Elin Sabelstrom
Libbie S. Seaborg-Jaedecke
Hildur Elida Stahlberg-
  Steinbrecher
Ivy L. Stone-Babcock
Lucy R. Wood-Mead

## 1909

Estrid A. Bergman
Fannie Boman
Olive E. Ermey
Laura Field-Caldo
Mayme A. Gunderson-Halvorson
Marie Gustafson-Landry
Marie E. Holmberg
Ruth B. Hall
Anna M. Johnson
Johanna R. W. Law-Hackbarth
Helen C. Liljegren-Rundquist
Gerda Lindberg
Hannah E. Magnuson-Bloomquist
Annie C. Munson

Freda E. Munson-Whitehead
Alma M. Odman
Elizabeth Proctor
Hanna H. Peterson-Hughes
Sadie A. Ross-Baker
Elvira Rosengren
Alga D. M. Renius
Helga K. M. Rasmussen
Ellen C. Simonson-Gustafson
Florence T. Sellergren
Esther M. Uldine-Bodine
Agnes M. Wallberg
Theresa Weninger

## 1910

Elizabeth C. Alm-Smith
Helen C. Anderson
Sarah C. Engquist
Julia A. Johnson-Baur
Selma O. B. Johnson-Lindsey
Hulda Alfreda Johnstone-Sibbald

Marie Nelson
Amelia E. Peterson
Susan B. Rogers
Margaret Saenger
Alma Alida Tolin
Alma C. Walters

## 1911

Amanda Anderson
Thyra V. Anderson
Cora E. Bensen-Elstad
Selma J. Bloomberg-Rose
Anna M. Conradi-Peterson
Augusta Eklund
Anna M. Gustafson
A. Olivia Johnson-Todd
Mary H. Larson-Hauser

Ella M. Linder-Godtneid
Amelia H. Loehrke
Mary E. Nelson-Freeman
Clara M. Pedersen
Euphemia Peterson-Stewart
Edith C. Peterson-Kuhn
Elizabeth Sakrison
Julia M. Swanson-Shuran
Hilda C. Weltzien-Jampolis

## 1912

Ellen M. Anderson-Fromholz
Hilma Anderson
Hilma A. Anderson-Strand
Anna W. Anderson
Elida C. Bayard-Samuels
Amy B. Chamberlain
Emily J. Christenson-Cleven
Ella M. Clauer-Franks
Alice M. Crone-Smith
Grace E. Defenderfer-Ryan-
  Hixson
Mabel M. Dimmick
Mollie E. Erickson
Amy Gustafson-Simonson
Jessie M. Grant-Nueremberg
Nettie G. Hoff-Johnson
Minnie A. Jack-Goldberg

Amanda J. Johnson
Josephine G. Jernstad-McCornack
Jennie C. Johnson
Fern A. Johnson
Laura G. Juel-Porden
Laura Jensen-Thompson
Isabel F. Kellman-Crosby
Louise A. Knauer
Anna C. Nord
Ida C. Olson-Whittaker
Elsa A. Odman
Ada L. Palmer
Edith C. Sandeen-Lindeen
Marie Sveeggen
Elizabeth A. Urbach-Yates
Myrtle Vallentin-Lovci
Janette F. Warner-Porlier

## 1913

Josephine Berglund-Rovelstad
Alma F. Crone-Nelson
Myrtle N. Ettinger-Butte
Emily Gerhardt
Maude E. Harlow
Elvira Hartvigh-Nickel
Esther A. Hellgren-Madsen
Louise A. Jensen
Esther J. Julian
Selma C. Lindell
Esther A. Magnuson-Frei

Ellen Neddermeyer-Marquardt
Gretta Nesheim-Opheim
Minnie W. Nelson-Benson
Selma V. Olson-Little
Harriet W. Olson-Holmgren
Hilda A. Pearson
Clara C. Peterson
Sadee Sawyer
Mabelle T. Sundblad
Adele Speck

## 1914

Elsie M. Aageson-Heidner
Florence Andersen-Marlow
Jessie May Arzberger-Goddard
Anna E. Berg-Packard
Mathilda Carlson
Lydia M. Frykholm
Hannah Hansen-Brownlee
Gerda Hedstrom-Eakins
Sara H. Hoesley-Tearnan
Edith B. Hokanson
Jennie E. Jacobson
Emily Johnson-Ley

Gunhild G. Johnson
Sara Elizabeth Liljegren
Jennie A. Larson
Clara Lawson
Carrie E. Maakestad
Anna S. Olson
Augusta J. Olson
Ellen Charlotte Peterson-Whaite
Esther M. E. Pohlson
Elsie A. Skoglund
Hilda Sundin-Dickinson
Ruth J. Vallentin

## 1915

Mathilda Eugenia Anderson
Pauline H. Atwater
Mabel Adelia Carlson
Ida A. Ehman
Laura A. Ericson
Julia Otteson Flikke
Aino Cecelia Gustafson
Mattie Hammerstrand-Trump
Laura Caroline Hartvigh
Fannie R. Holmgren-Rundstrom
Hilda J. Hultquist-Olson
Jennie Ethel Johnson-Weaver
Jennie E. Johnson-Gillespie

Alida Lindahl
Pauline E. Louko-Korhonen
Lillian Olsen
Betty A. Peterson-Botvidson
Martha A. Rohrbeck
Amanda Elizabeth Rundquist
Viola M. Smith-Brown
Jennie Strand
Leila A. Swanson
Ruth Johnhild Swanson
Christine Van Liere-Wilke
Selma Gerafia Johnson

## 1916

Mabelle S. Bayard-Lindholm
Agnes C. Bergh
Ruth Bonander
Ruth V. Carlson-Raymond
Emma S. Carlsted
Edna Marjorie Chapin-Quist
Ragnhild M. Christophersen-
  Petersen
May Lucille Cratty
Eva A. Edstrom-Miller
Laura Fisk
Blenda Louise Frisk
Hedvig Grund-Hannmann
Mathilda Gustafson-Strand
Cecelia A. Hillstrom
Clarissa T. Johnson-Drach
Edith C. Johnson

Myrtle W. Johnson-Behm
Naomi C. Johnson
Sarah Johnson-Schumm
Anna C. Lewis
Rosalind Lindstrom-Johnson
Sonja Lundholm
Helga Melby-Barrett
Lillie H. Nelson
Ebba Ohman-Bergh
Helen E. Olson
Hannah Elizabeth Swanson-
  Swanson
Florence M. Sundblad-Palmer
Anna C. Trulson-Goodall
Amy Weeks-Richie
Ingeborg Martha Yngve
Elsa E. Yoerg-Tearnan

### 1917

May C. Aagaard
Elsie May Burkhardt-Walther
Gladys Ferne Apker-Sanders
Gertrude Annette Burnson
Anna Victoria Carlson
Alice Casperson-Leeman
Anne Cleven-Wilkins
Florence Colson-Jones
Jennie Olive Fursett-Hagen
Malvina Gitzlaff-Craner
Esther Cecelia Goethe-Thomson
Vera June Hall-Barr
Clara Edith Hartman

Anna Hillstrom-Allen
Lailla Holmstrom-Green
Anna V. Johnson-Rylander
Christine Kroyer
LaVerne Morley-Schneider
Mabel Nelson-Mackey
Lois Hermina Pammel-Blundell
Olivia S. Peterson
Maria Siebrandts-Heiser
Ingeborg Silverson
Vivian M. Sjogren-Peterson
Lulu Belle Spencer-Roth
Louise M. Sunstrom

### 1918

Mabel Charlotte Burke-Anderson
Ida Burkhalter
Olivia Orilla Carney-Cratty
Mabel Eckstrom-Life
Esther Marie Erickson
Martha Rutlin Gaulke
Camille Guthormsen-Curtiss
Alma Marie Hokanson
Mabell E. Holm
J. Annyce Hummel
Elizabeth A. Juhl
Ellen Elizabeth Larson
Kersten Lindman-Ring
Amanda E. Mellin-Williams

Jane Mulder-Murphy
Anna M. Nilsson
Josephine J. Nilson
Signe Nordgaard
Gertrude J. Ritter-McBride
Mabel Rylander-Swenson
Katherine Seatvet-Gluck
Clara Marie Swahnberg
Ophelia Eschudy
Bertha Tweeten-Fradkin
Nannie V. Youngren
Wendla C. Youngren
Elvera 0. Youngert-Gannon

### 1919

Frances Ahlene
Ebba M. Anderson-Larson
Susan Ethel Bohon
Ellen A. Brodahl-Slama
Ruth Victoria Erickson-Branlund
Signe Adehl Fredrickson
Irene Lillian Gunderson-Gasser
Lyda L. Hartvig-Bessander
K. Esther Holmgren-English
Ida Louise Johnson-Dahl
Ruth Olga Lindstrom-Rogowski
Joan K. Mutschmann Faille
Esther Eugenia Nelson-Unis

Ida Carolina Nilson
Julia Nilsson-Baggesen
Ruth Olive Ohlson-Bredemeir
Minnie Olson-King
Helen M. Pearson-Courtney
Hilma J. Peterson-Wenzel
Helga Marie Sandberg-Wagner
Marie Sanwick-Paulson
Edna M. Schmidt-Anderson
Sister Evea Stark-Surrell
Agnes Ingeborg Wagner
Ellis J. Walker
Sophie Yoerg

## 1920

Florinda O. Abrahamson
Edna Marie Anderson-Rood
Edith Bergeson-Swanson
Lena Birkeness
Judith Marie Blomgren-Kerr
Lily J. Christopherson-Boregaard
Caroline I. Duffield
Alma Dorothy Eliason
Hedvig E. Hanson
Florence Marie Harold-Flourie
Lulu K. Jacobson-Quinn
Hazel C. Jensen
Vendela Marie Johnson-Olson
Helen Marie Johnson-Fritz
Hulda E. Johnson
Lillie Johnson-Badt
Linna Keeblatt-Schrep
Thyra D. E. Larson-Lindstrand
Sara J. Larsen
Anna Jeannetta Lemin
Elizabeth E. Machiels
Anna Kirstine Madsen
J. Anna Martin-Frandsen

Selma M. Mikkelson
Anna S. Nelson-Nelson
Anna Sophye Nyquist
Pauline E. Nelson-Splinter
Marie K. Peterson-Sorenson
Rachel Marie Reitan
Lydia Simon
Naomi Schmogrow-De Brisey
Trine Schmidt-Pond
Amanda W. Soderberg-Machlin
Madeline Sorenson-Deney
Rosie F. Strom-Otto
Lillian Oletta Stanke-Jasinsky
Effie Deborah Strand-Parish
Eleonora M. Stromquist
Ruth C. Sundblad-Duffill
Amy Swenson
Alma Vaupel
Letha Jean Wessels
Helen Jane Yoerg-Tulin
Alma Zschaechner
Avis Zwisler-Lynch

## 1921

Esther C. Anderson-Pfab
Nellie Charlotta Gustafson-
 Williams
Ruth Kathryn Helland-Percy
Millie A. Jacobson
Rena P. Jensen-Juhl-Nielson
E. Amelia Johnson-Goff
Hanna E. Johnson
Maude Evelyn Johnson-Robinson
Myrtle Marie Johnson-Edwards
Clara Imogen Jones

Thyra Rebecca Lund-Paulson
Alice T. Mathre
Bertha A. Paulson-Landin
Nellie Josephine Pearson-Nelander
Ella Rutt-Good
Ruby Alice Seversen-Jasinsky
Emma Florence Simpson
Marie Sörensen
Marion C. Swanson
Myrtle Olive Thorson-Weir
Florence Helen Wesslund

## 1922

Dagmar C. Anderson-Eubanks
Evelyn A. Anderson-Mull
Louise Anderson
Vivian Merie Apker
Ethel Ashwell
Beatrice Carlson-Colvin
Maud Marie Champion-Gottchling
Esther Irene Cleven
Florence Mildred Cleven-Altman
Elsie T. Conrads-Hallberg
Florence Eleanor Fish-Jacob

Ebba Louise Hjerstedt-Prill
Alfie Elide Hokland-Percy
I Frieda H. Jahn
Effie M. Johnson
Ircne R. D. Johnson-Joranson
Edith O. Johnson-Gallagher
Pauline L. Klett Knoll
Edith E. Koskey
Paula H. Larson-Hilker
Bertha Blanche Lauger
Charlotte Irene Lilly

Estella L. Nelson-Rose
Clara G. Olsen
Edna Mabeline Petersen-
    Shefveland
Johanna Marie Peterson-Olson

Emma Elizabeth Rydell—Hauberg
Ruth Rydman-Elliot
Vera S. Sifford-Schultz
Pearl M. Youngberg-Webster

## 1923

Grace Agnes Anderson-Svenwol
Selma V. Anderson-Wegner
Ruth H. Eckwall-Olander
Etta S. Erickson-Landstrom
Anna K. Hansen-Hansen
Sena Hansen Neilsen
Clara A. Hillstrom-Jasperson
Mabel Louise Hultgren-Danielson

Edidh L. Johnson
Edna L. Johnson-Nelson
Mabel C. Josephson-Huntley
Beda A. Lindberg
Elsie I. Ny Bloom-Larson
Esther M. Olander
Alma Swenson
Freda F. E. Youngren

## 1924

Emma C. Anderson
Ruth S. Atkinson-Howard
Clara Louise Bard-Perry
Eveline M. Beausang-Gustafson
Betty Olivia Benson-Doherty
Reta E. Beyer
Mildred M. Bolte-Barnes
Agnes A. Carlson
Marion O. Carlson-Michaelson
Lavinia P. Cleven-Knight
Marion C. Dreier-Bloecher
Pearl Louise Edwards
Mae Adaline Foresberg-Turner
Gyda H. Gunhus-Wright
Irene Juliana Gunnarson
Alma R. Mezel-Nerbos
Olivia S. Hirsch-Gross
Evelyn Marguerite Johnson-
    Swanson
Ida G. Kirstein-Christenson
Ruth Agnes Klar-Kallen

Agnes V. Kraase-Torgersen
Ellen K. Larsen
Vera H. Leaf, MD.
Alma Lee
Mildred I. Lenz
Edith Mildred Maakestad
Jenny Antonie Mathisen-Davis
Rose Meyer-Grill
Myrtle C. McIntosh
Margaret Elizabeth Naslund-
    Sprague
Dagney M. Nelson-Olson
Evelyn A. Norbom-Norup
Agnes Kristine Peterson
Helen Sailer-Sullivan
Elsie Laverne Sparkes-
    Hammergren
Sally Kristine Swanson-Hening
Cora H. Vinger-Thompson
Lillian Westerlund-Anderson

## 1925

Lulu I. Alberts
Olga E. Carlson
Harriett B. Carter-Becker
Grace Lorton Cooper-Woods
Gunhild Crown-Donaldson
Irene Friskopp
Muriel Greta Hanson
Dorothy G. Hanway-Hams
Esther G. Hooglund
V. Evangeline Isaacson-Hanson
Catherine E. Jensen-Mengers

Ethel M. Jones-Starck
Edna C. Kittleson
Helen N. Kolstad-McArdle
Bessie Kubec-Orillion
Edna R. Larson
Sophie A. Lund-Robertson
Wilmina H. Moran-Eckles
Eva W. Nelson
Naomi M. Nelson
Olga K. Nelson-Hall
Lillie M. Olson

Hazel E. Ottoson-Bierstedt
Lillian R. Radzom
Alma F. Rothkath-Sutterland

Signe I. Swanson-Sanford
Mathilda M. Westberg-Traner
Eleanor E. Wivagg-Efferding

## 1926

Elizabeth C. Algminowicz
Florence Osci Beck-Zohner-
  Swenson
Eleanor E. Berg
Frances- Hazel Burk-Lundahl
Edith Marion Carlson-Johnson
Margaret Elizabeth Chapin-
  Whitnall
Esther J. Ekstrom-Staudenrous
Emma Marie Erickson-
  Ruehrdanz
Ellen M. Gunderson-Merson
Della M. Hansen
Signe J. Hanson
Alice S. Holtan-Stillman
Marie M. Jacobsen-Petersen
Marie H. Jahn
Minnie J. Jensen-Uinther
Elna C. Johnson-Smith
Katherine D. Johnson-Rapp
Lulu Isabelle Kennedy-Sutter
Marie Ellen Latunen

Dagmar Helen Mathisen-
  Locklund
Wanda Clark Mead-Plasensia
Clara E. Megahan-Eckliff
Edith Nelson-Leaf
Gladys Darlene Nelson-
  Johnson
Luella May Omark
Evelyn H. Peterson
Mildred Evangeline Peterson-
  Bergquist
Norma Aurora Peterson-
  Rubrecht
Kathryn E. Potteiger-Behney
Eda Marie Ringstrom
Mrs. Nora H. Smith
Ruth L. Stohl
Florence Linae Strom-Stange
Carrie L. Twitchell
Bertha E. T. Wahlstrom-
  Carlson
Lila B. Winquist

## 1927

Anabel Alberts-Carlson
Clara E. Anderson
Gladys M. Anderson
Neta C. Anderson-Carlson
Lily M. Carlson-Schwendemon
O'Lafva Case
Beatrice Clark-Ziegele
Grayce C. Dotter-Call
Pearl L. Drake-Buhle
Grace S. Ferden-Espelund
Lydia J. Fredrickson
Genevieve Finnegan-Kaltoff
Ragnhild Gjestvang-Grotnes
Freda B. Grove-Schneiber
Aleda Halverson
Kathryn Hartong-Johnson
Gertrude Hass
Florence Hult
Esther W. Jensen-Johnson
Esther W. Johnson-McDaniels

Alta M. Johnson
Ruth Pierson Keating-Schneider
Irene List-Seaman
Constance M. Lundell
Emily I. Martinson-Garside
Ingrid M. Mattson-
  Schneidwind
Jennie Marie Nelson
Martha Nilsson-Ruzek
Edith L. Nyden
Genevieve K. Peterson
Mildred F. Pinkowsky-Nelson
Beda M. Ringdahl
Hulda Margaret Samuelson
Esther G. Seaberg
Evelyn L. Swanson
Della M. Ward-Bozdeck
Helene Waxvik-Damaecke
Mary Wegner-Bubb

## 1928

Marie Luella Abercrombie-Tea
Lenore Frances Alford
Merna Dean Amick
Evelyn Bernice Anderson
Lucille Alberta Anderson
Myrtle Christine Anderson
Gatha Baughn
Helen Black
Elsie Geraldine Carlson
Doris Mae Chenoweth-Kreitzer
Nina Bernhardine Dahl
Marjorie Elizabeth Davison-
    Baumann
Alexandra M. Fleming
Elsie Mae Fritz
Pauline Antonia Fritz-Burns
Beatrice Alphild Hartvigh-Manz
Edith Hedstrom
Elin Eugenia Henrikson
Gyda Jernstad
Alva A. Johnson
Ebba Ingeborg Johnson-Bergquist
Esther Helen Johnson-Nelson
Mildred Pauline Kratz
Ida S. Lindberg

Rose Evelyn Mord-Meikle
Esther Marie Nelson-Colliflower
Elsie Cecelia Nylund-Rodel
Clara Rachel Oberg
Marie Ohme-Franzen
Alma Olga Olsen-Newsom
Margit Elizabeth Olson-
    Anderson
Theresa Marie Olson-Johnson
Dorothy Paulson
Ellen C. Peterson-Johnson
Kathryn Marie Bawter
Siri Hildegard Persson
Helen Josephine Reistad-
    Jacobson
Cora Genevieve Trantow-
    Rackow
Irma Spalding
Dorothy Terese Swanson-
    Aranson
Margaret Swanson-Gustafson
Dorothy M. West-Knierim
Esther Evelyn Westerberg
Irene M. Wicklund-Bloomquist
Lucille Dorothy Young-Spetz

## 1929

Edna Hortense Ahlvin-Robinson
Adelaide Jeanette Alberts
Alice Marie Anderson
Dagmar Louise Andersen
Lynea Ann Back-Gately
Martha Virginia Bjorkman
Sigrid Johanna Carlson-Olsen
Lois Ruth Carroll-Fisher
Ruth Marguerite Cheney-Carrell
Florence Marie Danielson-
    Cavaney
Helma Eleane Davison-Schreiber
Mathilda Elizabeth Denef-
    Peterson
Marie Elizabeth Eckert-Hanson
Vivian Albertina Ekstrand
Helen Elizabeth Ekstrom-Genry
Ruth Ida Euler-Lorenz
Doris Hannah Friedland
Mildred Eleanora Gay
Laura Amelia Greason-Hinchman

Agnes Hanson
Alice Leone Hays
Augusta Jahn-Tilton
Edith Pauline Johnson
Svea Johnson-Matson-Anderson
Jennie Hazel Kirstein-Holbrook
Elsie Alina Koski
Bernice Yulande Larimore-
    Knight
Muriel Larimore
Mary Elfreda Lawson
Norma Caroline Leaf
Evelyn Mae Leslie-Hollatz
Helen Marie Liljedahl-Fredberg
Anaflo Argyle MacDonald
Viola Alice Molis-Nilson
Evelyn Margaret Morton
Elsie Ruth Nelson
Ethel Linnea Nelson-Crummer
Eleanora Julia Norling-Kelley
Esther Marguerite Nowack

Wilma Viola Pehrson
Eleanor Sophie Peterson-
 Hallquist
Jeanette Katherine Peterson
Luella Elvera Peterson-Lundin
Lillian H. Raisanen-Pollack
Bernadina Rehn-Johnson
Velma C. Sjogren-Marklund
Vernie Sjogren
Doris M. Staff
Edith Laura Stone

Julia Stortors
Helen Marie Swanson-
 McQueen
Ruth Linnea Swanson-Anderson
Esther Marie Templeman
Millie Marie Thuenen-Manley
Evelyn Eleanor Wallin
Astrid Mary Wickstrom
Mary Alice Wirt-Coleman
Lydia Winifred Wolle
Genevieve Agnes Zwicky-Gallo

## 1930

Dolores Abrahamson-McKean
Hildur E. Alm
Anna Marie Anderson-Boswell
Ethel Bjornstad-Atkins
Edna Marie Carlson
Linnea Carlson-Sciez
Esther S. Cederquist-Rogers
Borghilde Christenson-Toppila
Martha M. Dalin-Heath
Agnes G. Erickson-Anderson
Evelyn H. Erickson-La Pinske
Hortense B. Fortney-Behrens
Faye V. Fulton
Elizabeth E. Groom-Pautz
Linnea Genevieve Gustafson-
 Engberg
Beatrice Belle Henke-Cronin
Hilda V. Holmgren-Defner
Ruth E. Hult
Ethel Elizabeth Johnson
Dorothy Marie Keck-Roden
Chloe Milo Keith-Trammell
Hazel Kulp-Martin
Helene A. Klevos
Gladys Marie Krase-Bondi
Evelyn T. Larson
Eva Ilanda Mull-Roche

Gladys S. Nelson
Laila Eleanor Niemela
Emma E. Norell
Astrid L. M. Nygren-Carter
Laura W. E. Oak-Pratt
Gertrude M. Olson-Carlson
Roma M. Pearson-Lower
Olga M. Petersen-Hundtoft
Thelma C. Peterson
Marcella A. Raftshol
Valeda T. Reiter-Thiese
Naomi Lenore Roost-Hurt
Edith Marie Rummell-Claypole
Ila Elvira Saukko
Esther M. Schneider
Elsie E. Smith-Musson
Ruth A. Smith-Shellhammer
Sylvia Christine Swanson
Vera M. Swanson
Frances Thomas-McConough
Letha Wells
Mary E. Williams
Edna V. Wilson
Margorie Louise Wood-
 Ackerman
Hilda Andrea Zwicky-Cogswell

## 1931

Virginia Ann Anderson
Elfie A. Arvidson
Irene M. Allyn-Bush
Clara Belle Anderson-Sandquist
Leona H. Bergstrom-Smith
Bernice Dorothy Brandt
Clara S. Brocksh-Teets

Jessie L. Bauer-Getschman
Ruth S. Benson-Olson
Dorothy J. Carlson
Anna Elizabeth Colburn-
 Rosenau
Hermine J. de Leeuw
Marit Moe Droivoldsmo

1931 (Con't.)

Ellen Margaret Eliason-Schrank
Charlotte Helen Gerlach-
  Barkhausen
Ellen Lillian Graf
Cecelia Marie Goodman-
  Flickinger
Eleonora Anna Goodman
Marion C. Hanson-Hanson
Berit Helene Haukass
Alfhild J. Johnson-Gotz
Alvira C. Jensen -Kallman
Clarice Jahre
Eleanor Marie Jensen-Baysinger
Florence Louise Lindbloom
Elna Marie Laursen
Erma M. Leonard-Stacy
Hazel H. Lenz-De Vilbus
Karen Moilien-Shrader
Asta Augusta Mueller-Brooks
Ellen J. Nicholsen
Dorothy Noren-Anderson
Gladys C. Olson-Lawler
Anita Louise Olson-Barr

Martha E. Pearson
Edna Radies-Stoekmann
Eldrid Rasmussen
Prudence Elizabeth Rotramel-
  Dix
Ethel Alvira Rowe
Ethel M. Rundman
Ann Evelyn Salle-Hunt
Pearl V. Sayles
Esther J. Schreib
Estrid J. Seaholm
Miriam V. Sigfridson
T. Margaretta Silberg
Elsie Skyrud
Helen B. Steele-Lapinski
Esther Elizabeth Swanson
Phyllis Thompson-Cote
Selma Tornquist
Dolores Tusler-Zermuhlen
Johanna Wendel
Ruth Margret Wennermark-
  Leton
Ruth A. Williamson-Holmes

1932

Agnes L. Anderson-Peterson
Josephine H. Anderson-Ohlson
Eva Alice Beach-Reiter
Waverly Miller Bicknell-
  Tappendorf
Myra Elizabeth Brink
Nina Arlene Catey-Ewing
Mary Elizabeth Chapin-Burns
Stella Mae Conklin-Bittrich
Flora Lois Dorais-Potter
Violet M. Edmonds-MacNeil
Jeanette H. Ekwall-Morrison
Mary Elizabeth Falk
Gudrun Cecile Gerner
Marie Haurberg
Florence Gertrude Hedman
Evelyn E. Heidtke-Silco
Sadie W. Holm
Christine Elizabeth Johnson
Florence Charlotte Johnston-
  Lockwood

Bertha Larsen
Ethel S. Larson-Thorston
Joy B. Nelson
Hazel Elizabeth Nyblade
Signe Victoria Olson-Bellande
Martha Elaine Otterson
Helen Myrtle Peterson
Esther L. Peterson-Picken
Wilma Annette Peterson-
  Bomar
Marie Antoinette Skog
Esther G. Soderberg
Hazel Irene Spaulding
Grace K. Strasburg
Alice Marie Swanson-Lesh
Edna Thornblade
Elva Pauline Toepel-Nicholson
Edith E. Wesender-Steege
Mona M. Wightman

## 1933

Birdie E. E. Anderson
Thelma Katherine Borgstrom-Shirer
Ruth Cecilia Carlson
Andrea Bernice Clemenson-Bleeker
Clarice Louise Fritz-Grimes
Helen M. Ford
Elizabeth E. Gould
Laurine Ruth Grantz
Austa B. Hansen
Eva Elizabeth Helander
June Louise Holmgren-Kelley
Helen Hotvedt-Torgesen
Margaret Linnea Johnson
Sara Josephine Johnson
Ruth M. Kallhauge-Armstrong

Bertha Elizabeth Klauser
Evelyn Linnea Lambert-Shaw
Viana Catherine Laakson
Florence A. Lindquist
D. Marguerite Olson
Frances Jeanette Ostewig-Costigan
Anna Marion Payne
Pauline Ramsay-Marston
Amanda M. Rennhack-Fish
Helen Edith Rumsey
Esther Anna Sponberg
Mildred L. Stenlund
Margaret Arlene Swanson-Barden
Evelyn Sweet-Ahl
Sigrid Pearl Walback-Koven

## 1934

Bertha J. Anderson
Dorothy M. Anderson-Rennels
Loretta Anderson
Martha Blomgren
Selma Elizabeth Carlson-Johnson
Hertha Christensen-Wollum
Evelyn Grove-Weller
Viola Hawkinson
Josephine Hummel-Kalkwarf
Hildred Ivey
Catherine Johnson-Francis
Verdell Johnson-Pierce
Helen Kolste
Winnifred McNeil-Johnson
Elsie Mellin-Sundien

Florence Miller-Doolin
Verna Person
Jeanette Peterson
Mildred Raper-Boyd
Ethel Rose-Beck
Dorothy Rumsey-Shellorne
Esther Silas
Frances Sorensen
Myrtle Suttie-Miller
Miriam Vanni-Hammerberg
Mary Warren-Turner
Virginia Weingartner
Marion Wiles
Dorothy Wilke-Kracke

## 1935

Margaret Amble
Jane Sara Becker-Bauer
Aleda Bringe
Thelma Christine Dragge-Taylor
Gladys M. Engstrom-Schraffenberger
Mildred Gail Hahn
Marion Ruth Hollander
Eleanore G. E. Holmer
Leona C. Jensen-Thompson
Donna Olga Johnson

Helen Bernice Johnson
Rose Mae Kuchera
Margaret Alice Lutes
Virginia P. Moore-Busse
Margaret E. Nielsen
Esther Margaret Peterson
Ruth Dagmar Ryden
Muriel Marguerite Staffner
Isabella Stenman
Doris R. Warren

## 1936

Elizabeth R. Drotning
Maurine Forsmoe
Edna D. Goodman
Anita Graham
Sara Hedberg
Edna S. Hedstrom
Esther L. Holmer
Violet E. Jensen
Sylvia Lauridsen
Ina Magnuson

Bernice F. Markwart
Dorothy C. Mobeck
Inga G. Nielsen
Mia L. Pearson
Marian Perry
Esther E. Peterson
Grace C. Rehm-Connell
Helen A. Sampson
Margaret C. Swanson
Laura A. Winship

## 1937

Phyllis M. Beauvais
Antoinette E. Cardin
Mary Anna Cheever
Dolores Crudden
Pauline De Kiep
Marcella Edgren
Gudrun A. Engman
Velma I. Fisher
Helen E. Green
A. Myrtle Jackson
Helen J. Johnson
Helen Koivisto
Ruth L. Lindgren
Lucille F. Magnes

Florence M. Manley
Louise Mae Mosbeck
Mary S. L. Nelson
Ellen C. Norby
Lillian Ostrand
W. Irene Pehrson
Garna L. Peterson
Evryll E. Ring
Gladys M. Sahlmark
Julia Ann Sampson
Helen Schiesser
Janet Speidel
Irene Swanson
Thelma Thias

## 1938

Jeanette R. Anderson
Leona B. Backa
Eleanor C. Carlson
Beulah Virgene Ehle
Marion A. Erickson
Dorothy R. Fredrickson
Anne C. Glovatsky
Eva Ruth Godfrey
Dorothy Ione Hansen
Ruth Eleanor Hendrickson
Irene Marie Hildebrand
Florence L. Johnson
Lily O. Johnson
Lois W. Johnson
Clara T. Larsen
Esther Ruth Larsen
Esther A. Larson
Eleanore M. Malmberg
Harriet A. May

Alice E. McDaniel
Judith Mae Miller
Alfhild J. I. Moline
Dorodhy L. Mosiman
Evelyn J. Olson
Myrtle J. Paro
June Porlier
Elsie C. Rasmussen
Lethia L. Russell
Pearl M. Satre
Berdina M. Seegers
Charlene Shaw
Lillian Skagen
Marie I. Stotts
Beatrice M. Swanson
Ardis Tostenson
Mildred I. Wickman
Elizabeth M. Widen
Agnes Louise Wislander

## 1939

Hallie V. Amling
Doris H. Anderson
Jundine Anderson
June H. Anderson
Audray Arnold
Elsa M. Axelson
Winifred Backman
Caroline Blankshain
Elizabeth Caldwell
Ruth Ellison
Eva H. Erickson
Doris R. Espel
Gwendolyn Grams
Vera C. Gustafson
Edith C. Hammerstrom
Clara E. Harms
Mildred A. Helander
Marjorie Isaacson
Linda Jackson
Anne Jacobson
Fern A. Jensen
Sylvia V. Johnson
Grace Klingberg
Olga May Kmet
Dorothy E. Larsen

Marian Liebetreu
Edith Martenson
Ruth L. Monk
Marjorie Myren
Margaret A. Noteware
Myrl Olson
Betty Parish
Eugena M. Petersen
Linnea J. K. Peterson
Joyce Elaine Posey
Kathryn Prestegaard
Nora Roughton
Lois E. Saul
Ruth H. Schroeder
M. L. Sholander
Marjorie L. Starks
Avis Stinson
Flora I. Swanson
Edith L. Tang
C. June Vaughan
Helen B. Wagner
Ruth Wassberg
Louise Westerberg
Marion J. Williams

## 1940

Marion L. Ahlquist
Junis A. Anderson
Verna L. Bauer
Eleanor R. Broman
E. Jeanne Brumagim
Janet L. Bugner
Lillian Carlson
Ruth Christiansen
Edith Dedering
Marian L. Ekstrand
Florence V. Festerling
Anna Frang
Anna M. Geir
Kathryn R. Heggaton
Dorothy L. Herbert
Ruth W. Hopton
Gladys M. Hummel

Phyllis M. Igo
Viola M. Jacobi
Kathryn M. Johnson
Beverly Jones
Martha Larson
Alice M. Lilja
Viola C. Lofquist
Virginia Marks
Florence W. Noyce
Katherine I. Olson
Lillian Ostewig
Ruth E. Peterson
Evelyn Ranta
Anna J. Swanson
Dorothy E. Swanson
Elsie M. Tatch

## 1941

Ruth Marjory Alla
Bernadine Anderson
Helen L. Backlund
Oakie M. Baker
Edith A. Belden
Mary Oleta Bell
Olive Dorothy Benson
Jeanne Blank
Ida Lu Born
Frances L. Brinkruff
Christina Carlen
Mildred S. Carlson
Marion A. Cook
Agnes M. Dahlbeck
Vera H. Dexheimer
Grace Dillon
Stella A. Dytko
Grace L. Edmond
Pauline E. Fraser
Astrid Grunlund
Alene B. Johnson

Dorothy W. Johnson
Remola Johnson
Elizabeth Lindelius
Mary Nicholas
Harriet E. Nordstrom
Gladys A. Olson
Ruth V. Olson
Doris E. Pearson
Anlouise Rasmussen
Meta Schalinske
Ruth M. Schnabel
Alma Ruth Schroeder
Elizabeth J. Smith
Frances L. Stevig
Elsie M. Tuuri
Myrtle M. Vamgsnes
Anna Violet Vanni
B. Elaine Wahlstrom
Thelma D. Werner
Lillian H. Wilmer

## 1942

Dorothy Abrahamson
Wilma Baker
Dorothy Bergman
Leona Bottlemy
Elizabeth Brukardt
Naomi Callon
Helen Carlson
Juanita Castleberry
Lorraine Chalman
Grace Christensen
Helen Cook
Beverly Douglas
Frances Eash
Gertrude Eggers
Cleo Ellis
Dorothy Entz
Seiv Ericson
Ruth Fratzke
Edna Hedine
Edith Heide
Helen R. Johnson

Lois Johnston
Shirley Lembke
Annette Leonard
Margaret Leonard
Charlotte Lindborg
Irene Lomas
Betty Mathieson
Helen Myers
Helen Olson
Marjorie Osborn
Maryon Peterson
Dorothy Rewerts
Phyllis Sandgren
Virginia Sanford
Dorothy Shibley
Anona Sundlie
Joyce Syren
Gertrude Thomson
Geneva Wessels
Gretchen Zielsdorf

## 1943

Gail L. Ahlborn
Olive C. Anderson
Eleanor Brome

Kathryn E. Daugherty
Alyce Donkersgoed
Dorothy E. Drow

Lillian E. Eld
Maria E. Gilissen
Margaret Z. Goetz
Lillian G. Guttorm
Helen Heikkinen
Geraldine J. Henry
Mary A. Keech
Elizabeth A. Laakso
Barbara R. Leighton
Elsie M. Lindberg
Betty A. Lindholm
Virginia S. Liston
Karen M. Madsen
Jane H. Miller
Huldur Y. Modder
Florence I. Murdie
Hortense L. Nelson
Dorothea Nicholson

Margaret E. Nolte
Elizabeth M. Puhlman
Betty L. Randall
Besse R. Rummel
Caroline V. Schiller
Margaret F. Scott
Kate Seidewitz
Dorothy M. Shappi
Helen B. Sickles
Isabel S. Simpson
Vieno E. Somppi
Grace E. Strachan
Alice R. Swanson
Violet C. Swanson
Kathryn L. Thompson
Dorothy L. Tyler
Olive M. White
Elizabeth M. Zielsdorf

## 1944

Muriel Ackerson
Helen M. Andersen
Charlotte M. Anderson
Helen B. Anderson
Ruth Angerer
Harriet M. Arndt
Elizabeth R. Belitz
Jo Ann Bills
Marjorie C. Boswell
Charlien Bosworth
Marilyn C. Broman
Doris L. Brunell
Linnea Carlson
Marjorie J. Carlson
Anna N. Challberg
Esther D. Chamberlin
Ruth S. Cutka
Mary H. Elavsky
Lorraine E. Even
Kathryn A. Field
Bernice J. Flom
Ruby D. Goplen
Marion I. Grover
Ruth E. Grunlund
Ethel L. Gundberg
Sara M. Handford
Twila L. Hildebrandt
Helen I. Hill

Eleanor R. Johnson
Frances E. Johnson
Helen M. Johnson
Mina D. Kirkland
Florence J. Krajecke
Liesel Lackey
Hazel S. Lagerstrom
Mae J. Larson
Madge M. Martin
Julianne Meyer
Marian G. Morene
Jean H. Muchmore
Elizabeth M. Nelson
Ernestine M. Nelson
Marion G. Nelson
Helen E. Nord
Dorothy M. Olson
Geraldine A. Potts
Anna M. Quinlan
Shirley A. Roche
Betty J. Rothenberg
Ruth A. Schumacher
June N. Setterlund
Mildred D. Thorsen
Frances Vanress
Lavina M. Whitehead
Gladys M. Wood

## 1945

Lorraine Anderson
Marjorie Anderson
M. Boehlk
Ethel Bradac
Mary Ellen Brecken
Phyllis Byron
Annlizabeth Carlsen
Arlene Carlson
Betty Carlson
Ardythe Carlstadt
Kathryn Carpenter
Virginia Cassin
Winona Cassin
Lorraine Dallenbach
Bernice Didriksen
Elaine Engdahl
Hazel Erickson
Jeanette Fanshaw
Carol Fisher
Irene Fredericks
Eleanor Froberg
Ann Fuhrmann
Helen Gustafson
Jane Hammer
Burnell Hanson
Jeanne Hoffman
Charlotte Johnson
Marilyn Johnson
Dorothy Kemp

Beverly Kraft
Gloria Kuisti
Janice Larson
Clara Lima
Janet Luther
Dorothy Marinoff
Gladys Nelson
Jean Nelson
Phyllis Nelson
Nora Ottens
Marion Peterson
Margaret Ann Poyser
Adeline Riemenschneider
Betsy Ring
Marilyn Roelk
Patricia Rumbyrt
Eleanor Rytekonen
Bernice Samuelson
Joyce Schuette
Carolyn Schweer
Florence Serbin
Marion Skagen
Lillian Stetins
Anita Sues
Patricia Sweeney
Ruth Waterman
Eleanor Wille
Hope Williams

## 1946

Alice Anderson
Dorothy Anderson
Helen Andre
Marie Atkins
Margaret Beck
Sharleen Bennett
Charlotte Benson
Lois Benson
Grace Berger
Ruth Bergh
Marian Bohlmann
Doris Bruce
Ruth Buntrock
Dorothy Bystrom
Margaret Carlson
Mildred Carlson
Shirley Carlson
Helen Croffoot

Phyllis Diekman
Wilma Dubs
Virginia Duffill
Phyllis Engdahl
Phyllis Fahnestock
Patricia Garihee
Phyllis Groop
Jean Guest
Gail Gustafson
Laverne Gustafson
Lorraine Hanson
Mildred Hatland
Carol Holm
Harriet Johnson
Jean Johnson
Mildred Johnson
Dorothy Larson
Marion Larson

Ruth Lear
Signe Lindberg
Betty Jo Lower
Lorraine Lovgren
Ruth Martinson
Helen McCollough
Norene Melvin
Jean Metcaff
Florence Nordin
Virginia Nyce
Irene Nylander
Ruth Pearson
Irene Peterson
M. Audrey Peterson
Marie A. Peterson

Marjorie Rice
Dorothy Ritchards
Eloise Schmitz
Alice Schrader
Joyce Smeds
Traule Soetebier
Polly Stevens
Dorothy Strand
Helen Swanson
Lorraine Swanson
Margret Swanson
Ruth Teske
Leatrice Thompson
Lois Winquist

## 1947

Elaine Anderson
Florence L. Anderson
Marry L. Bakke
Ruth E. Bengson
Hildegard Benner
Catherine M. Bond
Bette Bruin
Hazel Corning
Dorothy Culbertson
Norma J. Drake
Mary I. Duncan
Leila Ehrenstrom
Marian L. Erickson
Muriel M. Fischer
Esther E. Fredrickson
Elda I. Gabeline
Marlene J. Georgeson
Margaret Gustafson
Violet E. Gustafson
Kathryn A. Hamill
Wanda L. Hayen
Beatrice E. Heikkila
Berniece B. Hess
Jean H. Hines
Marjorie Huseby
Doris A. Jeffries
Ethel A. Jensen
Gurlie G. Johnson
Joan C. Johnson
A. Marghat Johnston
Doris L. Koeck
Elsie Korpi
Betty J. Lapan

Geraldine Larson
Jeannette Lechler
Elaine Lind
Lucille E. Lindborg
Dorothy A. Lindstrand
Judith M. Lundberg
Mabel M. Mattson
Helen McLain
Tekla Nelmark
Joyce E. Nelson
Elizabeth Nicholson
Marion Northwall
Shirley M. Notter
Betty K. Olson
Ruth E. Olson
Anna Mae Peterson
Doris L. Peterson
Muriel Peterson
Ruth J. Peterson
Marilyn Pogemiller
Arlene K. Ring
Mildred R. Risold
Rena M. Scott
Iola L. Seger
LaVonne C. Seger
Marilyn A. Smith
Elouise M. Speener
A. Martha Sponberg
Norene Susanka
Goldie M. Swanson
Vivian A. Swanson
Shirley M. Wagoner
Ruth M. Warmbier

Pearl Wear
Dorothy L. Weidman

Lucille Williams
Constance Winegardner

1948

Caroline Anderson
Eileen Anderson
Elna Anderson
Irene Anderson
Shirley Apitz
Martha Bartlow
Louella Benner
Marilynn Benson
Lois Bergendahl
Kathryn Bodine
June Bohler
Edith Brookman
Elizabeth Brown
Mary Bulander
Mary R. Carlson
Lona Clauson
Virginia DeYoung
Pearl Dykstra
Delynn Eaken
Dorothy Eggen
Sylvia Frahm
Sylvia Freberg
Arlene Froelich
Ruth Fryksdale
Barbara Fuller
Evelyn Gebhard
Edith Goplen
Marjorie Gothe
Frances Green
Marilynn Gustafson
Pauline Hagenbuch
Elizabeth James
Carol Johnson
Jeanne Kiser

Martha Labda
Mary L. Latham
Gloria Larson
Vivian Londberg
Virginia Magnuson
Janet Malmquist
Inez Nason
Marijean Nelson
Lorraine Northup
Jeanne Olsen
Shirley Olson
Viola Pfeiffer
Joyce Rabausch
Eleanor Roehm
Eleanor Salow
Janet Scheel
June Schmeckpeper
Ruth J. Schmidt
Mary Schroer
Helen Schultz
Delores Seger
Erna Sigg
Barbara Spangler
Naomi Stengel
Ethel Stenlund
Elna Thorsen
Arla Vierow
Marion Wessels
Marilynn Wesson
June Wicks
Emma Wehman
Juliann Wiegel
Roberta Wilcox
Elizabeth Woodworth

1949

Carla F. Anderson
Ruth L. Anderson
Margaret M. Benson
Doris J. Blythe
Dorothy L. Bogren
Geraldine M. Brown
Nance B. Clark
Rita J. Clark
Helen J. Cowell
June Lois Een

Anna E. Enarson
Elaine L. Erickson
Margaret R. Falk
Kathryn Gerber
Gloria Hartman
Sara M. Hodney
Gladys Johnson
Patricia Juergens
Arletta J. Klages
Jeanne F. Knowles

Doris Koskela
Ruth S. Kridahl
Helen Krommenhoek
Jo Kurns
Audrey Kurz
Eleanor J. Larson
Leone A. Lindberg
Mary C. Lindbom
Mildred A. Lindroth
Evelyn Martin
Doris McGuire
Iva Lou McGuire
Carol Lou Miller
Carol Jean Molstad
Bernadette Noel
LaVerne Oerke
Jean Lois Orsett

Carolyn Peterson
H. Margery Plummer
Jean Richter
Eunice J. Ringquist
Betty Schlegelmilch
Mary L. Scobee
Mary Sievertsen
Betty Jean Smith
Marilyn J. Smith
Signe T. Sohlberg
Elaine Stubbs
Margaret A. Stumpf
Helen M. Sunblad
Beverly Swanson
Janet Thorpe
Margaret Wolbart

## 1950

Jeanne Anderson
Ramona Bauer
Eleanor L. Benson
Barbara Berg
Doris E. Bergstrom
M. Kathleen Cashion
Jessie Ann Cleare
Dolores Curtis
Georgina Daleanes
Patricia Faust
Audrey M. Fresh
Julia Fricke
Dorothy Garner
Dorothy J. Howe
Bettylou Johnson
Elvira L. Johnson
Lenore Johnson
Marian R. Johnson
Eileen E. Kangas
Betty Ann Klabunde
Lois M. Klinkhammer
Eileen Kors
Darlene M. Larson
Elsie H. Larson

Doris E. Leighton
Sylvia Lindquist
Ruth L. Mansfield
Dolores Miller
Shirley Morettes
Shirley Nelson
Margory I. Ness
Velma Neukomm
Mary A. Norkus
Eleanor A. Olsen
Caryl Anne Paarlberg
Joanne Paarlberg
Joyce E. Peterson
Marilyn E. Peterson
Lucille Primuth
Bonnie Jean Rogers
Nancy Ross
Janet L. Secor
Donnette Stennfeld
Ruth Mary Tatge
Phyllis Teteak
Edna Mae Thomas
Irene Winkka

## 1951

Darlene Adamson
Janet Anderson
Kathryn P. Anderson
Lois J. Barnett
Lorraine Barosko

Marilyn Jane Barrett
Beatrice Brown
Margaret E. Carlson
Marjorie A. Christianson
Patricia Cook

Dolores N. Fischer
Anita Freedstrom
Lily Garden
Edna M. Germann
Ardelle Hartman
Gloria Hermann
Marilyn J. Hornell
Alice Hugh
Janet Jennings
Ann Louise Johnson
Lois Ellen Jordan
Susan Margaret Keach
Carol Kellerman
Joan Kirk
Bernice Klingelsmith
Rose Mary Knudtson
Martha J. Kordewich
Evelyn Kraemer
Joyce Lane
Norma E. Larson
E. Janet Leeson
Marianne J. Leppiaho
Mimi Marcello

Helen J. Matthews
Henrietta E. McDonough
Darlene Miller
Betty Nelson
Mary June Nelson
Ruth E. Nelson
Lois Olander
Meryl Paulson
Frances Poole
Barbara M. Reardon
Donna Robinson
Bee Atrice Ruble
Anita L. Springer
Jean Stellmacher
Nancy Sutter
Lucille Timmerman
Charlotte M. Vanitvelt
Ruth Vanselow
Anna Mae Venne
Joyce Wallin
Elaine Wehrmeister
Dorothy Wells
Doretta E. Wobith

## 1952

Jean Ellen Bigler
Helen E. Bils
Virginia E. Bjork
Barbara M. Cook
Constance J. DeMet
Marilyn L. Fiedler
Frances L. Erickson
Annamarie Fjellstedt
Eloise L. Foster
Patricia M. Hallberg
Connie I. Hetrick
Doris C. Holmgren
Dorothy J. Johnson
Lois J. Johnson
Marcella J. Junker
Jeannette M. Kangas
Carol D. Koehler
Lois A. Kogler
Sophia M. Komadina
Margaret G. Koss
Shirley Lied
Marcella M. Miller
Marjorie H. Morse

Marilyn J. Myrmel
Carolyn A. Noble
Teckla Ann Person
Marilyn J. Peterson
June V. Peugh
Joan L. Rauschert
Elsie Reichl
Rosemarie Reiner
Patricia A. Richter
Claire V. Rousu
Betty Anne Sandberg
Gertrude E. Schleef
Irma H. Schnaufer
Norma H. Schultz
E. Kathryn Seawall
Mary Lou N. Shogren
Jean A. Stone
Dorothy F. Streit
Margaret M. Vogeler
Phyllis L. Westrom
Dolly Mae Wong
Gladys B. Wright

## 1953

Barbara L. Anderson
Ruth E. Anderson
Shirlee M. Anderson
Audrey A. Aubrey
Donna M. Bannon
Beatrice J. Bartanen
Ruth M. Birkle
Donna M. Bjorklund
Phyllis J. Bood
Norma J. Carlson
Lois M. Davis
Alice Eisenmann
Dorothea E. Eissfeldt
Corinne E. Engelhardt
Joan C. Faust
Virginia M. Froemming
Bonita E. Garvey
Norma J. Graefe
Dorothy M. Gratto
Marvella D. Gustafson
Leona M. Hedlund
Winefred M. Herndon
Natalie C. Kangas
Dorothy M. Karall
Margaret A. Karall
Carol J. Kaski
Elizabeth M. King
Carol J. Kinsman

Bertha D. Krueger
Marian I. Lamberg
Marilyn A. Larson
Carol A. L'Huillier
Charlotte Lindbom
Marion R. Lindgren
Lorraine A. Lund
Marion D. Lungren
Helen J. Molin
Mary C. Nicholas
Shirley A. Okerlund
Sue Parker
Pauline P. Parrish
Janet R. Peabody
Dorothy A. Pearson
Marlene M. Peterson
Carol J. Plautz
Anne C. Rakas
Lorraine E. Reid
Eleane J. Ridley
Arlene M. Selke
Patricia M. Shannon
Renetta Skiba
Janice E. Sutter
Ruth J. Thies
Ella M. Tienhaara
Carolyn M. Wilson
Ann C. Winkelman

## 1954

Ann Louise Adamson
Norma Allbritton
Gloria Anderson
Jeanne Balke
Eunice Berg
Nancy Beyrer
Marjorie Bils
Rosemarie Cangelosi
Nancy Cronenworth
Helen Danielson
Ellen Eby
Barbara Elmer
Barbara Harpster
Patricia Hoard
Ruth Hofer
Loretta Hotze
Anna Johnson
Alice Knaus
Shirley Knaus

Florence Koss
Sonya Lapp
Ingrid Larson
Mary Kay Leaf
Mary Louise Levine
Ruth Linstead
Norma Marks
Arlene Merriman
Jeanne Neilson
Joyce Neilson
Dorothy Neumann
Clarice Olson
Ann Osterman
Elda Peters
Carolyn Peterson
Lenore Pfeiffer
Jean Popelar
Rosemary Spicklemire
Ruth Stone

Betty Thies
Norrine Thomas
Louise Vogeler
Eulamae Watkins

Marjorie Weckwert
Lorraine Wirtala
Joan Wohfeil

1955

Josephine Anderson
Janice Anderzon
Joanne Anderzon
Helga Beck
Karen Benson
Violet Bergwall
Janice Bjork
Betty Bowers
Marjorie Carlson
Alice Chen
Carolyn Dow
Faith Dzurowcik
Carol Eklund
Judith Elam
Constance Engel
LaVerne Erwin
Beverly Gumz
Patricia Hanson
Eleanor Hine
Thelma Hollingsworth
Alice Ivan
Barbara Johnson
Patricia Kaufman

Shirley Knulty
Helen Kurringer
Audrey Lindstrand
Elsie Mackie
Dorothy Moeller
Ann Morgan
Joan Mueller
Jean Neitzel
Jean Nordstrom
June Odmark
Alice Olson
Anne Olson
Shirley Osborn
Darlene Peterson
Marian Rasmussen
Maryann Rosenau
Patricia Ruff
Sally Rushford
Jane Smedman
Doris Ummel
Jean Vehnekamp
Beverly Wehman
Joan Winkler

1956

June Baer
Luella Arnett
Joan Borchert
JoAnne Castelli
Caroline Christensen
Joanne Cyganek
Mary Jo Decker
Kathryn Dicks
Barbara Eldh
Bonita Emhoff
Donna Fasse
Mary Lou Forey
Ronelle Fort
Marilyn Ganzer
Ruth Gelinski
Vivian Gidley
Jacklyn Hayes
Rita Hackstock
Joanne Hedin

Florence Isaacson
Alice Jasperson
Arla Johnson
Jane Kaiser
Elaine Kentzel
JoAnn LaComb
Claudia Langebartels
Virginia Larsen
Alma Larson
Dolores Mansch
Lois Meyer
Barbara Miller
Marilynn Motzer
Audrey Nelson
Judith Oesterreich
Anita Ollikainen
Ingrid Persson
Carolyn Peterson
Karen Peterson

Mildred Peterson
Aileen Roder
Catherine Roderick
Doris Saari
Edythe Scheffler
Janet Schroeder
Carol Selke
Charlotte Semper
Margaret Skrabak
Ilene Smith

Patricia Smith
Phyllis Smith
Betty Soderquist
Gwendolyn Sparrow
Brenda Vogel
Eunice Warnke
Carlene Warren
Betty Wertz
Janice Westerlund
Ruth Wirtala

## 1957

Jill Anderson
Joyce Beckman
Dolores Bradfute
Mary Buitenwerf
Nancy Bystrom
Florence Elson
Doris Franks
Margareth Franks
Shirley Gibbons
Caroline Gunsallus
Carol Gustafson
Joyce Hendrickson
Wanda Hollub
Nancy Holmberg
Ruth Holmen
Sally Ihamaki
Donna Jacobson
June Johnson
Marilyn Johnson
Jane Kojiri
Jean Kojiri
Margaret Krupa

Martha Levine
Diane McLaren
Catherine Mudd
Lois Nelson
Marlene Nulf
Dorothy Nurmi
Carole Nystrom
Evelyn Parsons
Marilyn Peterson
Kristine Phillips
Bonnie Rapson
June Ritchey
Janice Roen
Barbara Romo
Anne Sandstrom
Ann Sarkela
Shirley Vicklund
Gayl Weber
Carol Westerberg
Lois Williams
Sally Williams
Josephine Witthoft

## 1958

Ann Ahlstrom
Sally Allyn
Joan Berg
Paula Biesmann
Linda Boers
Ardell Bohl
Judith Bond
Andrea Borg
Karen Brown
Anita Bush
Sally Carl
Mary Lou Carlson
Sandra Carlson
Alverna Cavallo

Phyllis Crayton
Madge Danielson
Judith Escher
Margaret Fergin
Kathleen Fiedler
Mary Fostveit
Madelyn Gabrielson
Cora Hanks
Nancy Hoefle
Janice Holtz
Janet Isaacson
Betty Jacobson
Carole Johnson
Sharon Johnson

Helen Karall
Donna Kelley
Dorothy Knol
Marie Kranner
Shirley Kuhr
Jacqueline Langlois
Nancy Larson
Karen Latola
Carol LeMieux
Lila Moen
Betty Monticue
Janice Moyle
Janet Murray
Sheila Musgrove

Carol Nelson
Nancy Nevala
Beverley Ninnis
Nancy Obergefell
Carol Rehfeldt
Hildburg Richter
Constance Robertson
Cynthia Ross
Nancy Schleitwiler
Shirley Schmutte
Nancy Seng
Julie Suzuki
Diane Wilhelmson
Barbara Wolf

## 1959

Karen Ahsmann
Karole Ahsmann
Donna Anderson
Doris Anderson
Inga Anderson
Gail Arden
Judith Barrett
Joanne Barrowman
Mary Beauvais
Mary Berg
Bonnie Borchers
Lorraine Carlson
Mary Carlson
Hildegard Chaveriat
Sue Christenson
Dorene Dawson
Marion Drake
Joan Driskall
Ilona Ellefson
Barbara Erickson
Betty Erickson
Helen Granskog
Sharon Guy
Sheila Haarman
Marlene Hill
Barbara Holmgren
Joyce Johnson
Marjorie Johnson
Karen Keenan

Sandra Kampainen
Carol Knopf
Sharon Korpi
Eleanor Larson
Margot Larson
Marcia Lindahl
Ruth Lockner
Fern Logeman
Carol Maloney
Nancy Mangold
Eleanor Meinheit
Maxine Miller
Barbara Nelson
Patricia Norton
Suzanne Nuske
Anne O'Hare
Arlene Ohr
Katheleen Peterka
Karol Peterson
Susan Roberts
Norma Sorensen
Dorothy Splinter
Nancy Szilagui
Arlene Thompson
Karen Voelker
Barbara Wiedeman
Geraldine Witthoft
Janet Wright

## 1960

Frances A'Hern
Karen Alexander
Carol Andersen
Jane Anderson
Darlene Marksity Bach
Carol Childs
Martha Dehaven
Barbara Denecke
Nancy DuFour
Myrna Erickson
Donna Steuerwald Gizewski
Judith Honkala
Jean Howard
Donna Jones
Judith Juntunen
Kay Kantor
Judith Katzke
Dolores Keto
Jacqueline Komlenich
Judith Lauer

Mary Lindner
Judith Maki
Maila Veber Mallett
Marilyn Martin
Lucille Banick McCoy
Carole Palm
Sandra Patterson
Kay Helston Prideaux
Jane Rosenquist
Vivian Rosenthal
Linda Keffer Rutter
Barbara Swanson
Kay Swanson
Joyce Tonyan
Rosemary True
Gloria Ulvila
Anna Wainio
Mary Ann Welton
Kathryn Wright

## 1961

Carol Jeanne Anderson
Ruth Eleanor Anderson
Kay Kuusisto-Autio
Valentine Stecenko-Belous
Linda Jane Berry
Janet Kay Boelcke
Miriam Susan Cizmar
Margaret Frances Curran
Lynda Jo Dougveto
Karen Martha Enkro
Judith Karen Enoksen
Patricia Jane Farber
Sandra McDowell-French
Jeanette Ann Frounfelker
Carolyn Kumpf-Gaertner
Barbara Kucik-Gullikson
Jean LaVerne Haan
Carolyn Louise Hacker
Joanne Helen Hammerberg
Roberta Winifred Howlett
Sharon Verleen Isom
Janice Victoria Johnson
Jean Katherine Johnson
Susan Christine Johnson
Sharon Loraine Kamin
Donna Delores Kempinski
Diane Lynn Kloske

Nancy Mills-Koke
Ruth Ann Lindberg
Margaret Redpath-Lindquist
Judith Ethel Lockwood
Bonnie Heather Lusk
Judith Ann Maples
Diane Kuhrt-McCarthy
Kathleen Anne McCarthy
Marie Hinds-Mead
Margaret Ellen Middleton
Edith Elizabeth Miller
Grace Darlene Minor
Janet Ann Mossberg
Marilyn Mae Nasberg
Sandra Lee Nehlsen
Sandra JoAnne Nelson
Janet Mary Newhouse
Ann Louise Nielsen
Diana Lee Olson
Karin Victoria Olson
Jacquelyn Lu Peacy
Joan Claire Petersen
Jane Viola Rapson
Sandra Kay Reid
Phyllis Jean Richie
Jean Eleanor Schaffer
Kaija Gertrude Setala

Marcia Joy Smith
Signe Bellande Specht
Karilyn Susan Sterrenberg
Judith Irene Strook
Vivian Lee Thomas
Ruth Mildred Tronet
Mavis Marie Turpeninen

Judith Anne Vandlik
Diane Katherine Whitney
Beverly Jane Wiening
Karen Ellen Wigg
Diane Kay Zettle
Barbara June Zemek

## 1962

Judith Lynn Anderson
Robinette Lynn Anderson
Barbara Cheryl Andrews
Carolynn Marie Beech
Margaret Louise Bidwell
Marilyn Jo Bradley
Carol Ann Klinger Carlos
Brenda Kay Weimer Carlson
Ingrid Elizabeth Carlson
Janice Brooks Carlson
Patricia Ann Cowley
Marjorie Elaine DeWitt
Norma Jean Drogule
Carol Elaine Ebert
Janice Kay Rider Erkenswick
Judith Forslund
Eileen Agnes Gavert
Carol Ann Gidel
Carol Immonen Gorsuch
Sue Ellen Grana
Karen Jean Green
Sandra Marie Harrall
Marjorie Jane Heavyside
Diane Della Henderson
Mary Lee Hendrixson
Ellen May Hetrick
Mary Hunt
Bonnie Lee Hydorn
Nancy Marie Johanson
Celjie Ailien Johnson

Gail Louise Johnson
Joanne Lillian Johnson
Penna Jean Johnson
Diana Mae Johnson Kia
Heidron Kilian
Barbara Ann Kreiter
Sharon Julette Kujanen
Beatrice Ruth Lang
Claudia Larson
Lucia Leonard
Karen June Lepske
Dale Mary Manthey
Sue Marie Marks
Sally Lee Maxwell
Diane Mary Meyers
Sharon Lee Nikunen
Ruth Marie Oxley
Joanne Carol Allen Palumbo
Marjorie Kay Polk
Sharon Lee Poppen
Rita Rasmussen
Judith Sak
Martana Patricia Sarnecke
Sallyann Catherine Schiemann
June Yvonne Sheetz
Emily Ann Sotak
Barbara Ann Carlson Sullivan
Judith Marion Vander Kamp
Patricia Ann Winterroth

## 1963

Cheryl Marie Aigner
Caroll Ann Anderson
Susan Lee Anderson
Carol Gertrude Baltzer
Karin Eleanore Berg
Janice K. Bjorn
Marilyn Carol Boettcher
Bonnie Jean Burr
Carolyn J. Carlson

Mary Jean Coyle
Penelope Cecelia Crosh
Judy K. Dillow
Verna Beth Feline
Phylis Meilner Foster
Susan Carol Gepperth
Carolyn Pauline Gliege
Alexandra Constantina Grivas
Dianne Beverly Gromek

Doreen C. Gromek
Carol Jean Hartzke
Carla Rae Harvey
Christine Lorraine Hilgert
Judith Linn Jehm
Jeanette Agnes Johnson
Karen Evenson Johnson
Sharon Gaye Kats
Carolyn Kay Larson
Sonja Elizabeth Lindbergh
Faith Ann Lindstrand
Karen Frances Manssen
Mary Ann Masters
Harriet Jean Mattes
Kathryn Ann Mayry
Ardith C. Nelson

Nancy Louise Nelson
Margaret Joan Pretzel
Rosemarie Richter
Clare Rizer
Kay Marie Sauer
Carol Joan Schmidt
Sandra Kay Sines
Carol Jean Stegall
Karen L. Stratton
Judith Aitken Swanson
Lynne Carol Terpstra
Betty Ann Thomson
Evelyn Patricia Wekenborg
Janet Loraine Wendt
Kathleen Ann Wessel
Marcia Eenigenburg Wilk

## 1964

Lois Jean Ahrndt
Elizabeth Ann Argall
Marcella Ruth Ashland
Shirley Jeanne Behrends
Karen Ann Bischoff
Gloria Ann Bruch
Mary Melby Childress
Katherine Janet Clark
Pamela Bachi Cudworth
Julia Ann Ferris
Anne Fortuin
Sharon Bradley Fuller
Bonnie Carol Granger
Dolores Marie Gregor
Diane Marie Haddon
Janice Louaine Hanna
Joan Myrna Harlow
Ann Hall Herbert
Patricia Eileen Herlihy
Elberta Kay Hofer
Judy Lee Jackle
Helen Marie Kinnunen
Karen Marie Koelling
Sonja Eleanor Johnson
Deborah Julia Lytikainen
Susan Joan Mabie
Karen Sue Marchetti

Beverly Joy Meyer
Roberta Ann Moore
Sharon LaVerne Neland
Margaret Elma Nicholson
Karen Sue Nyberg
Ingrid Marie Olson
Ruth Ann Helen Olson
Barbara Jean Olszewski
Kathleen Rose O'Neill
Irene Carol Puder
Susanne Nadeau Puder
Judith Esther Rosten
Joanne Heft Rowell
Patricia Ruttkay
Karen Jean Scharp
Sharon Groeneveld Schuette
Ellen Dene Seyferlich
Kristine Olsen Smith
Mary Elizabeth Tank
Elizabeth Genovese
    Twietmeyer
Nancy Lou VanBeck
Priscilla Anne Weeg
Roberta Seibt Welch
Margie Barrett Wong
Joyce Bennink Zipse

## 1965

Virginia C. Anderson
Sandra K. Breymeyer
Carla J. Bruce
Elizabeth L. Choy
Ellen R. Christensen
Charlene M. DeSimone
Edna G. Ewing
Carol N. Geegan
Janice D. Glanz
June P. Gonzales
Joan M. Gruetzmacher
Beverley A. Hanson
Marilyn G. Hecht
Jane S. Helmboldt
Judith A. Hines
Beverly J. Jensen
Sandra L. Kainrath
Susan L. Karoly
Kathryn J. Kittelson
Suzanne M. Klug
Elizabeth A. Koehne

Carole A. Larson
Karen T. Lind
Lynda R. Lott
Lois A. Malinsky
Nancy J. Massow
Charlotte B. McCorkle
Susan H. Muehlschlegel
Carol J. Oliva
Hazel L. Patterson
Phea A. Prophet
Diana J. Rich
Darlene J. Rood
Marsha A. Salmon
Regina S. Seyer
Jacqueline J. Sneed
Dolores A. Terborg
Joyce C. Thomas
Judith A. Weidman
Bonnie L. Wernquist
Grace M. Wilson

## 1966

Mary Jo Barter
Jean A. Bellamy
Catherine A. Brown
Joan E. Carpenter
Joan M. Doxtater
Diane L. Draudt
Anita D. Ebert
Beverly A. Ellens
Isabel J. Gibson
Dianne L. Herrmann
Susan M. Horn
Cleo L. Hoverman
Jill E. Johnson

Linda R. Kusik
Elaine Kuzma
Joanne Numsen Miller
Linda L. Nelson
Joanne L. Oesterreich
Delles A. Ovens
Ilona M. Sinickas
Janice Beckman Sirk
Diana Bellus Smith
Jacquelyn Witthoft King
Karen J. Wojtun
Eileen C. Wuschke

## 1967

Carolyn Anderson
Louise Autio
Mary Lou Bellamy
Loraine Bruemmer
Suzanne Burdsall
Sheila Churchill
Janet Dykstra
Joan Harrisville
Janice Hook
Elizabeth Kauke
Kathleen Krueger

Susan McCourtie
Karen Outland
Nancy Pawlicki
Marilyn Peltonen
April Petkus
Isabella Seppa
Karen Sleziak
Lois Tellinghuisen
Jeannette Turk
Violette Vlasaty
Patricia Whipple

## 1968

Janet Carol Amraen
Lee Anne Loek Biewer
Diane Esther Cole
Delores Kay Dewey
Sharon Lee Harris
Dolores Elizabeth Henk
Nancy Ellen Kelson
Mary Lou Klein
Linda Elaine McCombe
Linda Diane Mock

Nancy Ann Murley
Carolyn Crockett Naylor
Teresa Christine Peters
Janet Claire Radtke
Cheryl Ann Recker
Betty Ann Havlik Shotten
Joyce Marie Swenson
Connie Lou Welch
Beth Lee Youngs

## 1969

Marsha Bridges
Penelope Butler
Susan Carr
Linda Casella
Kirsten Fahlund
Kathleen Fawcett
Carol Gellert
Cheryl Guth
Shirley Heitschel

Dorothy Holmblade
Penelope James
Joy Jeschke
Kathleen Harding Leonardson
Carol Meyers
Patricia Miloch
Connie Spangler
Emma Kubassek Soto
Lydia Tanner

## 1970—3 Year Class

Judith Bailey
Judith Camera
Ann Cole
Mary Conti
Kathleen Duis
Janolyn Fickas
Cathy Ford
Sherry Giebel
Donna Haugen

June Hutchens
Linda Larson
Dona Miller
Barbara Revis
Lois Schmalz
Barbara Seelman
Linda Surin
Karen Welden
Beery Whitfield

## 1970—2 Year Class

Barbara Bergh
Gwen Domina
Barbara Dumont
Natalie Farris
Kathleen Fritz
Sandra Gruell
Christine Johnson
Lois Kohnert
Deborah Logsdan
Sheryl Moore
Susan Mueller
Roberta Novak

Mildred Olsen
Kathryne Rhodes
Nina Rowan
Rhonda Schulz
Susan Sefrhans
Linda Singletary
Fannie Smith
Pamela Spina
Deborah Swanson
Nancy Trotter
Diann Williams
Miriam Wittman

## 1971

June M. Arbogast
Joyce O. Arrington
Cora Blank
Odell W. Coleman
Marcia B. Durham
Colleen N. Easoz
Carol D. Frye
Barbara J. Kalder
Cheryl A. Leake
Dorothy L. McCaffrey
Fabrienne C. Kreft
Maryetta Mahoney
Candyce A. Marzullo
Judith L. Massey

Cynthia G. Mrakovich
Diane M. Novak
Sharon L. Owens
Kathleen L. Pipes
Deborah A. Quinn
Linda M. Roos
Judith K. Rose
Joyce A. Sanders
Judy M. Terreberry
Patricia A. Tetzloff
Patricia J. Van Auken
Kathleen J. Warnock
Angela Wedekind

## 1972

Josephine Bakos
Catherine Baldwin
Martha Berg
Matlyn Blanchard
Anna Blum
Wilsie Corner
Charlene Flahaven
Janice Gallagher
Lucinda Glover
Mary Griffin
Patricia Gorman
Debra Heatley
Janice Heller
Roseclair Hesler
Shirley Jackson

Beverly Kilbert
Karen Laird
Adrianne Cacciatore Leonard
Beth Lexau
Janet Loucky
Mary Merrill
Sharon O'Neil
Beatrice Rosado
Linda Schuetz
Maria Smith
Donna Trilk
Laurie Tuke
Deborah Vyverberg
Sylvia Wardisani
Cynthia Welgatt

## 1973

Diane Armstrong
Barbara N. Brock
Jackie Bucalo
Madalyn Decancz
Isabella Fortier
Judith Frankel
Roosevelt Gallion
Karen Granback
Tina Lee Hall
Sandra L. Harvey
Rose C. Jackson
Janet Johnson
Penny Kursewicz
Eileen Magrath

Kathleen E. Marcoux
Marcelline Martin
Debbie Mead
Janet Miller
Marguerite Murnane
Marilyn Nolan
Nancy Nowak
Michele Rizzo
Diana Santelli
Barbara C. Sexton
Laurence Van Dyke
Jean Vasquez
Laura Watt
Eileen Zucarro

## 1974

Barbara Alderson
Roger Arquilla
Janet Blindauer
Lucretta Booker
Sharan Buchacz
Diane Bukowski
Georgianne Butz
Ruth Carlberg
Ruthanne Carlisle
Nancy Cronin
Sharon Crouch
Catherine Czernia
Jill Danzey
Deborah Ernst
Alethea Fidone

Mary Hartung
Kathleen Laffey
Erika Lochner
Martha McDonald
Roger McGhee
Lynn Race
Becky Ray
Marcia Schafer
Christine Solberg
Karen Sturges
Terry Takemoto
Carolyn Uczen
Elizabeth Ulvilden
Mary Joanne Watson
Kim Westerberg

## 1975

Kimberly A. Anderson
Carin Baren
Virginia M. Boehme
Lia Buscemi
Diane Bylut
Paula E. Crossen
Patrice Edmunds
Peggy Jo Fawcett
Gloria R. Guichard
John F. Hamrick
Lynn D. Hannula
Roberta Horcher
Anita Larson
Joan Maass
Jeanne B. Magill

Marilee Mazurek
Kathleen Ann Mulvey
Kathryn L. Olson
Wayne C. Nagel
Nancy S. Nelson
Helen Neylon
Fran Ric
Beth Rick
Nancy Ryan
Patricia Schuetz
Debbie Jo Schwartz
Rebecca Semrol
Carol Sweeney
Sally J. Weisman

## 1976

Mary Althoff
Julie Backstrom
Patricia Ann Basiletti
Meredith Claus
Candace Collins
Elaine Connery
Laura Farroli
Mary Gamman
Loida Garcia
Ann Hasier
Dan Hendricks
Barbara Holthaus

Sandra Houchen
Debbi Ivanor
Vicki A. Keating
Amy Mattes
Claudia Morse
Dorin Polys
Anna Siler
Melissa Stumpf
Barbara Whitten
Sharon Wilson
Patricia Wright

## 1977

Susan Anderson
Ellen Berggraf
Debra Blomstrann
Jon Brierton
Mrs. Jon Brierton
Stacy Bryant
Janet Burman
Mony Carter
Janis Center
Barbara Grand
Charlie Hardy
Maureen Holcomb
Jeanne Holper
Martha Hyde

Dorothy Lindsey
Stella Loukas
Janet Moryl
Karen Noelle
Douglas Passett
Maria Lourdes Ramirez
Zee Rodado
Cynthia Schmidt
Sandra Siuciak
Eileen Smith
Diane Stevens
Patricia Tajiri
Barbara Travis

## 1978

Karen Anderson
Christine Aubert
Victoria Bacon
Kathleen Berry
Asta Brazionis
Shirley Chisolm
Margaret Fitzgerald
Rebecca Graham
Gay Grom
Diane Hales
Sondra Horton
Cheri Johanson
Jane Kalas
Kathy Larsen
Dory Manalo
Marilynn Markwald
Cynthia Martin
Rosa Moist
Sharon Morgan
Patricia Murray

June Ostertag
Gloria Palmer
Carole Ramai
Jametta Ray
Susan Ray
Nancy Revennaugh
Maureen Roberts
Fran Rudolph
Helen Schneider
Mary Beth Scully
Jesusita Sepulveda
Bay Sittler
Catherine Siwinski
Linda Sterba
Sheila Stranc
Peggy Stumpf
Joyce Swanson
Nancy Swanson
Rebecca Weber

## 1979

Leslie Aaserude
Linda Abbinanti
Gayle Andrae
Cindi Barrett
Melodee Bartel
Sharon Bukowy
Faye Centeno
Sally Clark
Roland Davis
Ruth Etherly
Tanya Frazier

Helen Gallo
Dorcas Haque
Lynn Hoellerich
Cindy Hopkins
Maria Hunter
Eric Jacobson
Robin Kielp
Jerry Lama
Yudie Leibovitz
April Levka
Joan Lohan

Mary Lukes
Anne G. McBride
Barb Mochocki
Susan Moelter
Esther Morales
Karin Oehring
Joan Pfingston
Nancy Rech
Dorothy Rittmueller

Roberta Beckert
Otistine Blackmon
Julie Blake
Joanne Dynek
John Eherenman
Karen Fredriksen
Iluminada Gutierrez
Mildred Hartnett
Mattie Harvey
Mireya Hobbs
Wilhelmina Houston
Maureen Kelly
Paulette Klarin

Margaret Blake
Mary Jane Borg
Mary Brennan
Dixie Cartwright
Pam Colletti
Robin Custer
Barbara Davis
Genevieve Best-Dickson
Desiree Gimse
Colleen Holcomb
Frances Howard
Mark Isaily
Simone Jahnke

James Daniel Bozora
Sheneill Bland Bryant
Karen Lynn Casey
Elizabeth A. Castro
Stella Cotsialis
Mary Denise Davis
Sheila DeNeal
Julie Ann Devaney
Carolyn D. Everett

Terry Royne
Donna Ryan
Debbie Saari
Joyce Sklamberg
Linda Tober
Maria Velez
Donna Woodruff
Willie Young
Karen Zeason

## 1980

Edwin Kopytko
Robert Lant
Susan Lindstrand
Elizabeth Mandik
Kathi Mastro
Katherine McDonald
Peggy Morgan
Janice Olson
Lynne Poshepny
Cynthia Schmidt
Roberta Smith
Lisa Stevens
Petrina Swanson

## 1981

Maureen Lehman
Patricia Littlejohn
Rosemarie Mazzie
Brenda Melander
Judy Quevedo
Judith Quinn
Karin Scimeca
Andrea Stollenwerk
Jacquelynn Tillett
Patricia Togher
Amelita Tolentino
Jeannie Villegas

## 1982

Melba T. Ferina
Isabel Gallardo
Inge Gazer
April Grason
Pamela Hannah
Joan Harasty
Maryloo McNear
Audrey D. Moorer
Carmen Murillo

Cynthia Ordinario
Pamela Phillips
Edna L. Ramos
Olga A. Salcido

Migdalia Sosa
Patricia S. Tellers
Gwendolyn L. Williams
Joyce Winters

### 1983

Elba Maria Alva
Agnes I. Castleman
Margaret M. Cincotta
Joseph C. Dankowski
Pamela J. Dati
Susan K. Dean
Dorothy Jean Dobbins
Candace P. Greiner
Pamela J. Hanus
Veronica Elaine Heming
Julie Ann Hoekstra
Linda Marie Howell

Priscila R. Inawat
Margaret E. Jackson
Pamela Miller McGraw
Trudy V. Mincey
Charmaine M. Owens
Kenneth W. Perry
Laurie Ann Quinn
Leslie M. Rodriguez
Francine Watson
Karyn A. Wesley
Bonnie J. Williams
Betty Zausner

### 1984

Pamela Brebis
Lisa Coulson
Susan Dawson
Mary Beth Dubrick
Patricia Edwards
Kristi Erickson
Cathy Ether
Yolanda Glenn
Mary Hartray
Susan Kinsman

Diane Krawczak
Debra McLaughlin
Kim Mullins
Mozelle Ratliff
Renee Reade
Theresa Rucker
Edward Schubnell
Susan Scott
Adriana Teran

### 1985

Elena Arreola
Anna Maria Aza
Theresa Blangin
Patricia Boykin
Margaret Boyle
Kathleen Deck
Cheri Gimse
Sheri Gordon
Michelle Madda
Ronald J. Martino
Ann Miller
Cheryl Mondoux
Cynthia Murray

Mary Nichols
Jeri Olsen
Mariana Paladines
Michelle Rock
Steven Rush
Gloria Simonelli
Roger Skebelsky
Britt Steinhoff
Brenda Swanson
Nora Tacderas
Leslie Thomas
Rita Verheggen
Mariola Wesolowski

## 1986

Margaret Abernethy
Marta Fernandez
Kimberly Harrison
Felecia Horton
Elsa Pacete

Jyl Palomo
Kathleen Santiago
Emily Torres
Chandra Wells
Cynthia Yabes

## 1987

Lisa Buthman
Kathryn Heath
Carla Rone

Romaine Rothstein
Emily Torres